The Complete Guide to Traditional Thai Massage

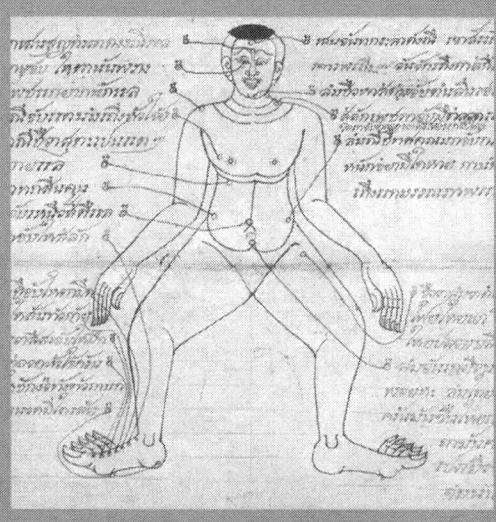
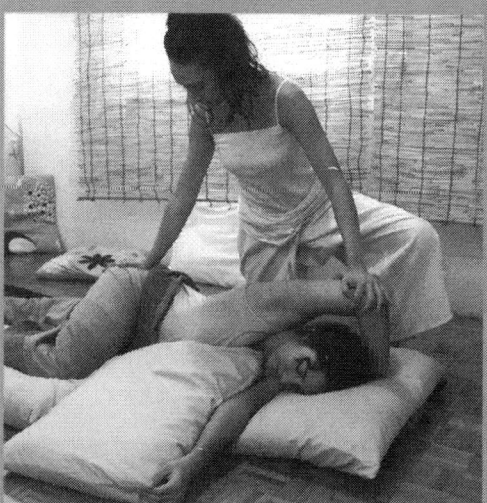
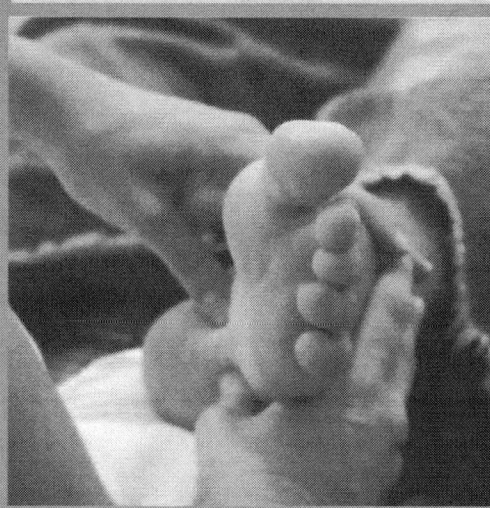
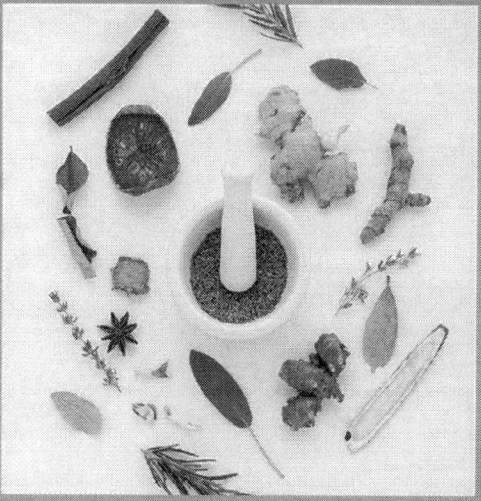

Elefteria Mantzorou

history - sip sen - tok sen - luk pra kob - 4 positions
100 + photos - 200 + techniques

The Complete Guide to Thai Massage

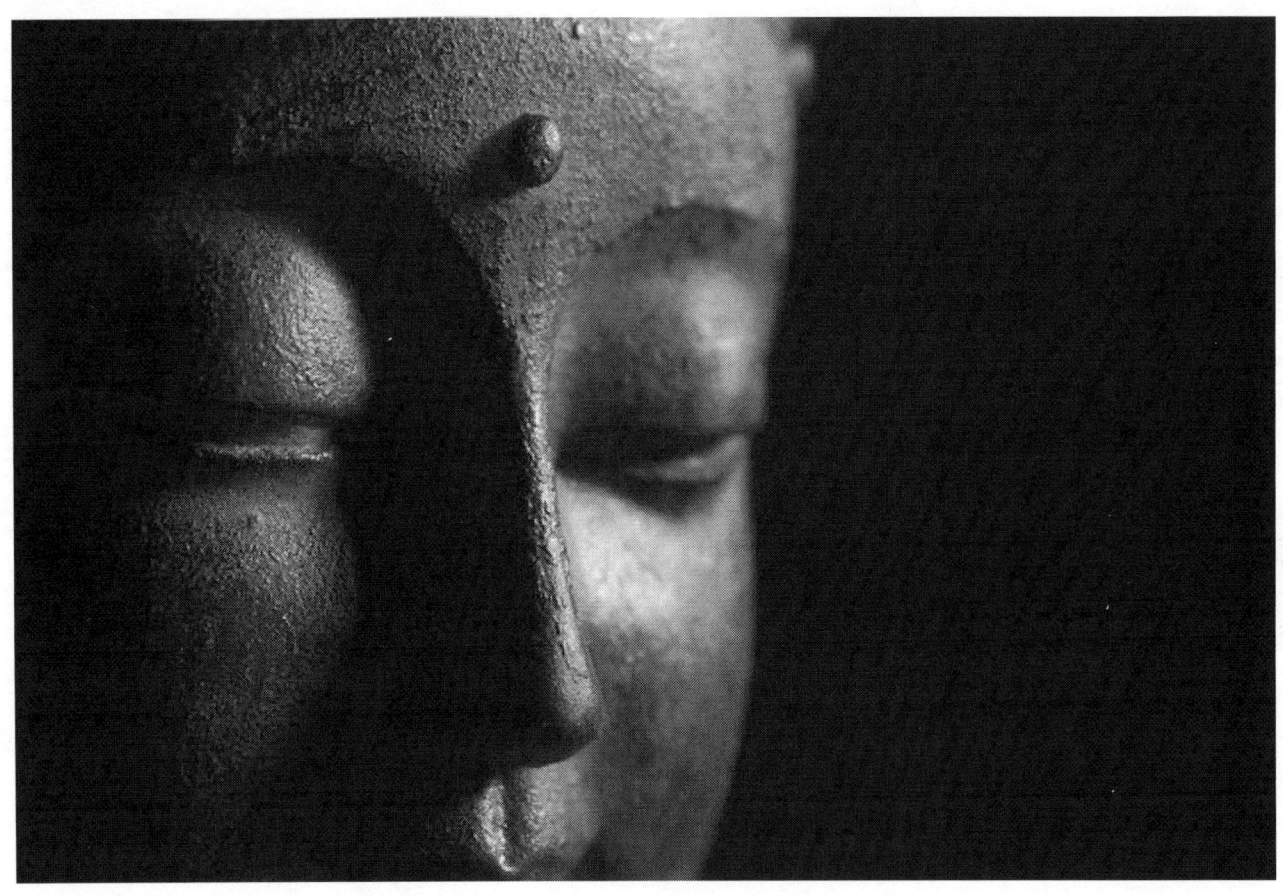

Elefteria Mantzorou

Although the author and publisher have made every effort to ensure that the information in this book was correct, the author and publisher do not assume and hereby disclaim any liability to any party for any loss, damage, or disruption caused by errors or omissions, whether such errors or omissions result from negligence, accident, or any other cause. This book is not intended as a substitute for the medical advice of physicians. The reader should regularly consult a physician in matters relating to his/her health and particularly with respect to any symptoms that may require diagnosis or medical attention.

All rights reserved by Elefteria Mantzorou © 2015. No part of this book may be reproduced or utilized in any form or by any means – electronic or mechanical, without the explicit written permission of the author. Unauthorized use will be prosecuted.

contents

about the author 4

the theory
introduction & history 5
methodology of Thai massage 7
principles of Thai Royal Medicine 8
the mantra of Jivaka 10
contraindications & precautions 11
space & hygiene 11
sip sen: the Thai meridians 13

the techniques
Jap Sen: working on the energy lines 25
how To Stop The Blood Flow 32
the feet 35
what lies underneath 48
leg techniques 52
    single leg techniques 54
    two legs techniques 78
    what lies underneath 95
trunk - abdomen & thorax 99
    what lies underneath 111
arms & hands 114
    what lies underneath 134
side position 137
prone position 173
    what lies underneath 206
    Thai massage and lumbar disc degeneration 210
seated position 212
    what lies underneath 228
face & scalp 230
    what lies underneath 243
tok sen 246
luk pra kob 250

epilogue
blending it all together 258

about the author

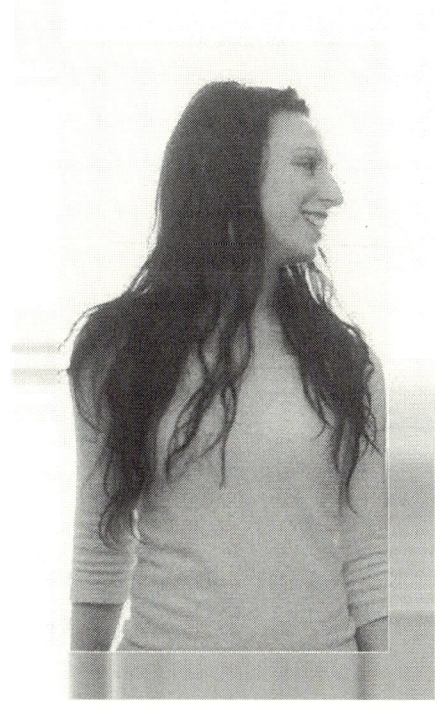

My name is Elefteria Mantzorou. I was born in Athens, Greece. From my childhood I felt attracted to herbal medicine and alternative treatments.

Disregarding any common sense, and following the flow of events without any conscious decisions, I found myself in Thailand many times. There, I studied Thai Massage, Thai Foot Massage & Thai Herbal Compress at the Old Medicine Hospital, and at the school of the unforgettable Mama Lek and her son Jack Chaiya. I also met personally Tai Chi instructor, Tew Bunnag.

For several years I lived as a backpacker. I went to many places in Europe and Asia, working as a volunteer, studying, staying in ashrams, or simply traveling. I worked as a volunteer in wildlife sanctuaries, and have treated countless wild animals. In these sanctuaries, I also worked as a surgeon's assistant. Another experience that has remained indelible in my memory is my acquaintance with Masanobu Fukuoka and natural farming, as I had volunteered in one of his projects in Greece.

In between my trips, I studied alternative medicine (aromatherapy, herbal medicine, Swedish massage and anatomy, physiology and pathology) and was certified as a medical translator. I also attended courses on osteopathy. I started teaching in 2004, and since then I have trained hundreds of people.

In 2013 I opened my own school, FLOW, in a quiet neighborhood of Athens. Well, until I start travelling again, you might find me somewhere here:

FLOW - Wellness & Training
8, Milona str., 11363 Athens
Website: jointheflow.weebly.com

Be always well!

introduction & history

Thai Massage (or *nuad thai*, as is its traditional name) is an ancient healing art of Thailand. It is largely influenced by Indian medicine, Ayurveda, and Chinese medicine, as well as by various indigenous traditions.

Anthropologists have no unanimous view on the exact origin of the «Thai» people. Some argue they are indigenous, others that they emigrated from more northern areas. However, it seems they originate from prehistoric peoples that inhabited Southeast Asia, central and southern China 40,000 years ago.

In Thailand, the "father" of their traditional medicine (and therefore of Thai Massage) is considered to be a historical figure named Jivaka. Jivaka was supposed to the doctor of Buddha, and had studied next to one of the most famous healers - teachers of his time, Atreya. These three persons (Buddha, Jivaka and Atreya) lived and taught in India.

The affinity with the Indian tradition is more than evident. For example, the main meridians of Thai Massage *Itha & Pingkala Sen* remind strongly, both in their name and in their course, the Indian *nadis Ida* and *Pingala*.

In Thailand, medical knowledge was preserved in Wat (Temples). Monks-teachers taught the traditional medical knowledge to young monks-students orally. The ancient texts of Thai Massage were considered equally valuable with the religious Buddhist texts, and were kept in the palace of the King in Ayutthaya, which was then capital of Thailand.

The first international reference in Thai Massage was done through a report of the French officer Simon de Loubere, who lived in Thai royal court in 1661. In particular, he said "When someone in the Kingdom of Siam is ill, he entrusts his body in an experienced person who steps on him with his feet".

The Burmese invasion of Ayutthaya in 1767 resulted in the destruction of valuable part of Thai tradition. And because the medical texts were not copied, a large part of them was lost. The Burmese were expelled by King Taksin after a few months. In 1832, Emperor Rama III ordered the last remaining medical texts to be engraved in stone. The inscriptions were placed in the temple Wat Pho, which is still located in Bangkok, the present capital of Thailand.

In 1906, during the reign of Rama IV, all the surviving records of the ancient medical sciences were translated in the current Thai language. Most importantly, the royal medical book *Tum Ra Pade Sard Songkroah* (Chabub Luang), which describes the process of Thai Massage, was written down.

There are two main schools of Thai Massage in Thailand - Northern (practiced in Chiang Mai and surrounding areas), and Southern (represented mainly in school-Temple Wat Pho.

The differences between these two schools are small. The theory is essentially the same. The main difference lies in the Jap Sen methodology, the emphasis on stretching (primarily found in North School) and the focus on acupressure points (primarily found in South School).

In the early 20th century, the traditional Thai medicine was declared illegal and unscientific. However, in the mid-1990s, the government decided to support traditional treatments again. Now they are incorporated in the modern health care system, and the corresponding studies are approved by the Ministry of Education of Thailand.

Thai Massage and Anatomy

The inscriptions which are now displayed at Wat Pho, demonstrate images (60 totally) of the meridian *sen* lines. 30 of them demonstrate the anterior part of the body, and 30 of them the posterior.

These inscriptions have serious anatomical inaccuracies. This is due to the fact that the dissection of corpses was forbidden until the 19th century.

methodology of Thai massage

Thai Massage is an integral part of Thai traditional medicine, which is an autonomous system. According to the principles of this healing system, the human body has some meridians through which cosmic energy flows. These meridians are called Sen (= line). One of the main goals of Thai Massage is the balancing of these meridians.

Thai Massage is traditionally practiced on a mat. The receiver should wear light and loose clothing. The therapist uses his thumbs, palms, elbows, forearm, knees and feet (or sometimes his whole body) to perform the techniques.

Thai Massage methodology includes:

• Stretching. These stretches are the most distinctive feature of Thai Massage. The goal is to decompress and give space to the body. Some of them are passive applications of yogic asanas (postures).

Stretching may restore the relationship of the protagonist - antagonist muscle groups, thus contributing to relief from chronic musculoskeletal problems and chronic pain due to the gradual shortening of muscles.

• Adjustments, resembling the low and medium velocity techniques of osteopathy. (Note that Thai Massage techniques are not as specific as the osteopathy techniques). Some advanced practitioners may apply high velocity techniques as well (thrusts). In some countries / states this may require a special license.

• Massage techniques. These include the typical kneading and tapping of Swedish massage. However, all Thai Massage techniques are dry, since there is no oil involved.

• Work on Sen lines. This is done by a specific protocol (to be explained shortly), which mainly consists of presses with the thumbs and palms. This technique purifies and balances the subtle electrochemical system of the body. This is one of the reasons that Thai Massage is considered sacred.

• Hot herbal packs (luk pra kob). These packs contain muscle relaxant and anti-inflammatory plants. They are steamed and then placed on specific points. Using them relieves muscle pain, detoxifies the body and provides a deep feeling of relaxation.

principles of Thai Royal Medicine - phaet phaen thai

In Thailand there are two main traditions. One is called "medicine of the rural areas" and the other "Royal tradition". The latter is so called because the records were kept in the royal palace. Those trained in this art worked mainly in the king's court. The other tradition is found in various nomadic tribes living in Thailand (mainly in the north) and contains many shamanic elements. Certainly, these two traditions have influenced each other.

It is believed that the human body consists of 42 factors, which are classified into four elements (Earth, Water, Air, Fire). In Thai language they are called *thaad* (reminds me of the Sanskrit word *tattva*, which means *element*).

The **Earth Element** consists of 20 factors: 1. Hair, 2. Body hair, 3. Skin, 4. Muscles, 5.Tendons, 6. Ligaments, 7. Bones, 8.,Bone marrow, 9. Teeth, 10. Brain, 11. Heart, 12. Lungs, 13. Liver, 14. Pancreas, 15. Kidney, 16. Spleen, 17.Chyle, 18. Stool, 19. Stomach, 20. Intestines.

The Earth factors are solid and compact.

The **Water Element** consists of 12 factors: 1. Tears, 2. Phlegm, 3.Mucus, 4. Saliva, 5. Sweat, 6. Blood, 7. Lymph, 8. Urine 9. Bile, 10 Pus, 11. Sebum, 12. Fat.

The Water factors are characterized by moistness.

The **Air Element** consists of six factors that actually operate in three systems: 1. Breathing (inhalation-exhalation), 2. Blood circulation (blood flow towards the heart and out of it – arteries and veins), 3. Digestion (urination and defacation).

The Air factors exhibit mobility.

The **Fire Element** consists of 4 factors:

1. Digestive Fire: Something like the *Agni* of Ayurvedic medicine. It controls the digestion and absorption of food.
2. Body Heat: Controls the heat of the torso.
3. Temperature of the extremities: Refers to the heat of the hands and feet.
4. Age Cycles: If the element of Fire is in excess, the person tends to get angry more easily. It is believed that excessive anger causes premature aging, and the "age cycles" are accelerated (I would call that a form of oxidative stress!).

The Fire factors are associated with heat and temperature.

Thais believe that the Universe too consists of these 4 elements: Earth, Water, Air, and Fire.

It is also believed that human beings receive all these factors during pregnancy, from the mother's umbilical cord. This is the main reason that the navel is considered the center of the human body, and all *sen* originate from there.

A factor may become deficient or excessive because of environmental factors, stress or malnutrition. Factors can be balanced through proper nutrition, Thai Massage and herbs. It is worth noting that food is divided into four major categories: 1. Animals, 2. Plants, 3. Metals, 4. Herbs.

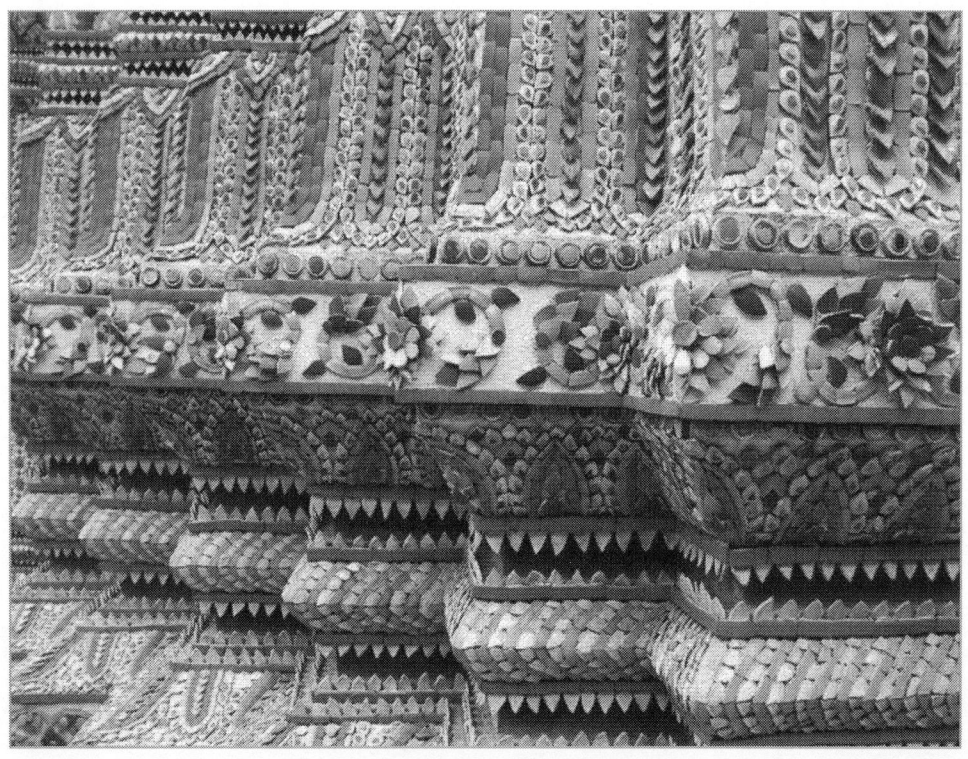

the mantra of Jivaka

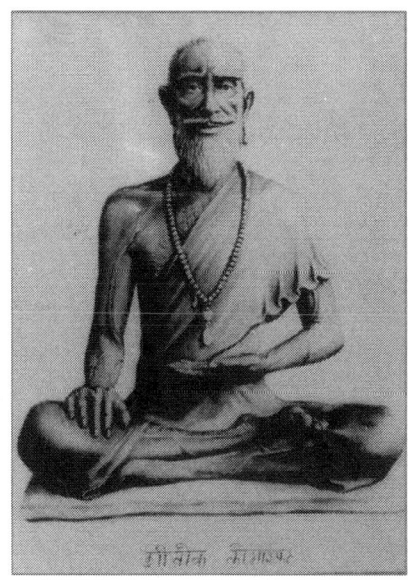

According to tradition, before the beginning of the session, the therapist offers a prayer to Jivaka, the father of Thai Massage, asking for help and blessings.

This is optional. If your religion does not allow you to do that, you may as well skip it.

This is the *mantra,* in *Pali* language:

OM NAMO SHIVAGO SI RASA AHANG
KARUNIKO SAPASATANANG O-SATHA
TIPA MANTANG PAPHASO SURIYA-JANTANG
KOMARAPATO PAGA-SESI WANTAMI
BANTITO SUMETASO A-LOKHA SUMANA-HOMI. (repeat 3 times)

PIYO-TEWA MANUSSANANG PIYO-PROMA NAMUTTAMO
PIYO NAKHA SUPANANANG PININSRIYONG NAMAMIHANG
NAMO PUTTAYA NAVON-NAVEAN NASATIT-NASATEAN
A-HIMAMA NAVEAN-NAVAE NAPAITANGVEAN
NAVEANMAHAKU A-HIMAMA PIYONGMAMA NAMO-PUTTAYA.

NA-A NAVA LOKA PAYATI VINA-SHANTI. (repeat 3 times)

We call upon our founder, Father Jivaka, to inspire us through his holy life. Please give us the knowledge of all the elements of nature, which is the true medicine. Through this mantra, we pray to you that you bestow us the light of knowledge, which is like the light of the sun and the moon. We pray that through our body, we will be able to restore health in the body of our client.

The Goddess of Healing abides in heaven, and mankind lives on Earth. In the name of the founder, may the heavens be reflected on earth, so that the whole world is healed. We honor you. We honor the Buddha. We pray that our client becomes happy, peaceful, and free from disease.

contraindications & precautions

- Thai Massage is contraindicated if the receiver has fever or any infectious disease.
- Do not exert pressure on inflammatory areas (e.g. with dermatitis or eczema).
- Thai Massage is contraindicated if there aneurysm, thrombophlebitis or any other serious cardiovascular disease.
- If the patient is suffering from cancer, we can work very mildly. Sen work is usually safe. Applying more dynamic techniques is possible only after at least 3 months after chemotherapy or radiotherapy. In any case, the consent of the oncologist is necessary.
- Thai Massage is contraindicated to clients with osteoporotic fractures (and any fracture that has not healed properly).
- Thai Massage is not recommended during pregnancy, at least during the first 4 months. After that, it is possible to apply some techniques, especially those of the side position. Avoid any deep work and pressure on the legs.
- The application of hot herbal packs in areas with varicose veins is forbidden.
- Thai Massage is contraindicated in people who have undergone organ transplantation. Thai Massage (in fact, any form of bodywork) may boost the immune system, and can therefore be harmful in this case.
- If the receiver has any health problem that raises doubts as to whether Thai Massage is suitable for that person, a doctor should be consulted.
- Always respect the receiver's physical limitations.

space & hygiene

Here are some rules for the area where the Thai massage is performed:

- Thai Massage requires much more space than classic Swedish massage, because of its stretches.
- The mat on which we place the receiver should be soft. The mat should be placed on a non-slippery floor or material.
- Have at least 3-4 pillows to support the body of the receiver correctly. It is advisable to have an extra pillow for your knees.
- The therapist and the receiver should wear comfortable, loose clothes.
- The room must be very clean.
- I recommend dim lighting and soothing music.

• The receiver should not have eaten a heavy meal at least two hours before a Thai Massage session. After the session, I tell my clients to avoid food for the next hour, to drink lots of water, and to bathe after 2-3 hours.
• The therapist should wash his hands before the massage.
• The sheet covering the mattress should be washed after each session. The same applies to the pillow.
• Herbal packs that contain fresh herbs can be refrigerated for 7-10 days. Dry herbs can be kept for 6-9 months. Be sure to keep them in a tightly closed plastic bag, otherwise their pungent smell will infuse the entire refrigerator!

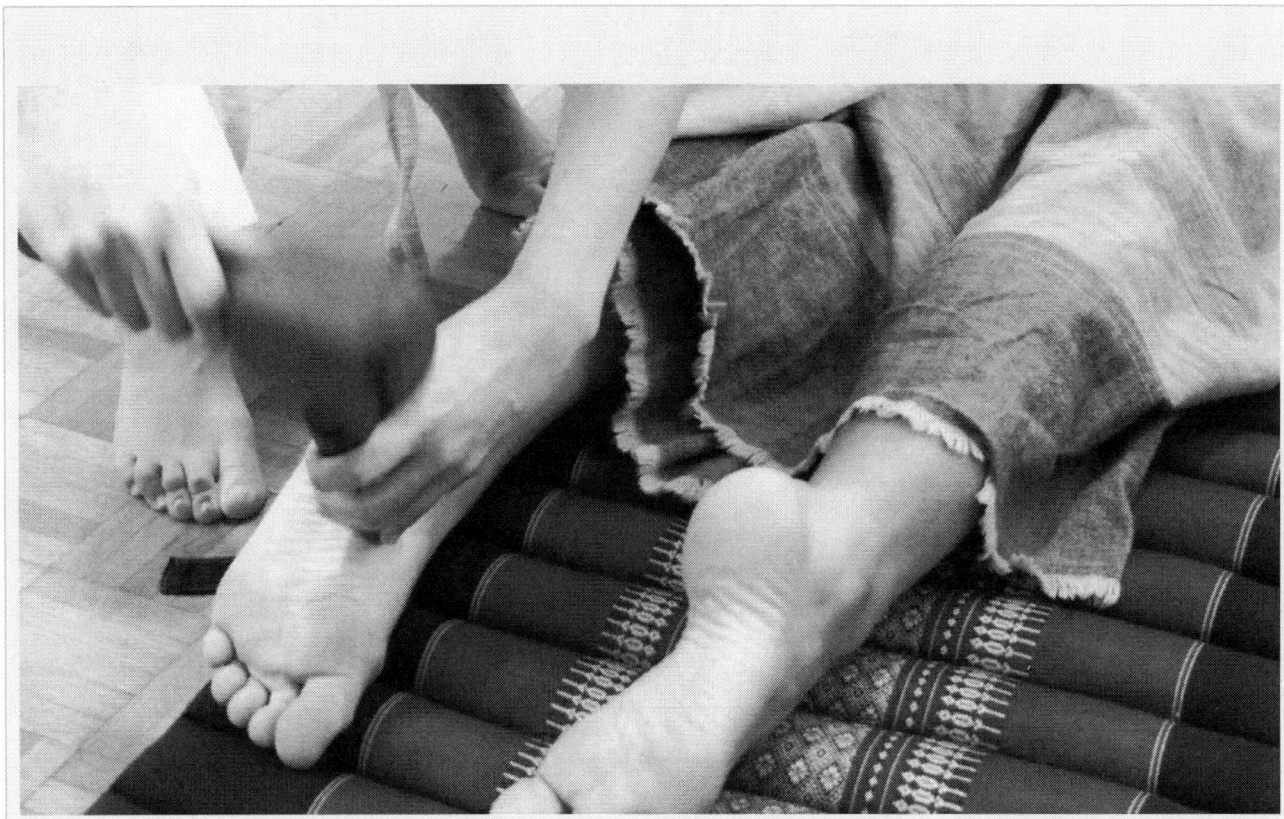

The Thai Massage mat should be soft and thick. This ensures that the client will be comfortable and safe, even during the application of techniques like the one shown in the photo.

sip sen:

the Thai meridians

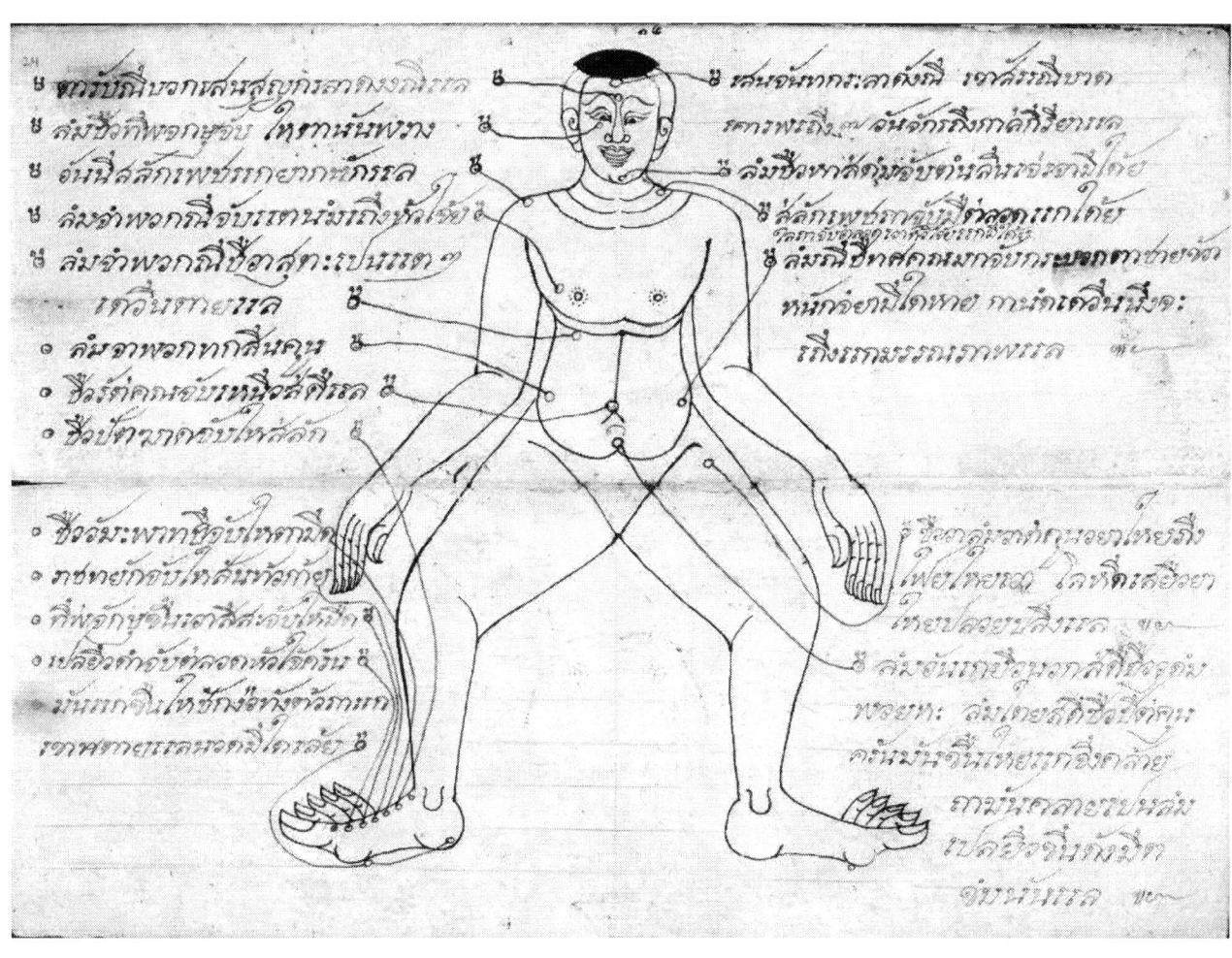

In the Thai language, *sen* means "line". The Thai meridians are called *Sen*, and in massage therapy, ten basic "lines" are used (*sip* means "ten").

The *sen* have more similarities with the Ayurvedic *nadi*, than with the Chinese meridians. The *sen* do not correspond to specific organs, like the Chinese meridians, and are indicated for problems that may occur across their course. Each sen has some acupressure points.

Sen work is called *jap sen*, and it is done in 5 steps:

1. Stretching (opening the line)
2. Walking with palms (warming the line)
3. Walking with thumbs (working on specific lines and points)
4. Walking with palms (warming the line)
5. Stretch (opening the line).

According to the traditional protocol, the therapist should start working upwards all sen lines – that is, from the feet towards the head, and from the hands towards the heart. Then, he should return to the starting point. Bear in mind that there may be some differences to this protocol, depending on the school.

It is not necessary to work all the lines in one session, and it is not necessary to work on the whole course of a line.

Jap sen should be applied after training with a qualified teacher.

There are many sen lines crossing the legs. There are three lines on the outer surface of the foot, and 3 in the interior.

In the following diagram we see the leg lines. Please note that the 3rd internal line is worked only in the prone position, since it passes from the posterior thigh muscles and the heads of the gastrocnemius muscle.

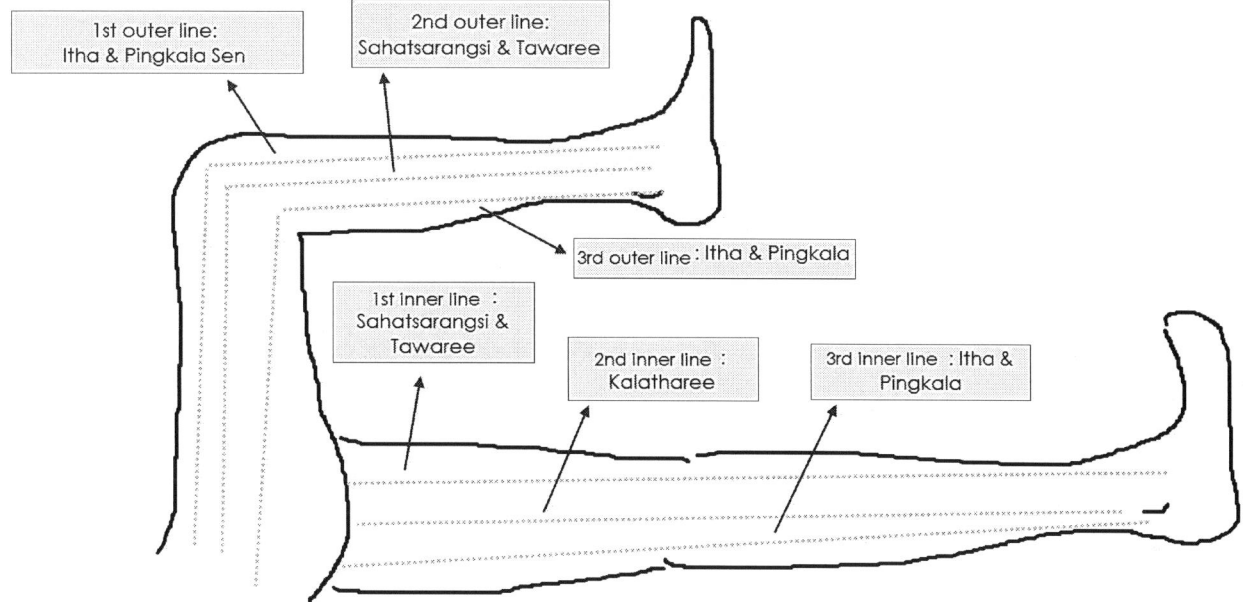

In the next pages of this chapter we will have a look at the 10 meridians. The words *sen, line* and *meridian* in this book are synonyms.

Depending on the school, there might be slight differences in the course of the lines.

1, 2. Itha & Pingkala sen

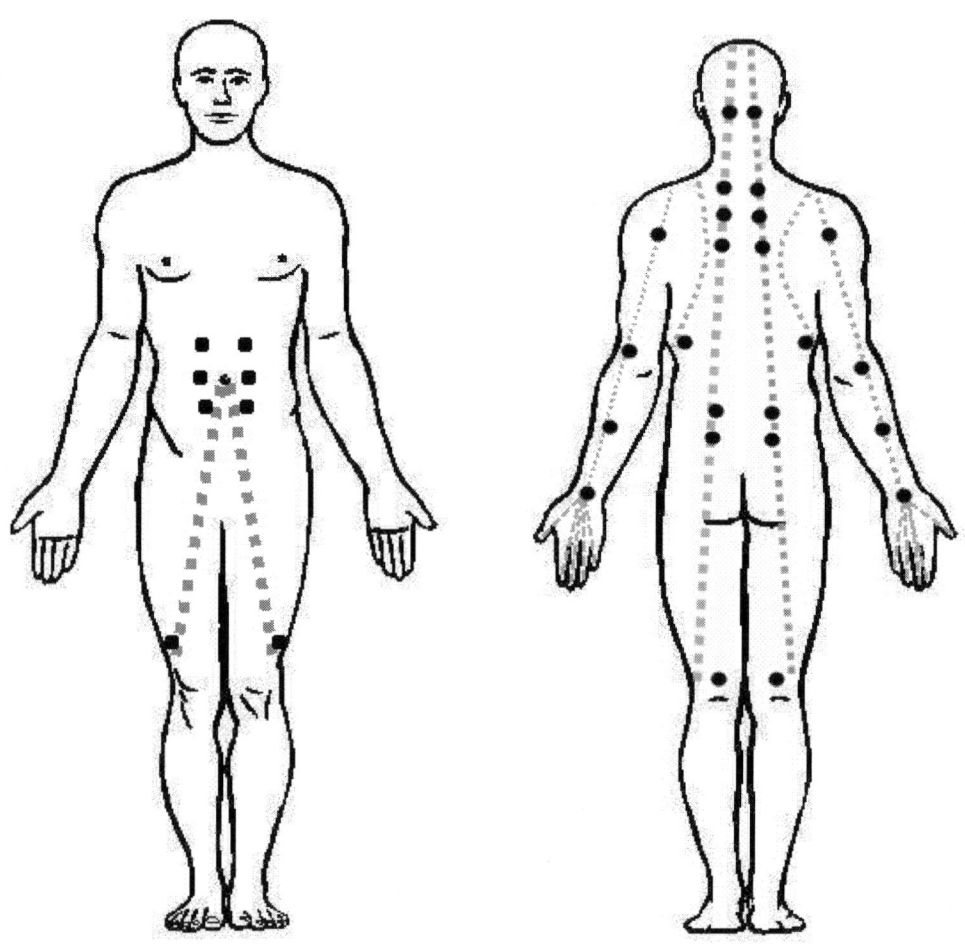

Itha originates from the navel and descends the anterior part of the left thigh, forming the first external line. Then it turns outwards on the left knee, and then follows an upward course between the heads of the posterior thigh muscles, forming the third inner line. It continues its course next to the spine, passes from the scalp and the forehead, and finally ends on the left nostril. Pingkala follows the same path, but on the right part of the body.

These meridians also have sub-branches.

- There is a sub-branch that continues until the toes of the dorsal aspect of the foot, and another that run between the heads of the gastrocnemius muscle (starts below the knee joint).
- Also, in the upper part of the thoracic spine, there is another sub-branch, which passes next to the scapula, crosses the anterior surface of the arm and the dorsal surface of the hand, and ends on the fingertips.
- Finally, there is a sub-branch above each eyebrow.
- Another sub-branch starts from the hip bone and runs down to the ankle, forming the third outer energy line of the leg.

Work on the Itha and Pingkala for these problems:

- Muscle aches (back pain, sciatica, neck pain).
- Pain in the knee joint.
- Carpal tunnel syndrome (work on the arm points shown on the photo).
- Sinusitis

The six points of the abdomen are used for digestive problems (refer to the section of abdominal techniques for the procedure).

These sen are connected to the sense of smell.

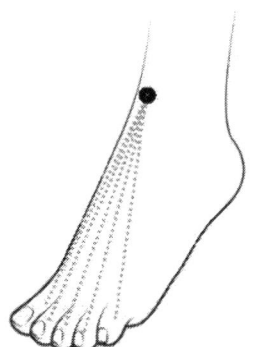

The Itha and Pingkala lines on the dorsal aspect of the foot.

3. Sumana Sen

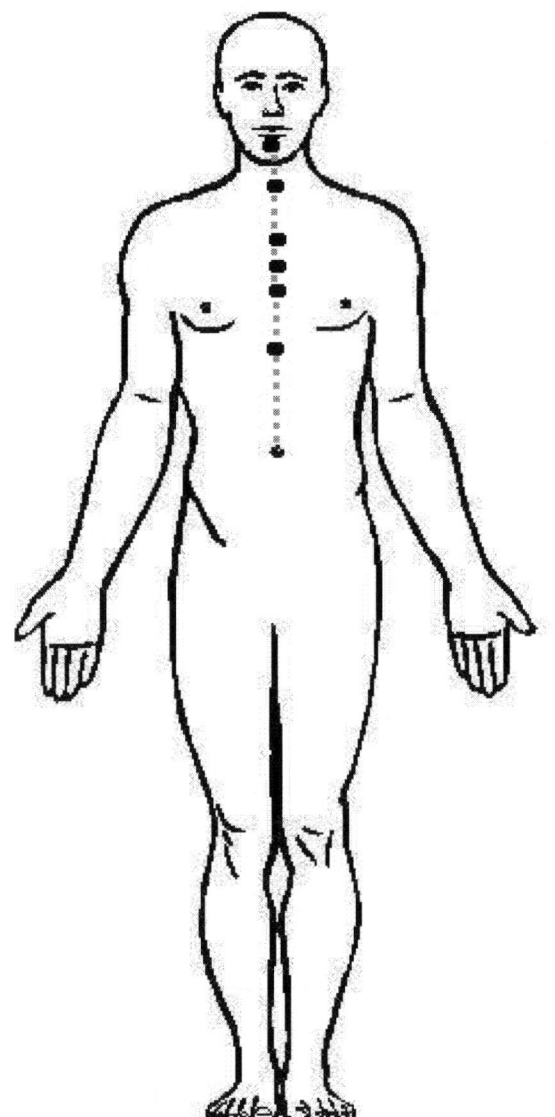

Sumana Sen originates from the navel, crosses the trunk, and ends at the root of the tongue. It is connected to the sense of taste.

- Work on Sumana Sen for disorders related to the respiratory system, and the mind (stress, arrhythmias, etc).
- The point below the xiphoid process is used for digestive disorders (dyspepsia, gastroesophageal reflux, etc.)
- The point above the sternum is used for hiccup.
- The point below the lips is used for nausea.
- The point at the root of the tongue is only used when we want to eliminate some toxic substance from the body via emesis. In order to activate it, the finger is inserted into the oral cavity.

4. Kalatharee Sen

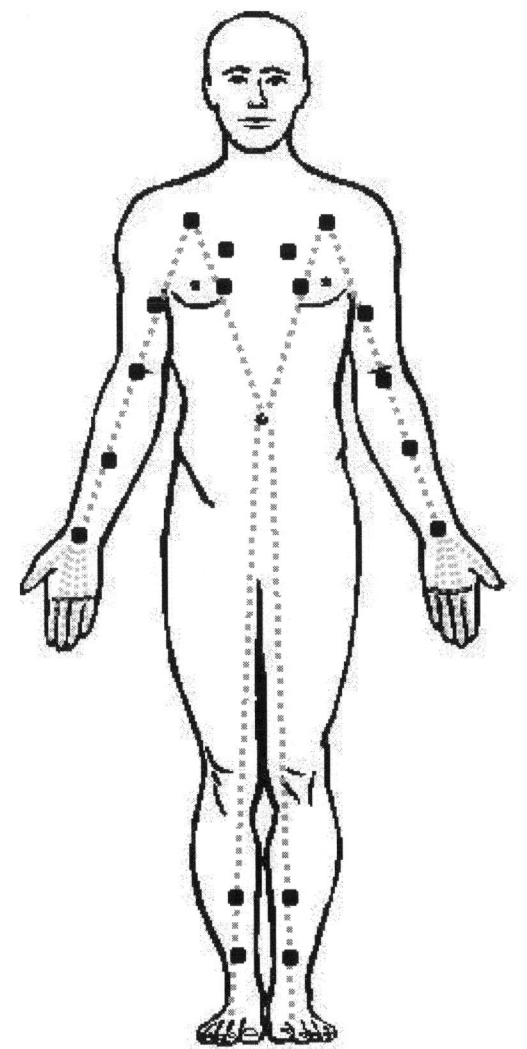

Kalatharee Sen originates from the navel and is divided into four major branches: two branches descend on the trunk, run on the legs (forming the second inner line) and end at the toes, on the plantar surface. The other two branches run upwards on the trunk, cross the arm (between the ulna and radius) and end on the fingertips, on the palmar surface.

Kalatharee Sen is used for problems in the arms and legs (pain, weakness, numbness, muscle aches, etc.). However, it is also the main sen indicated for arrhythmias and disorders of the nervous system.

Kalatharee Sen is connected to the sense of touch.

The points of the legs are shown in the illustration. One is located three fingers below the knee, while the other is next to the ankle.

The first point of the hand is near the axilla, the second in the center of the arm, the third in the elbow joint, and the fourth at the center of the forearm. There is also a fifth point on the wrist joint.

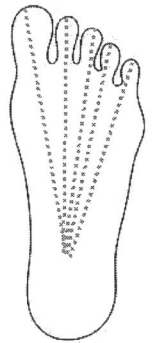

In this diagram we see the lines on the plantar surface. There is a definite similarity with the plantar aponeurosis.

5, 6. Sahatsarangsi & Tawaree Sen

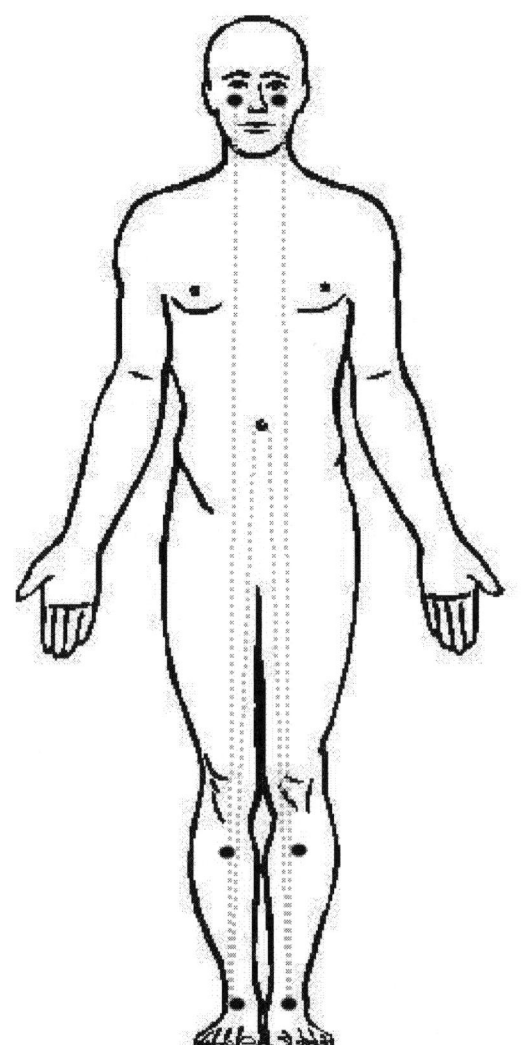

Sahatsarangsi Sen originates from the navel, descends at the inner surface of the left leg, forming the first inner line. Then it turns on the left ankle, forming the second outer line, and runs upwards to the neck. It ends below the left eye.

Tawaree Sen follows the same path, but on the right part of the body.

Both Sen are connected to the sense of sight.

These two sen are used for leg and eye problems. If there is an eye problem, work on the sen that runs on the opposite leg (e.g. if there is a problem on the left eye, work on Tawaree sen).

The first point is located three fingers below the knee, while the second is on the foot joint.

7. Nantakawat Sen

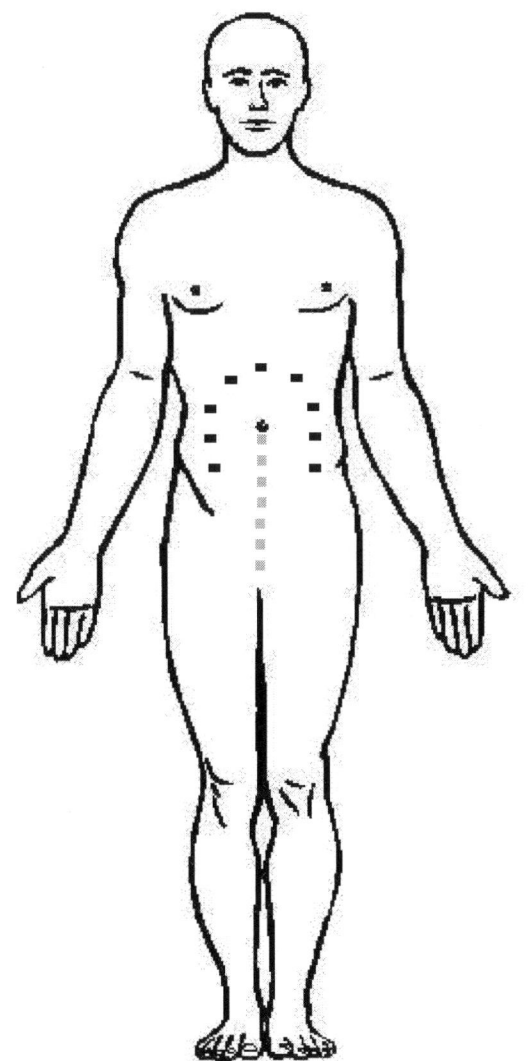

Nantakawat Sen originates from the navel and is divided into two branches.

The first is called *Sukumang* and ends at the anus, while the second *Sikinee* and ends at the urethra.

This Sen controls the absorption of food, the transformation of liquids and the elimination of waste substances from the body.

Nantakawat Sen is mainly associated with the processes of urination and defacation. Generally, it is used for digestive problems (constipation, irritable bowel syndrome, etc.).

In cases of constipation work in a clockwise direction, while in cases of diarrhea work anti-clockwise, on the 9 points shown on the illustration.

8, 9. Lawusang & Ulanga Sen

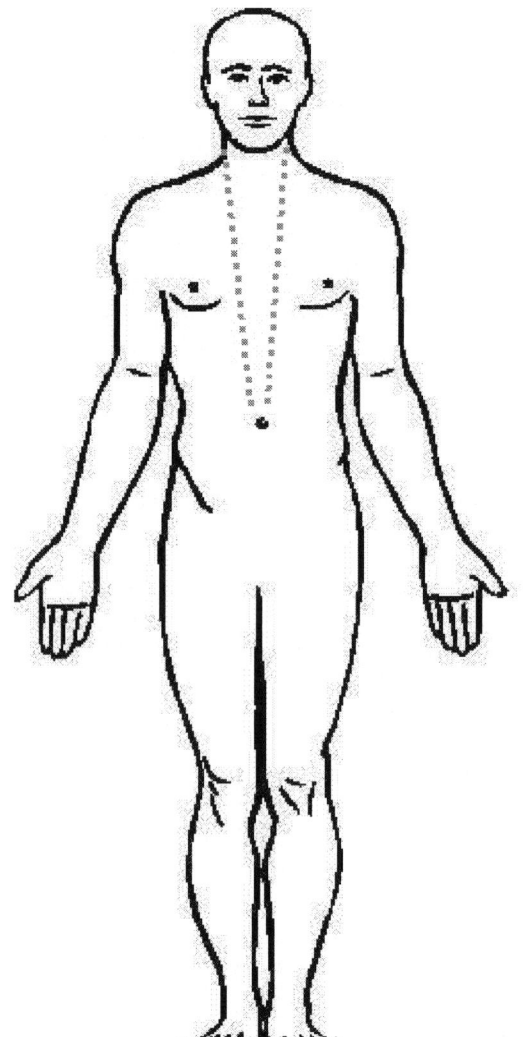

These two Sen have two alternative names in the Thai language. Lawusang is also called *Chantapusang*, while the Ulanga sen is also called *Luchang*.

Lawusang Sen originates from the navel, runs upwards on the trunk, passes next to the left ear, and ends on the temples.

Ulanga Sen follows the same path, but on the right side of the body. These two Sen control the sense of hearing.

Generally, they are used for pain on the face. They can be used for:

- earache and tinnitus (due to stress).
- any pain not due to acute inflammation (e.g. headaches).
- motion sickness.

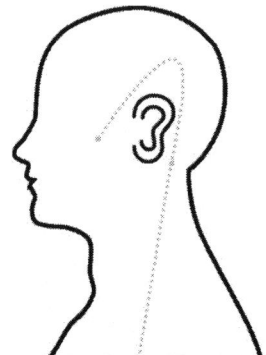

The course of Lawusang and Ulanga Sen around the ear.

10. Kitcha Sen

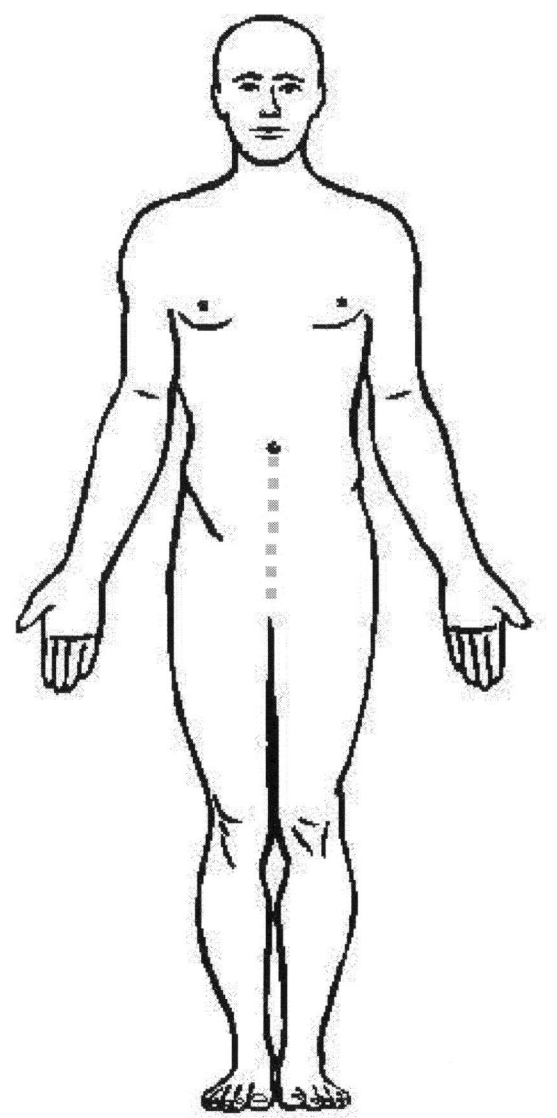

Kitcha Sen originates from the navel and descends to the genitals.

In women ends on the clitoris, and is called *Kitchana*.

In men, it reaches the end of the penis, and is called *Pittakun*.

Generally, it is controls sexual arousal, and reproductive capacity and function.

Kitcha Sen is used mainly in cases of sexual frigidity, erectile dysfunction, and also for disorders of the female reproductive system.

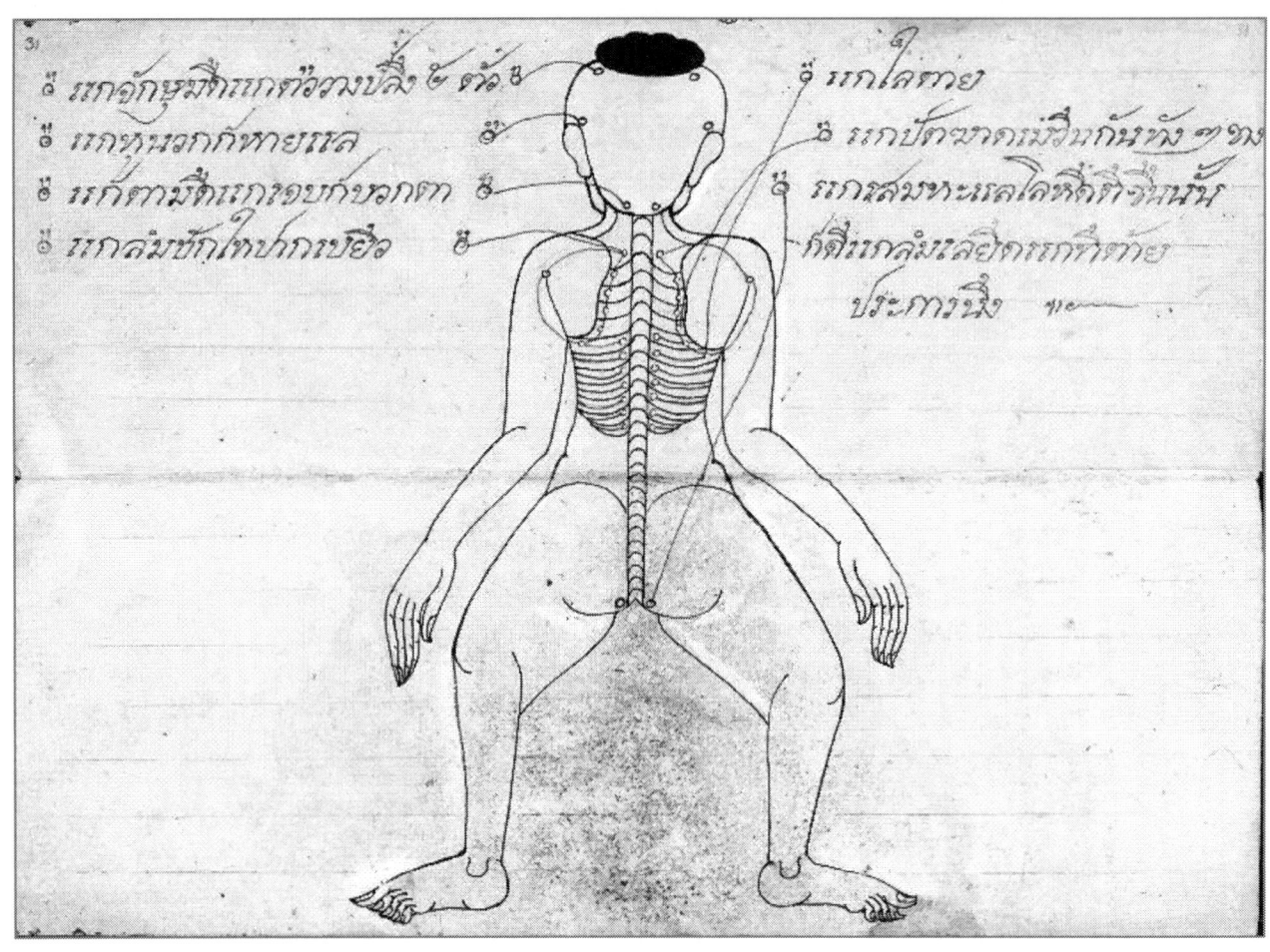

Traditional Thai drawing showing Itha & Pingkala Sen points.

Jap Sen: working on the energy lines

In this section, I will show you how to work the Sen – the traditional Thai meridians.

On the legs, we have 3 meridians on the outer side of the leg, and 3 on the inner side.

The following photos demonstrate Jap Sen on the legs. The same principles apply for any part of the body, like the arms, the back, etc.

In Thai, "Jap" means "work, and "sen" means "line". Hence, *Jap Sen* means "working on the lines".

Jap Sen is performed in 5 steps:

1. Stretching ("open" the meridian).

2. Palm walking ("warming" the meridian).

3. Thumb walking (focused work on each sen line).

4. Palm walking (same as Step 2).

5. Stretching (same as Step 1).

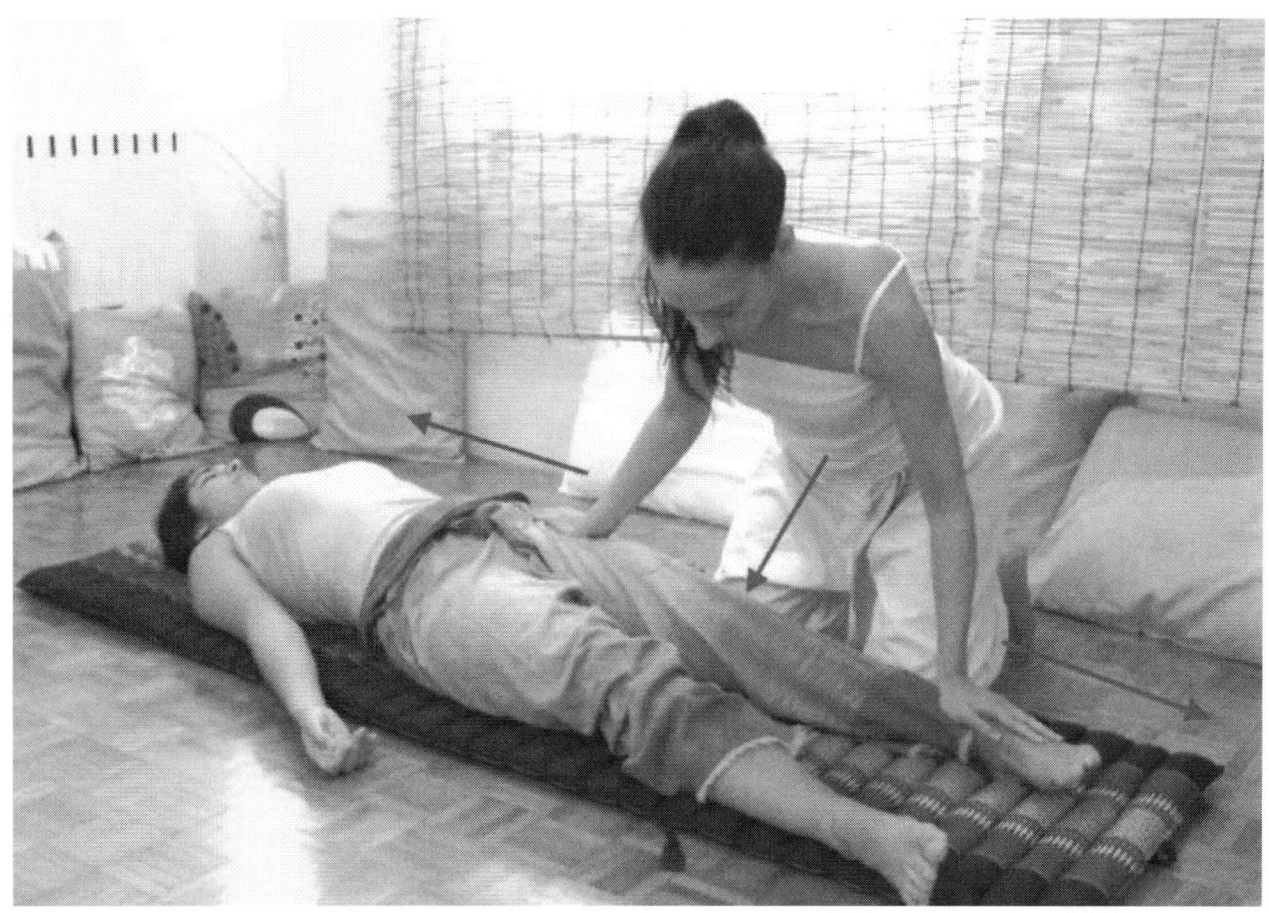

Start from the 3 outer lines. First stretch the meridians, by placing one palm on the receiver's ankle, and one palm on the quadriceps muscle. Breathe in. When you breathe out, use your body weight in order to apply the stretch.

This is Step 1 of 5.

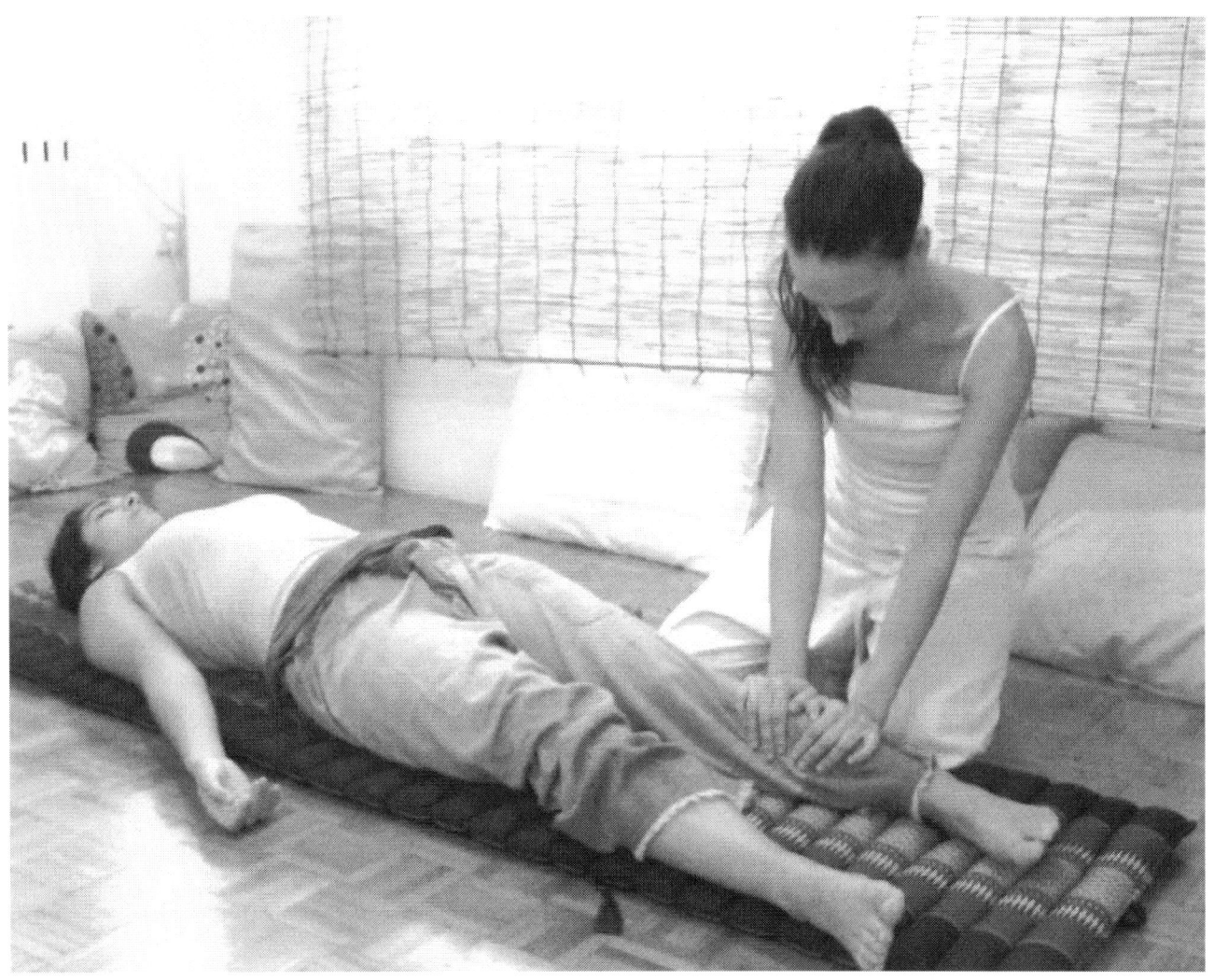

Then walk with your palms on the outer lines. This is supposed to "warm" the meridians. Skip the knee.

This is Step 2 of 5.

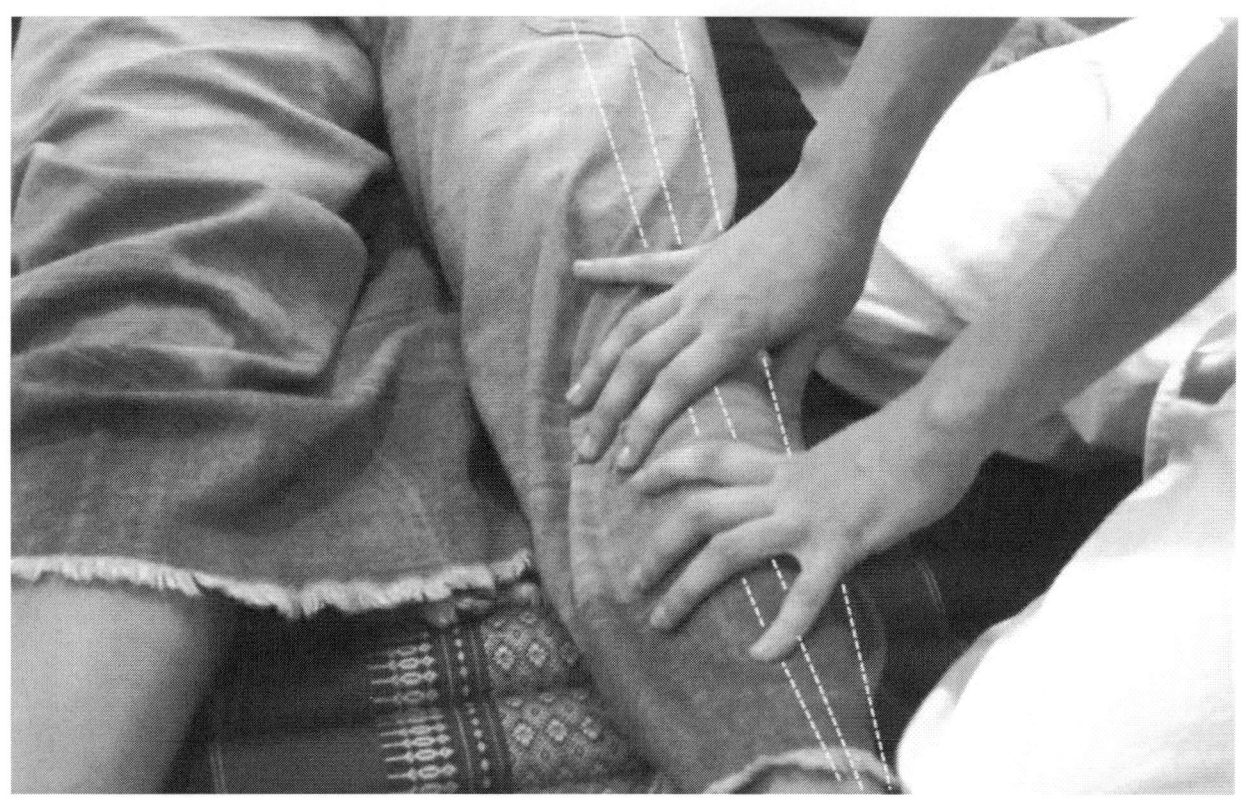

Then, using your thumbs, press the 3 outer sen. Work from the feet towards the hips, and then return.

This is Step 3 of 5.

Then repeat the warming (Step 4 of 5), and the stretch (Step 5 of 5).

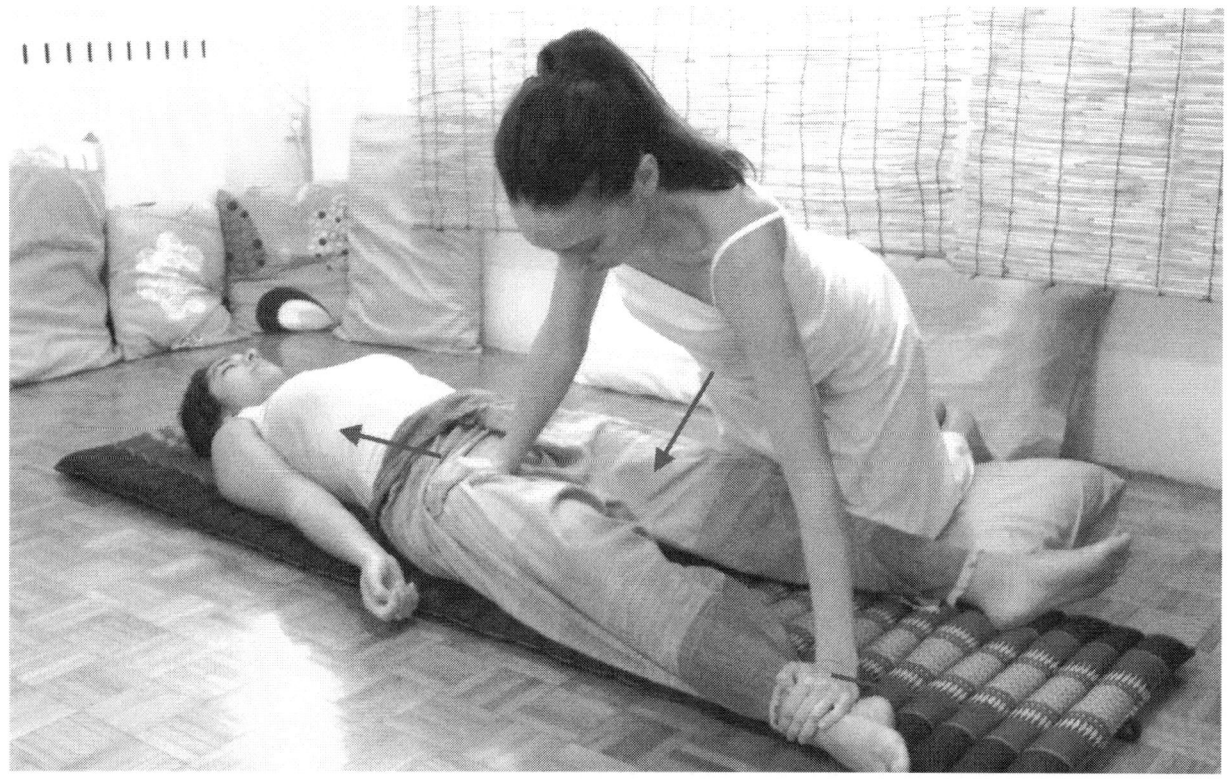

Then work on the inner Sen lines. From the supine position, it is possible to work only on the two inner lines.

Apply again the 5 Steps. The one shown in the photo is the 1st: Open the meridian by stretching it.

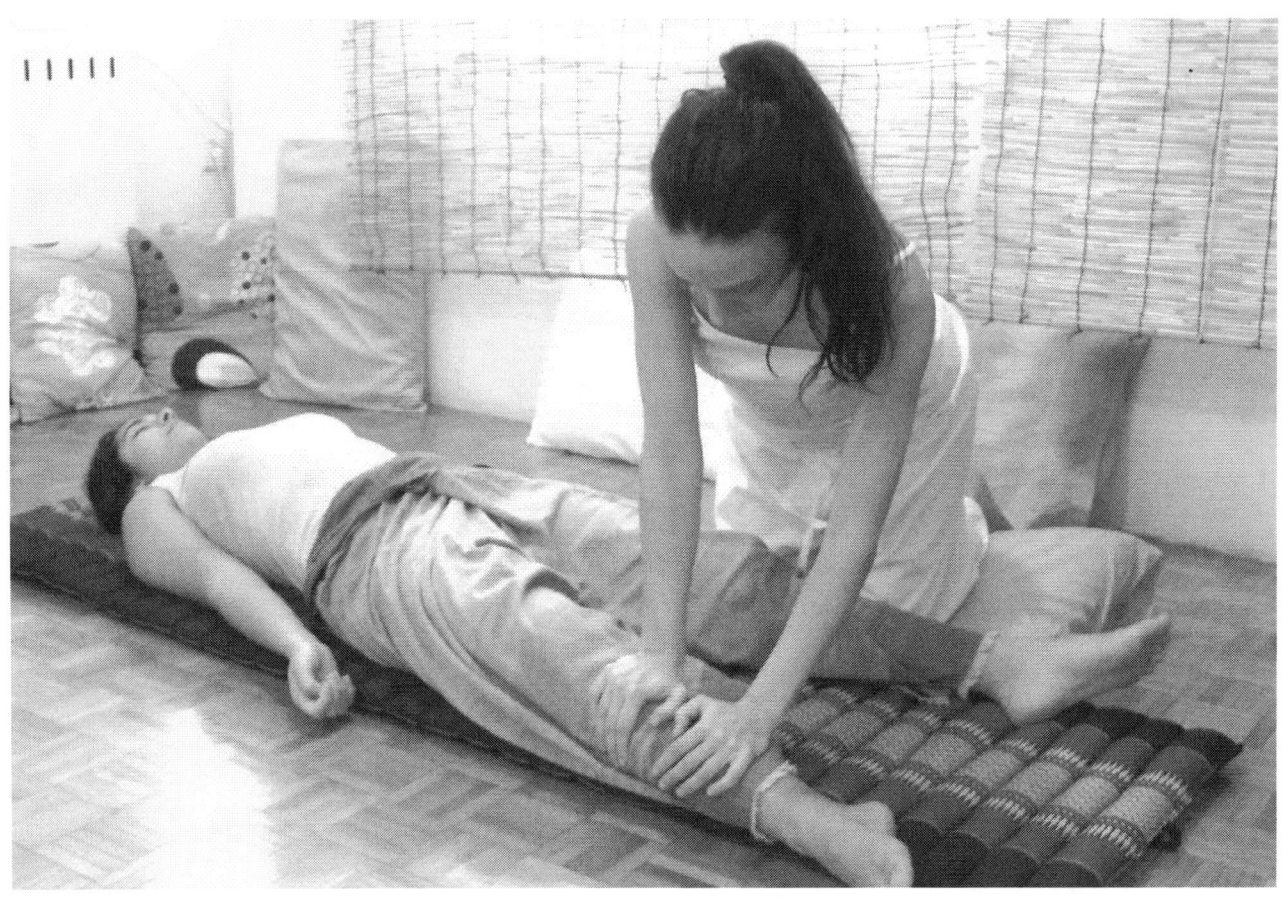

Then apply Step 2 of 5: Warm the meridians by palm walking. Again, skip the knee.

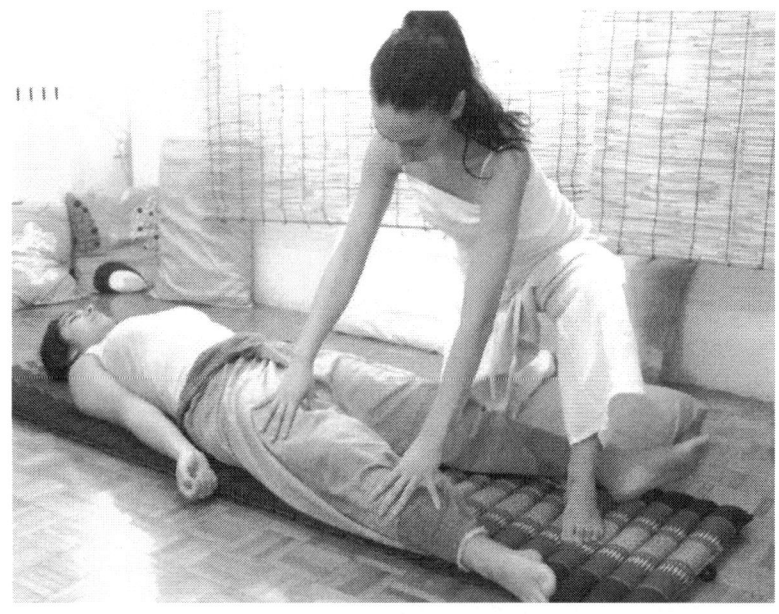

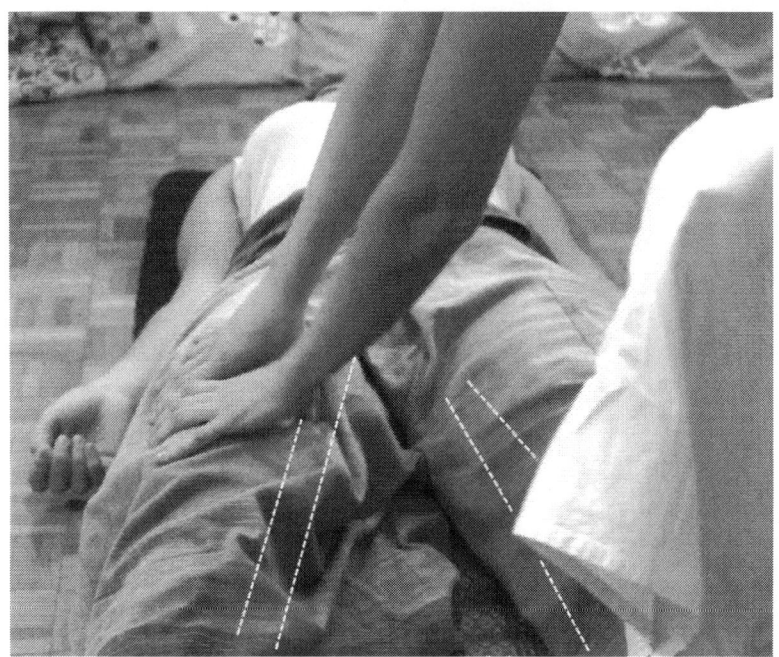

Then apply Step 3 of 5: Do Jap Sen (thumb walking) on the inner leg lines, Sahatsarangsi – Tawaree, and Kalatharee Sen.

Then apply again the 4th and 5th Steps.

How To Stop The Blood Flow

This technique is called "Stopping the blood", and it is optional. When done correctly, it leaves a pleasant feeling / rush of heat on the legs. It can also promote lymphatic drainage on the legs. However, it should never be done on people with cardiovascular disorders.

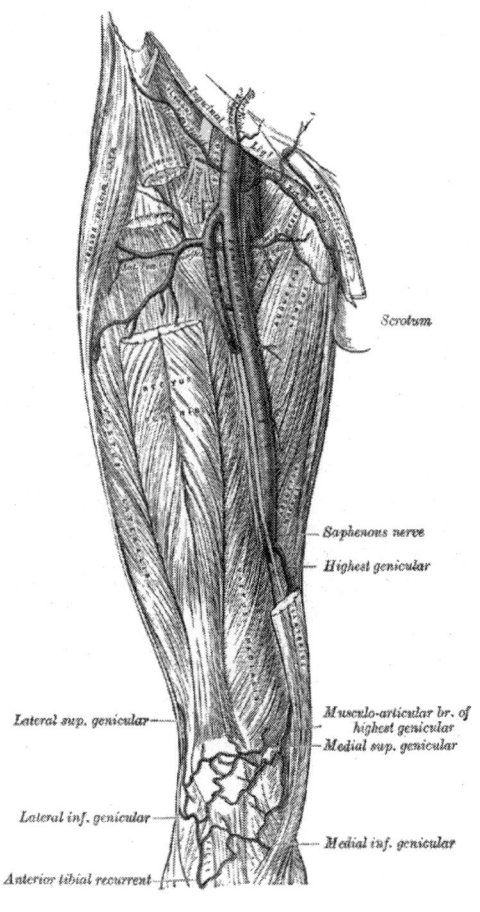

i. Femoral Artery

The therapist stops the blood flow on the legs for about 15-20 seconds, by blocking temporarily the femoral artery with his / her palm.

The femoral artery (see image at the left) can be palpated halfway between the pubic symphysis and anterior superior iliac spine. That's quite close to the genitals, so make sure the receiver is comfortable with this.

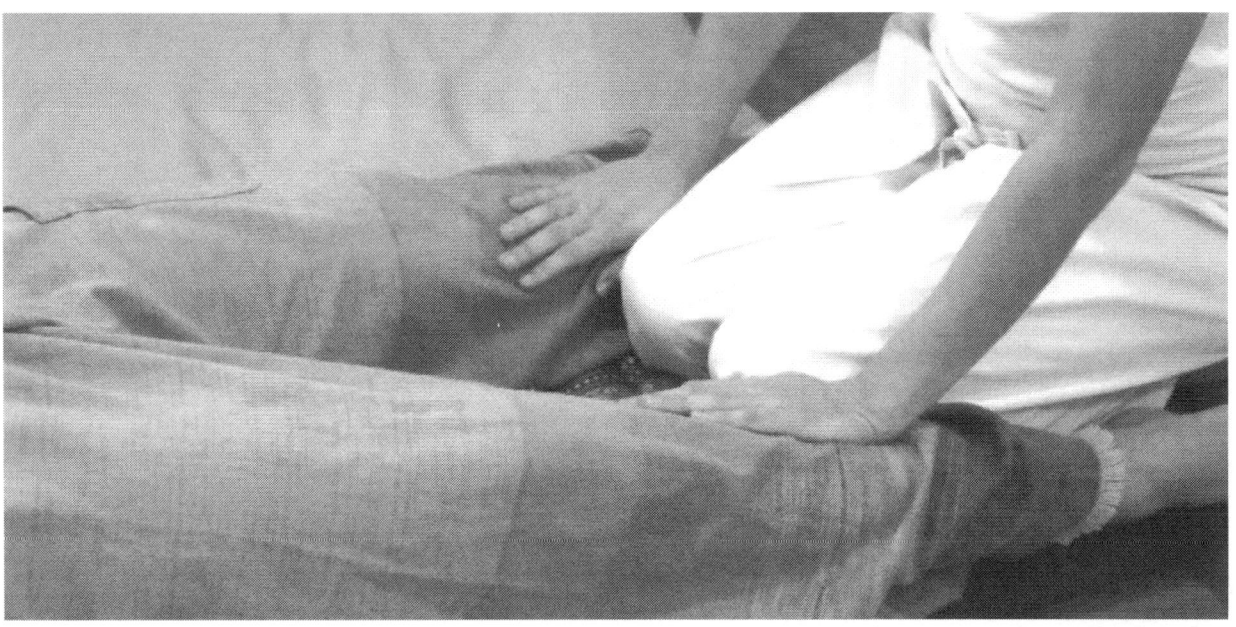

1. Using your hypothenar eminence, walk with your palms on the inner side of the lower leg. Do alternative presses and work slowly.

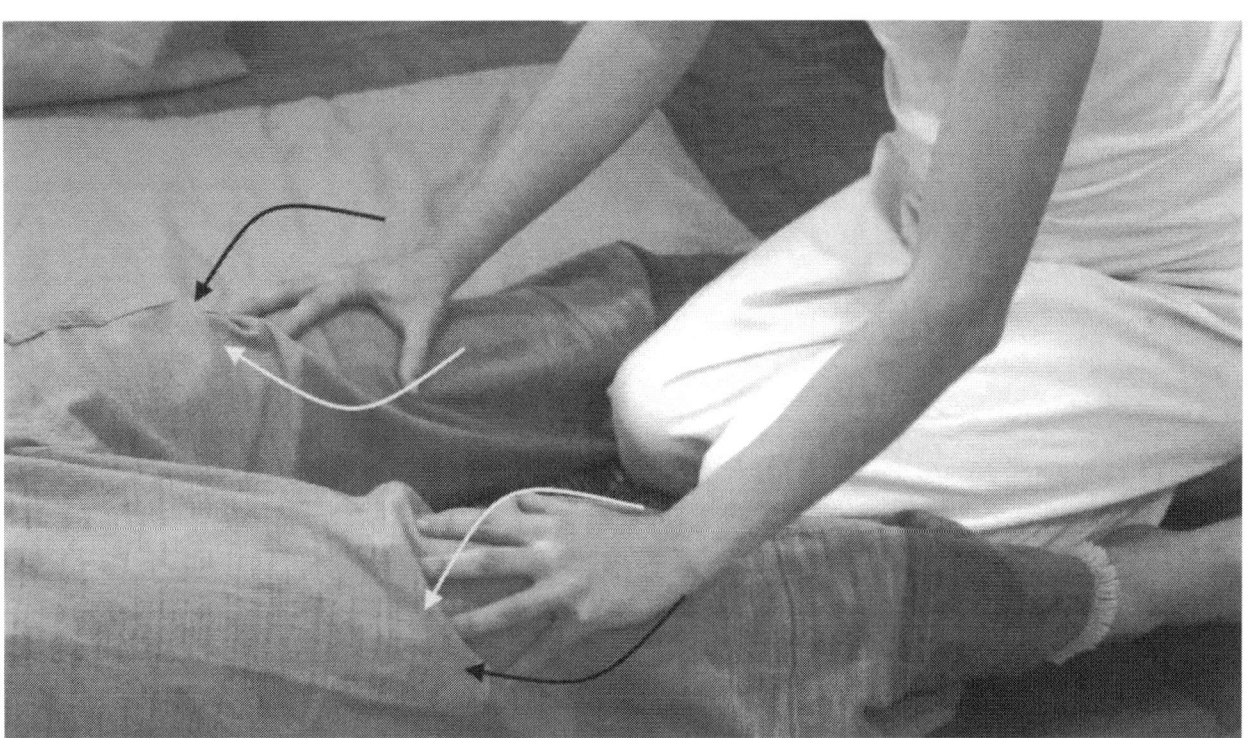

2. When you reach the knees, grasp them both and rotate the knee joint gently.

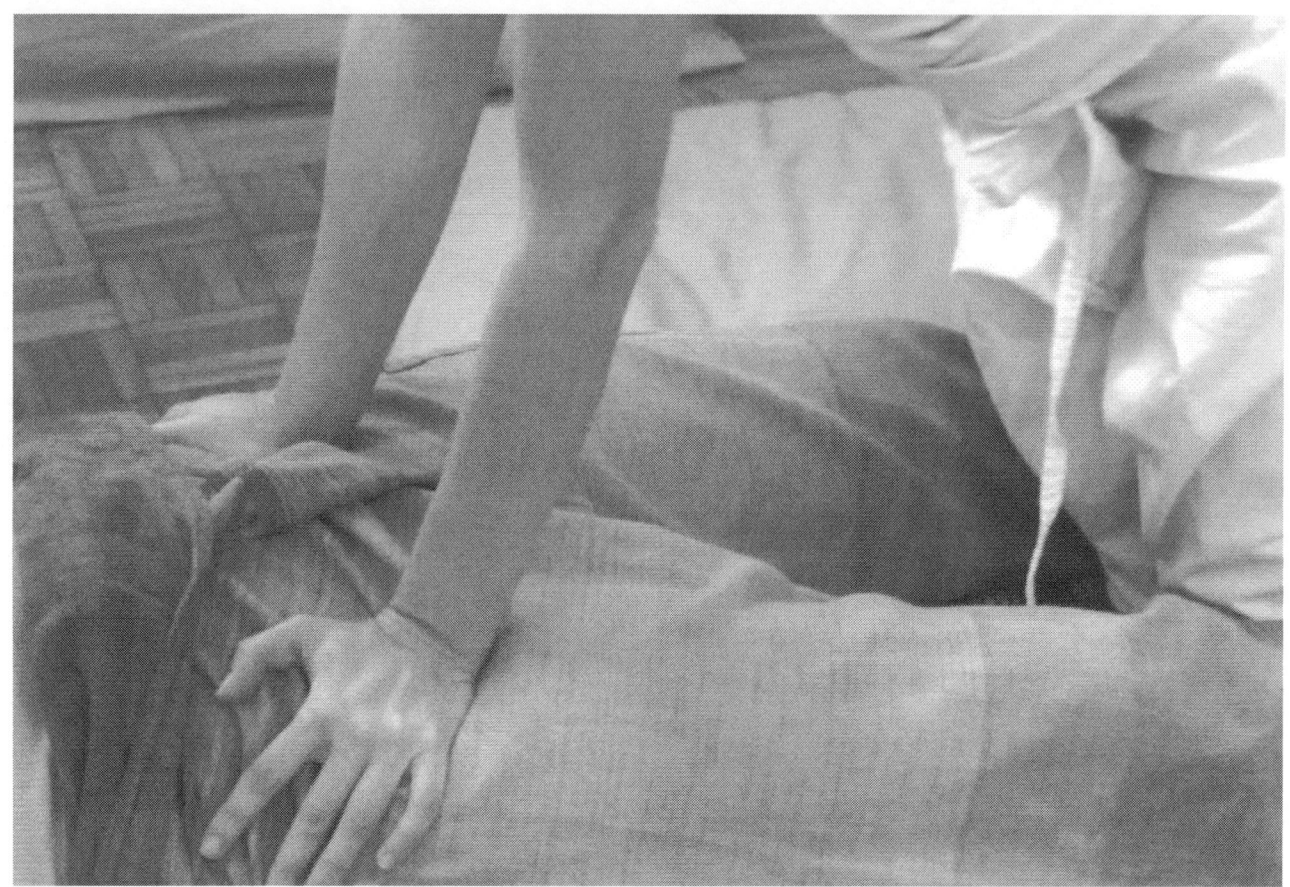

Then continue walking on the thighs with your palms. Look for the femoral artery pulse, and stop the blood flow with your palms. Press firmly for 15-20 seconds, and then release.

Return your palms on the receiver's feet, by repeating the previous techniques in a reverse way.

If you performed the technique correctly, the receiver will feel the heat (the blood, actually!) coming down her legs.

Let the receiver calm down for 4-5 seconds, and then walk back towards her feet, by repeating Step 2 and 1.

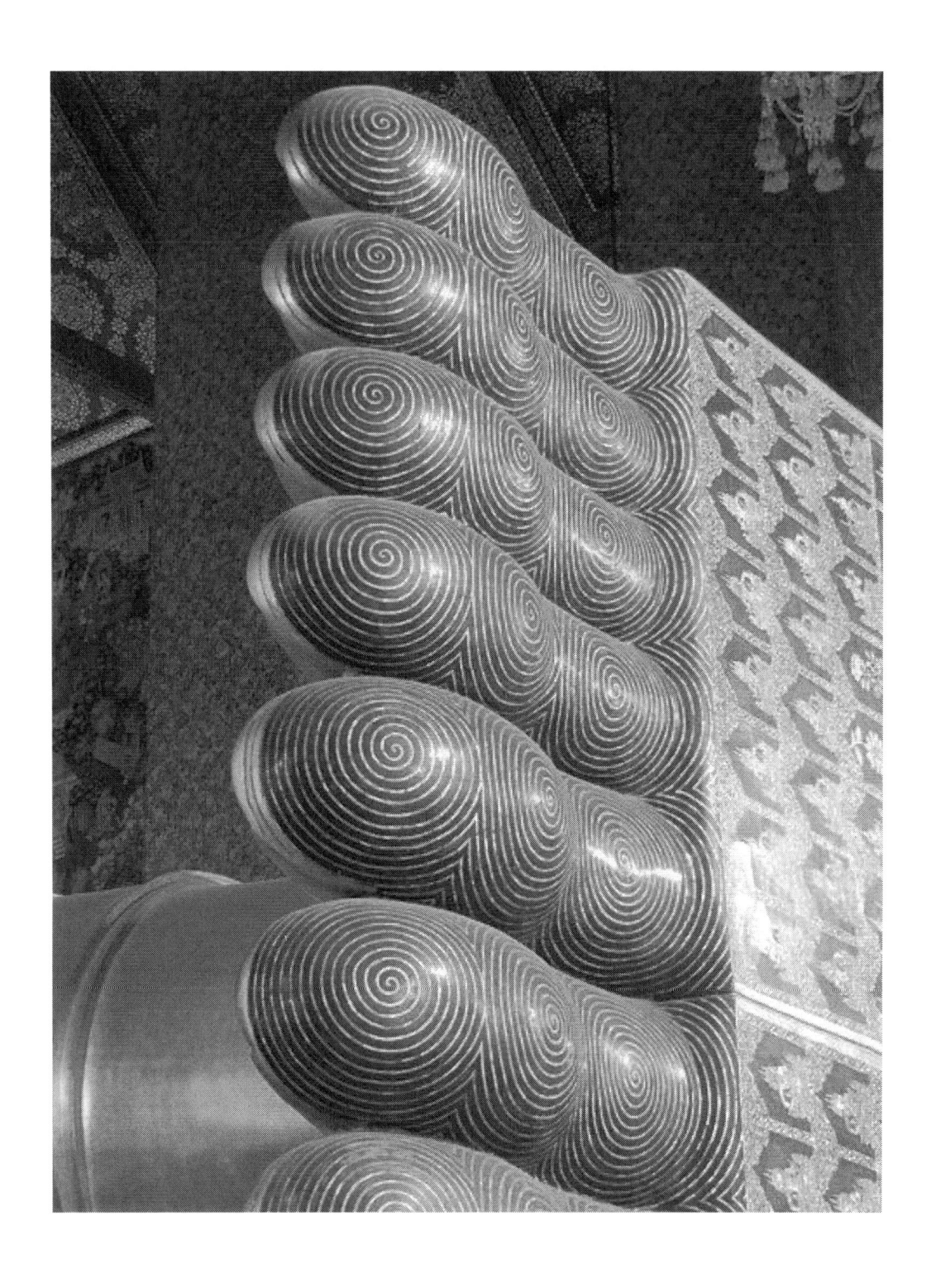

the feet

Traditionally, a Thai Massage session begins from the supine position. Actually, traditional Thai Massage has a protocol: The therapist moves from the receiver's feet to his head. Thus, the session opens with these techniques.

These techniques create a feeling of trust between the therapist and the receiver.

Also, as they induce a very pleasant feeling of relaxation, they help the receiver to "surrender" to the therapist, who will proceed with far more dynamic and interactive work in the next steps of the session.

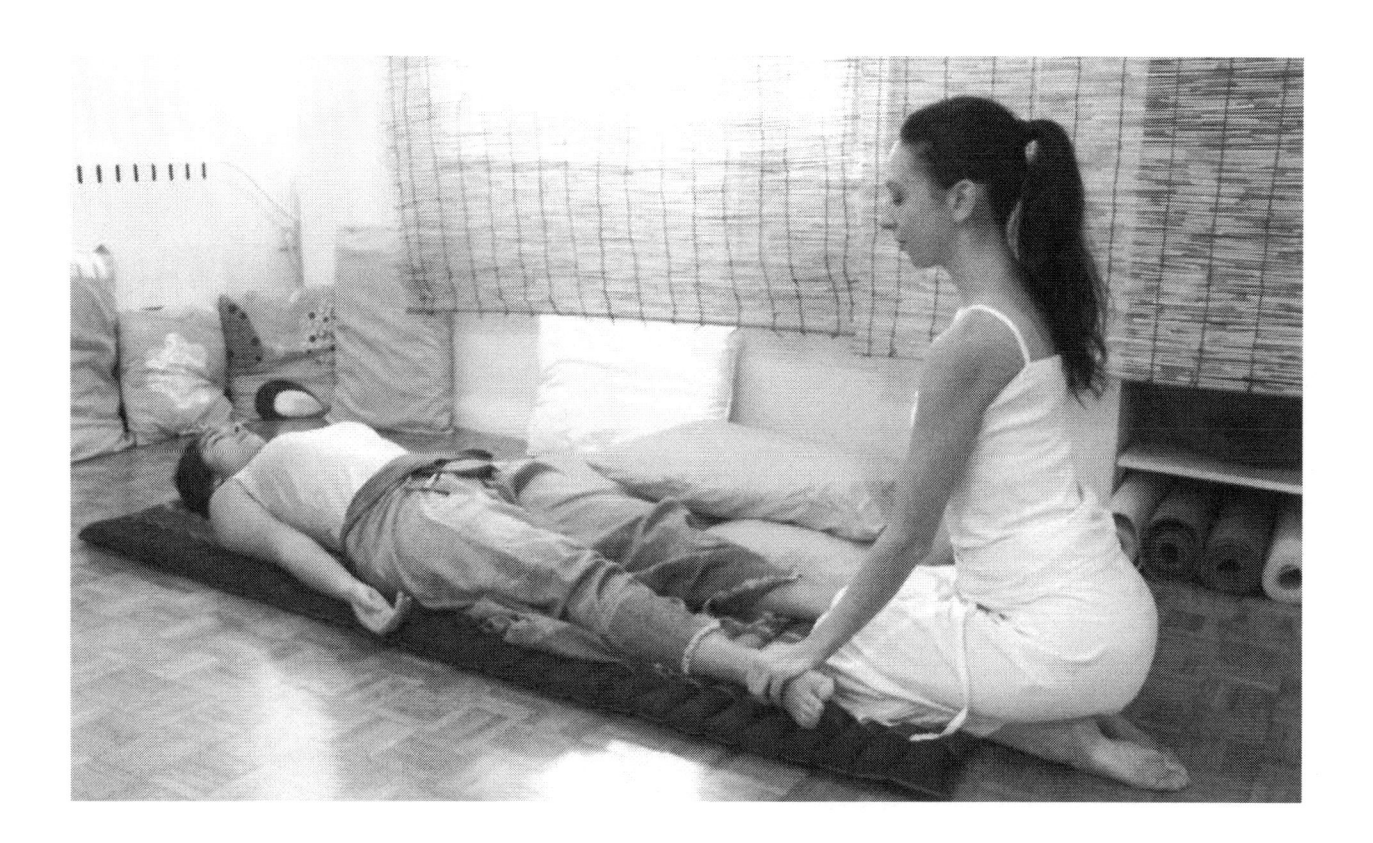

This is the initial position. The therapist should kneel in front of the receiver's feet, maintaining her spine straight and relaxed.

Open the receiver's feet at the width of her shoulders, and place the heel of your hands on her inner arch. If you feel that you should protect your knees, please kneel on a pillow.

Now you are ready to start.

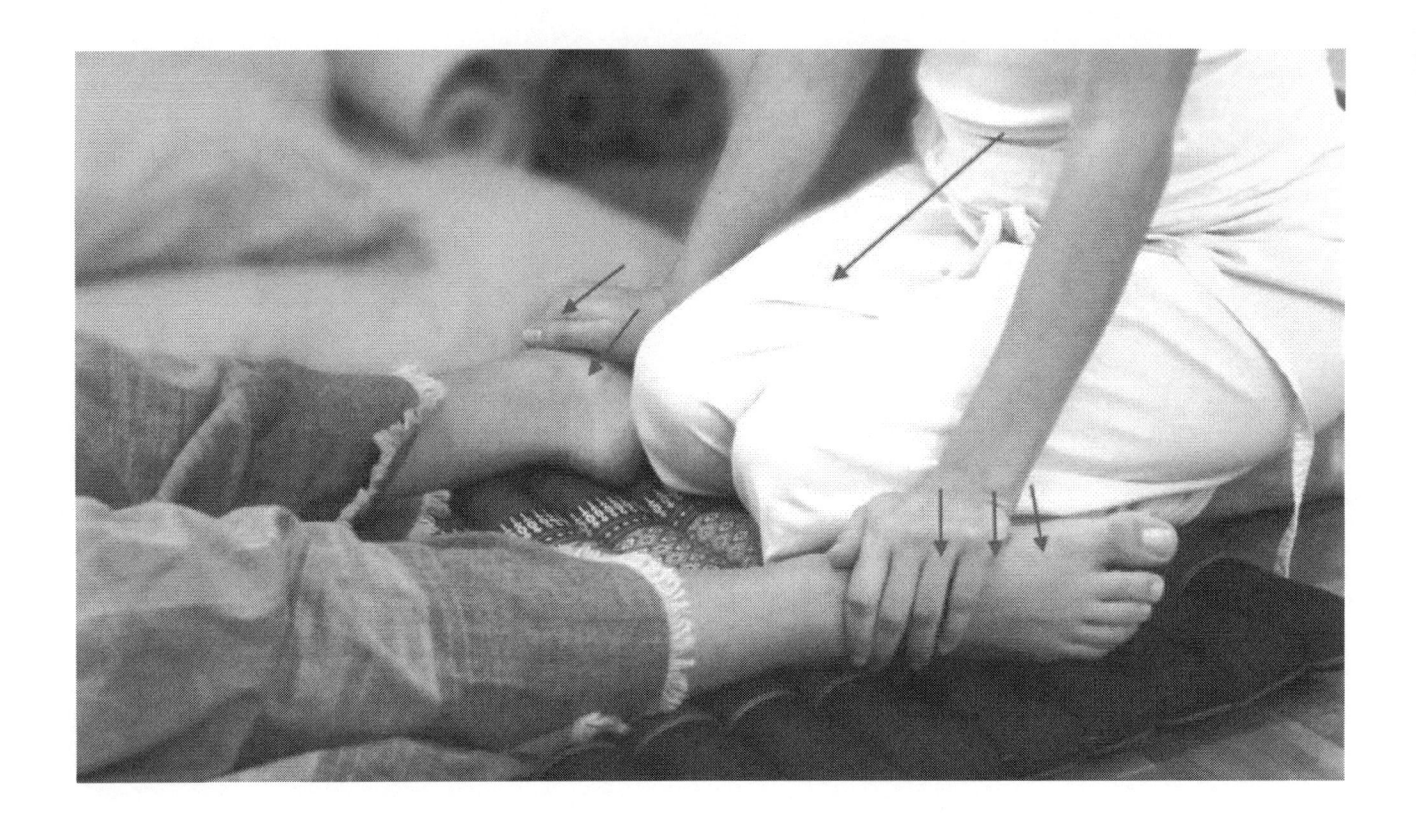

1. Walk on the inner arch of the feet with the heel of your hands. Work with your body weight – never apply pressure from your shoulders.

Press alternatively with each palm, and maintain the pressure for at least 3 seconds each time.

Be careful not to apply pressure on the metatarsophalangeal joint and the ankle.

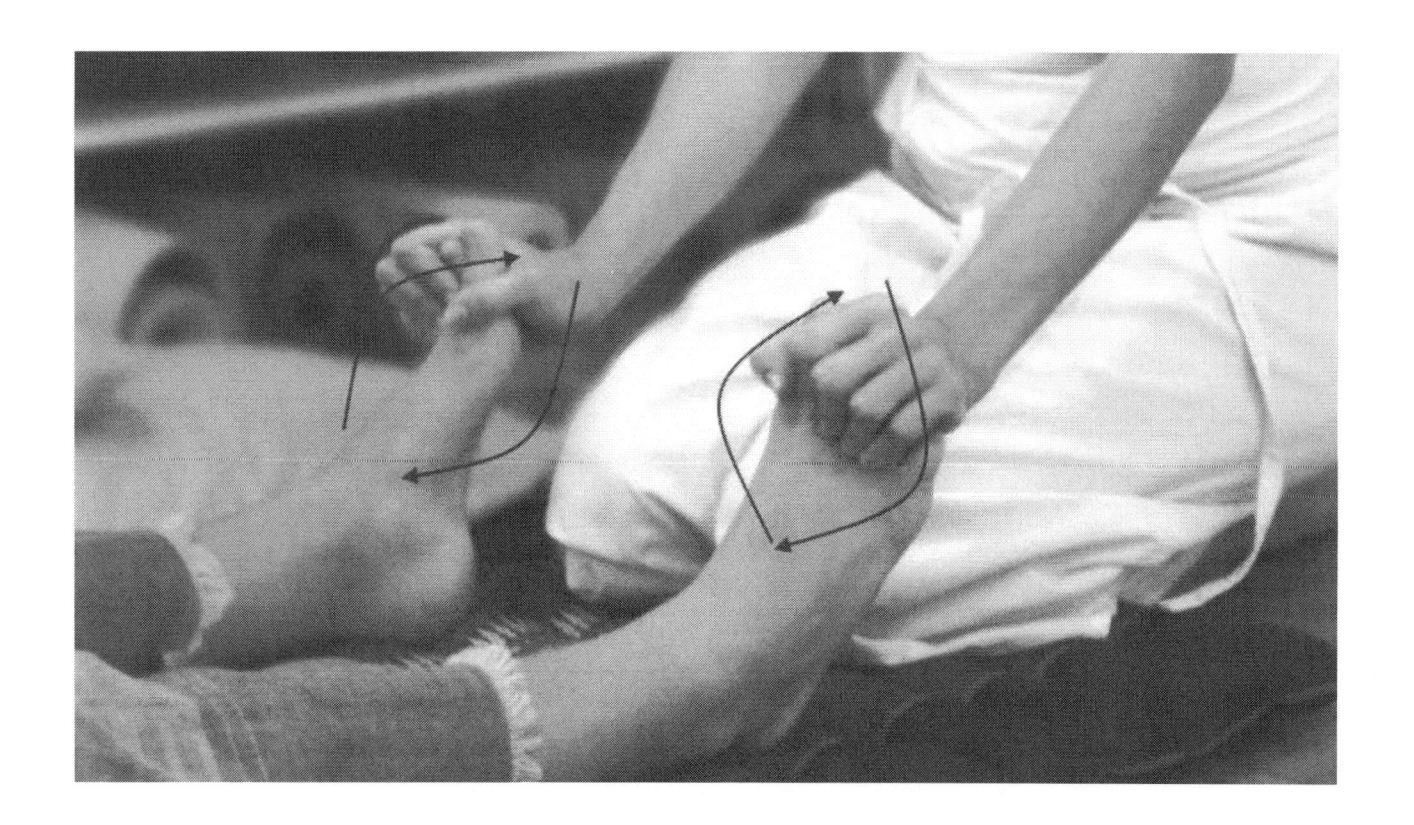

2. Grasp the receiver's feet and rotate them towards both directions. Be sure to cover the entire range of motion. Always work gently and slowly. Your grip should feel steady, but not tight.

At this point, you may perceive some sounds during the rotation, coming from the joints. This probably means that the receiver has loose ligaments and joint hypermobility at the feet. In that case, you should not apply any pulls that target the particular joints.

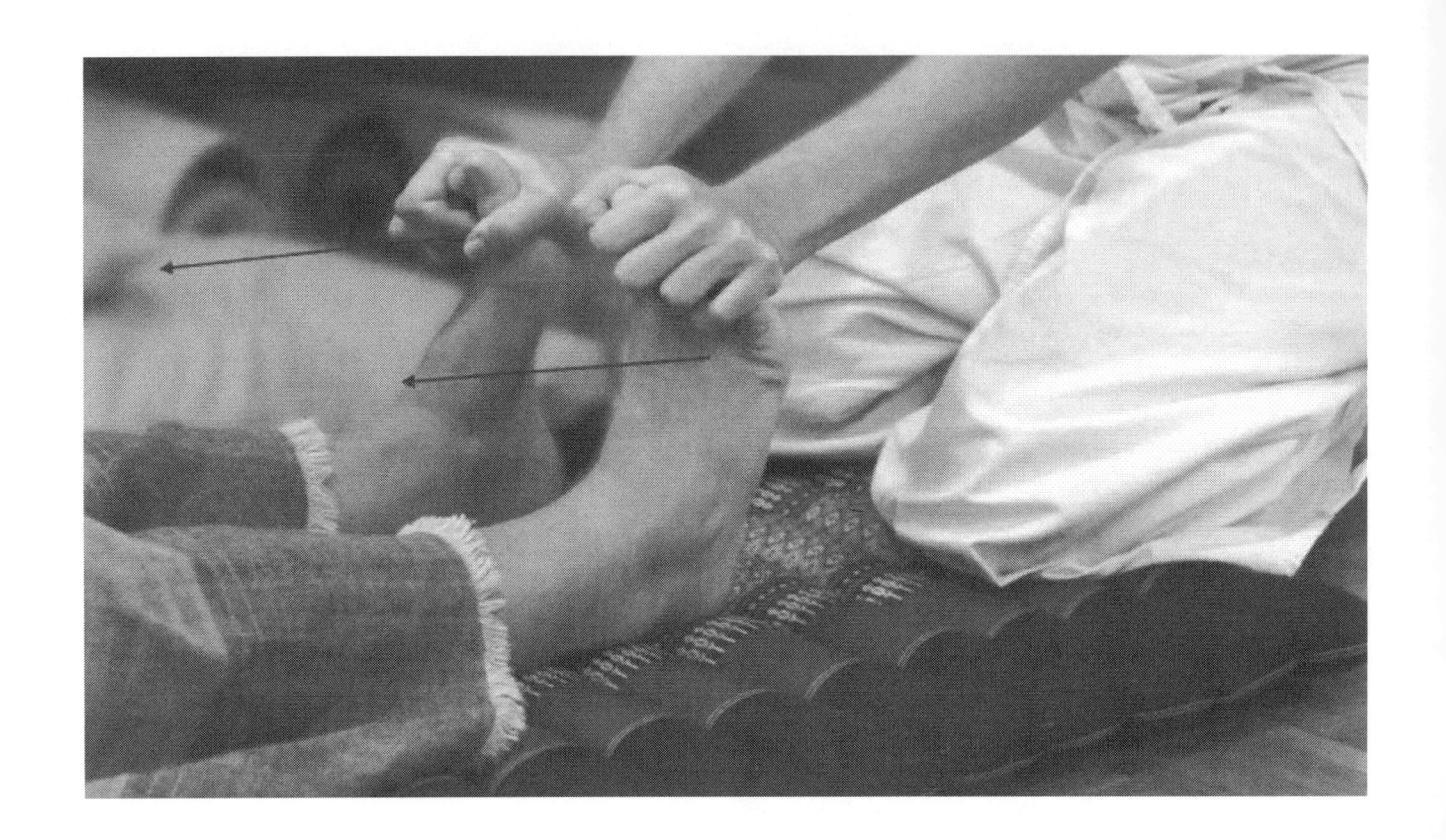

3. Bring the receiver's feet close to one another, in order to align them with the receiver's central axis. Now push the receiver's feet towards her head.

The stretch should be felt to the Achilles tendon.

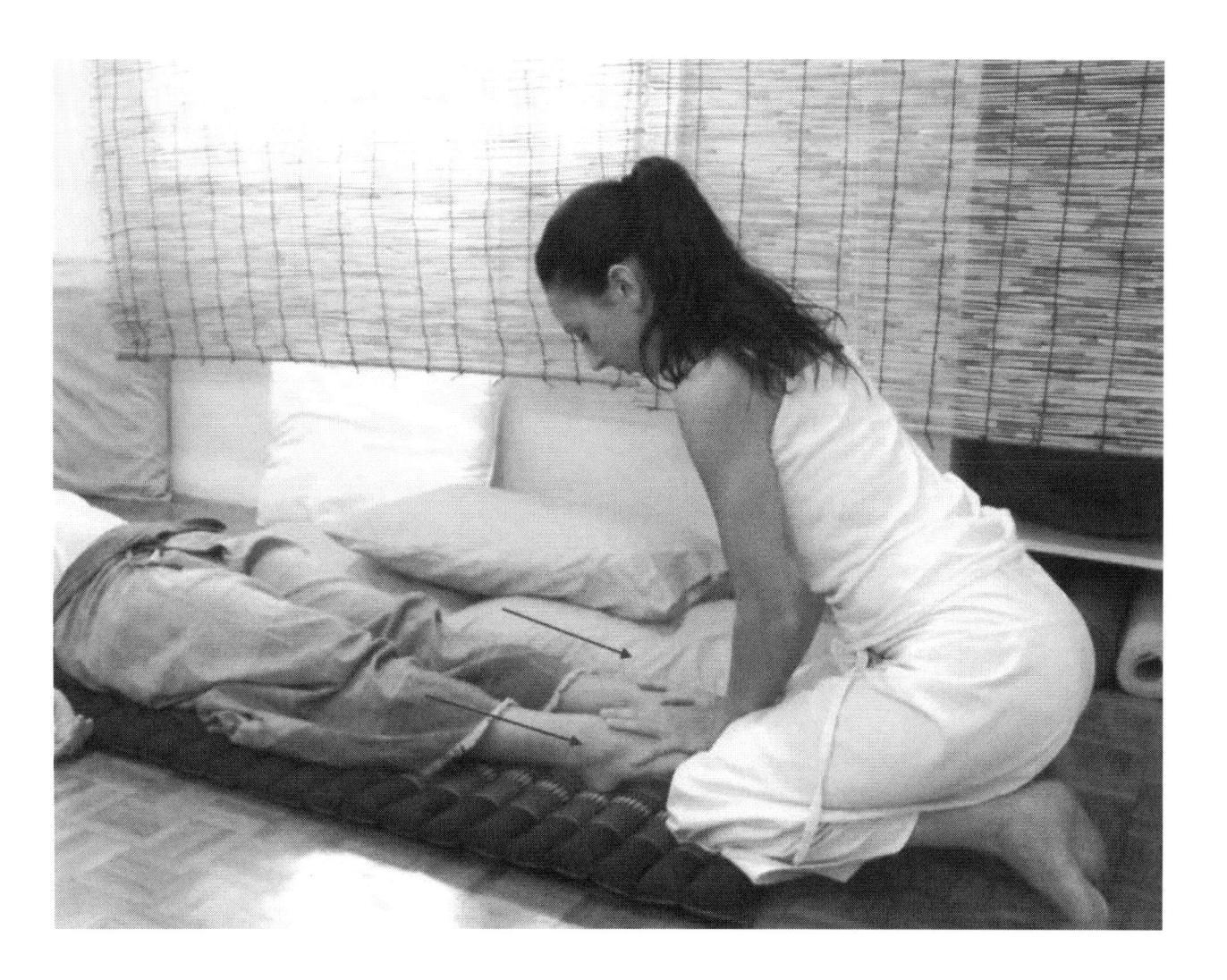

4. Place your palms on the spot where the metatarsophalangeal articulations meet the phalanges, and press the receiver's feet downwards.

The stretch should be felt mainly on the anterior muscles of the lower leg. However, this technique is a mobilization for the entire leg, as it is felt up to the hip.

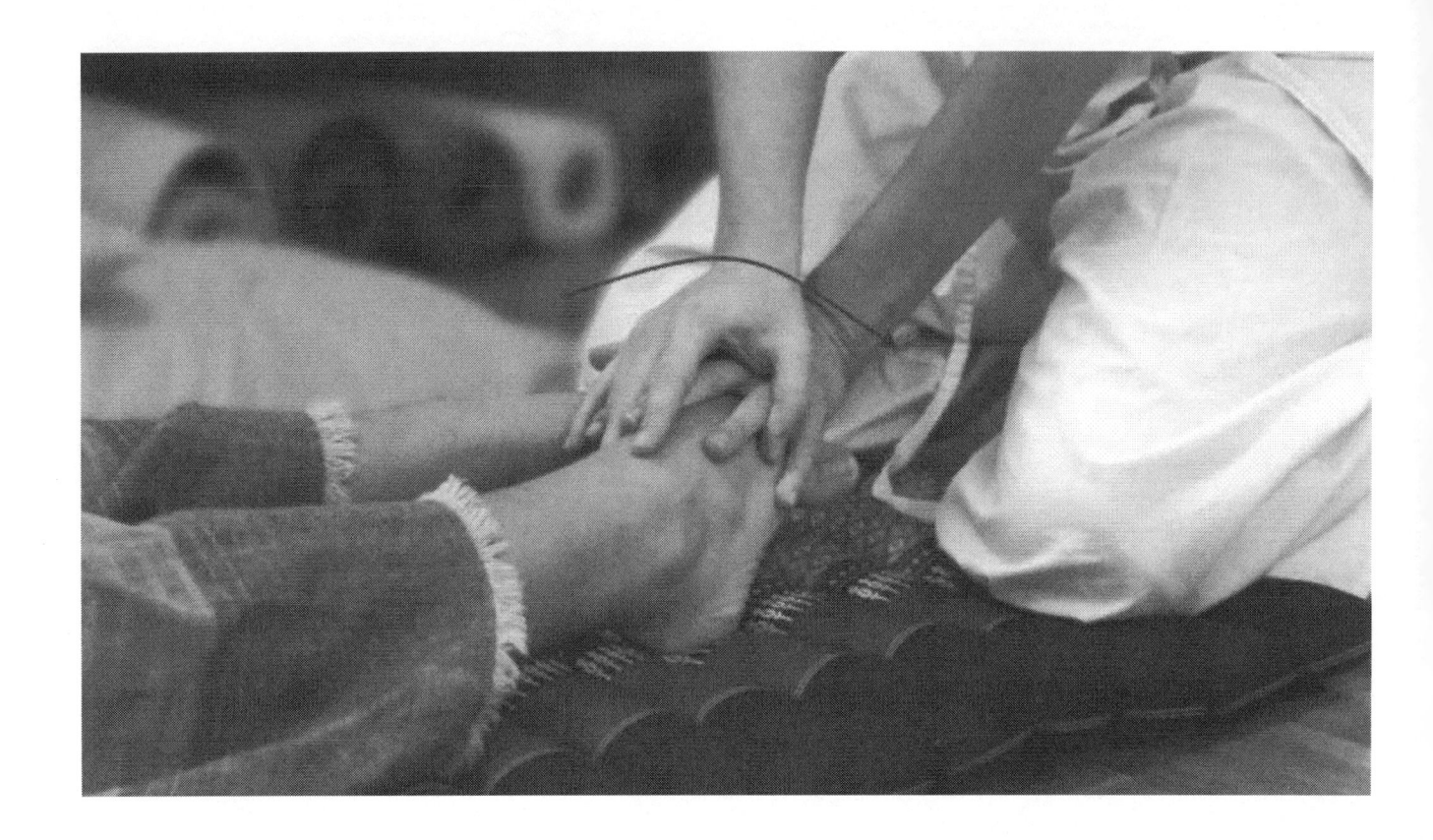

5. Place the one foot above the other, and press both feet of the receiver downwards.

Please do not perform this technique on osteoporotic women.

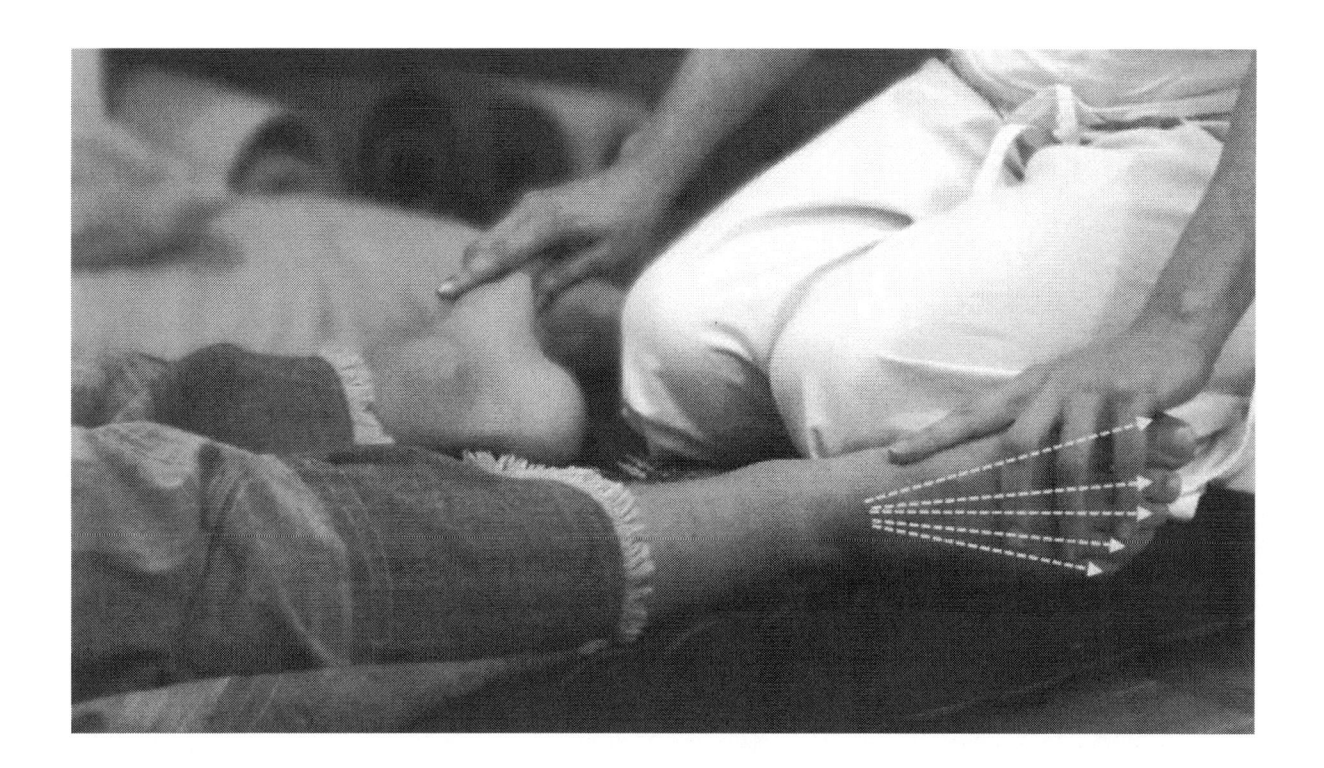

6. Place your fingers on the dorsal aspect of the receiver's foot, and your thumb on the plantar aspect. Using your thumb, apply pressure on the Kalatharee Sen. Do not apply direct pressure on the toe joints – just rub them gently.

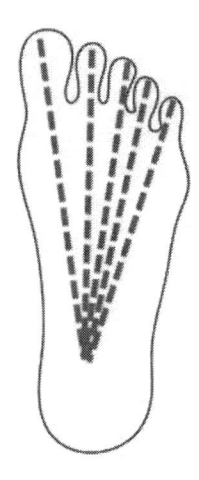

Work from the big toe towards the pinky toe, on 5 lines. At the end of each "line" pull gently the toes.

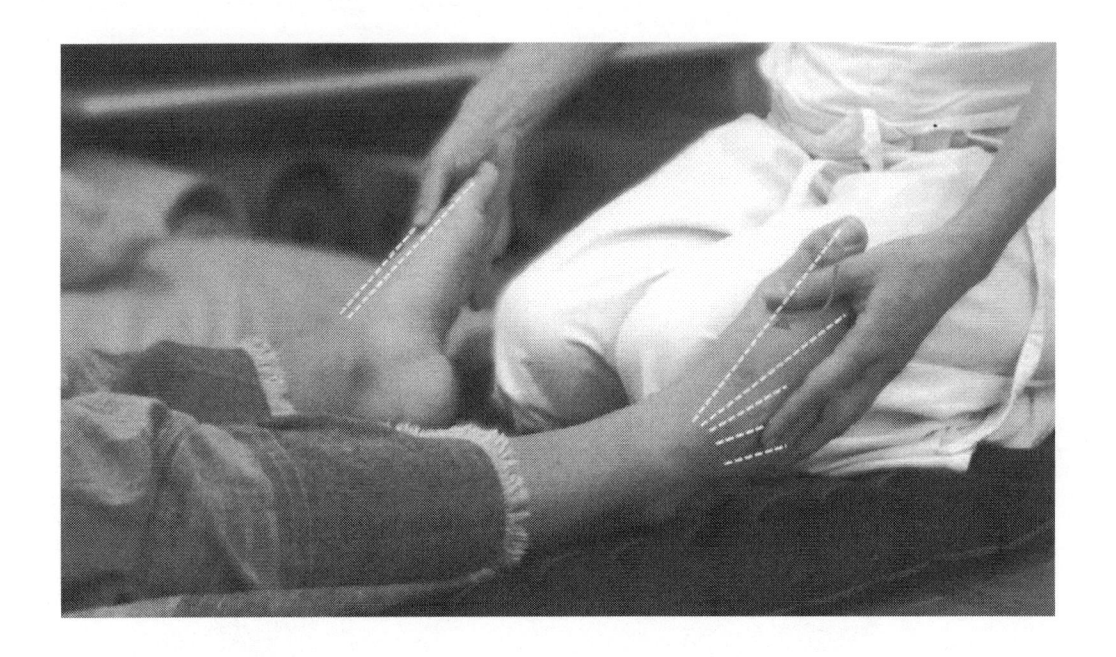

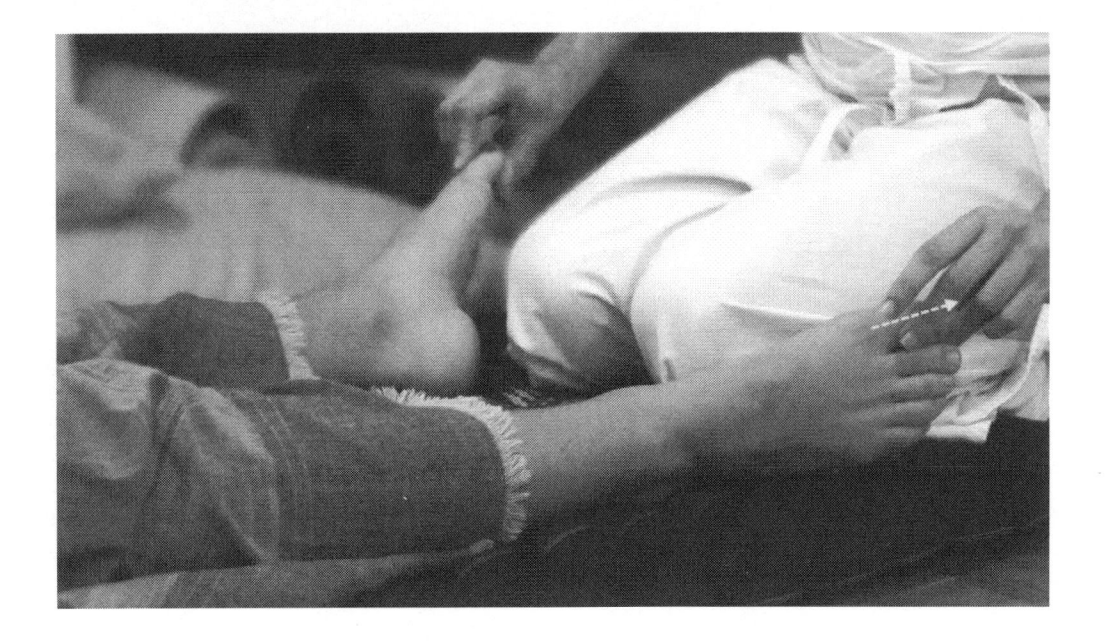

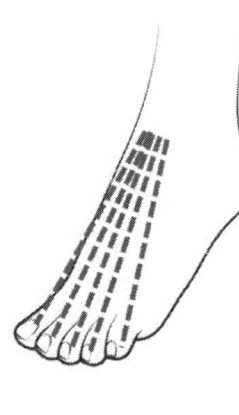

7. Now follow with your thumbs the Itha & Pingkala Sen lines on the dorsal aspect of the foot. Again, work from the big toe towards the pinky toe, on 5 lines. At the end of each "line" pull gently the toes.

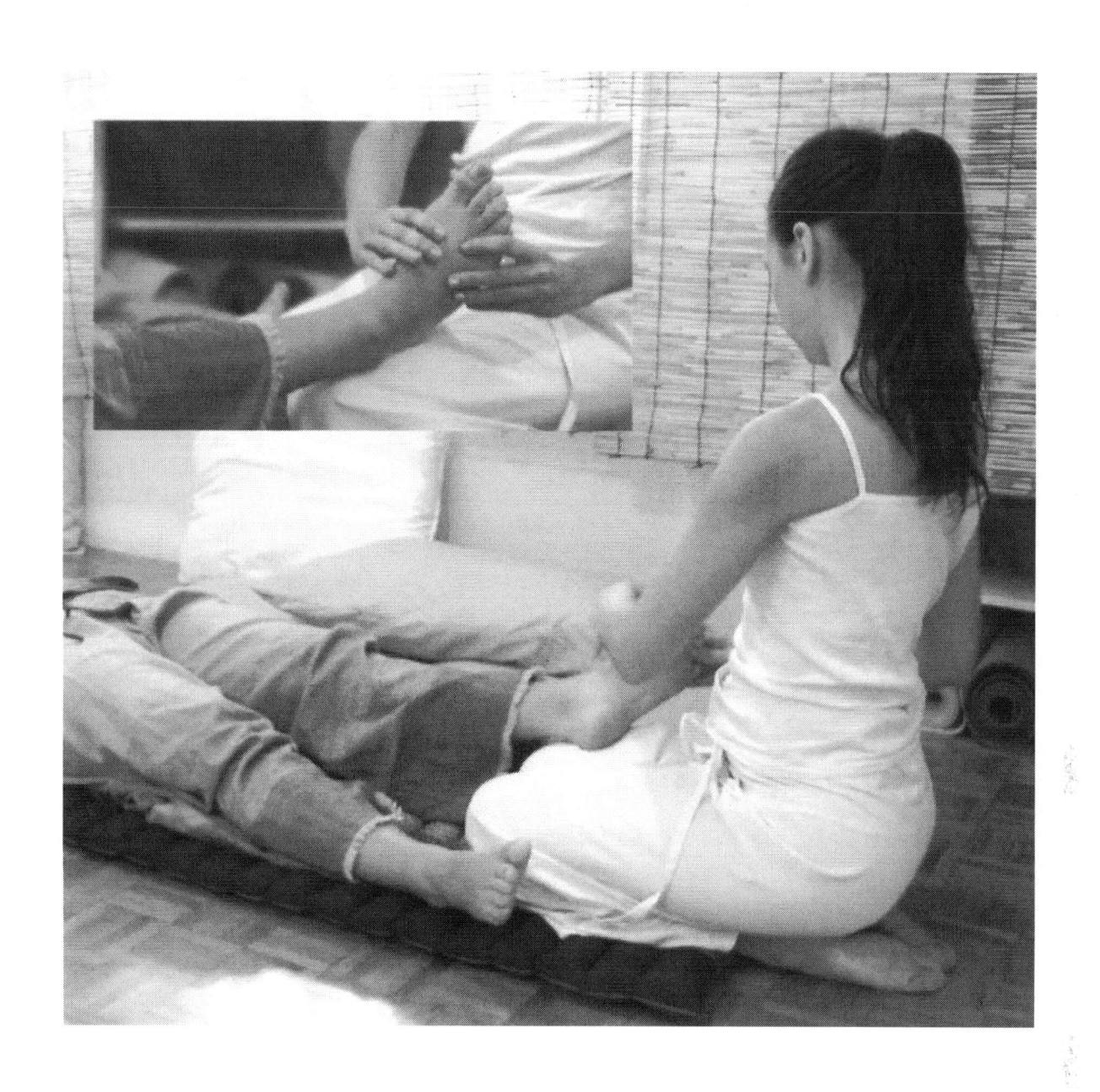

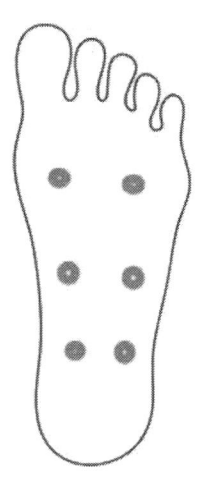

8. Place the receiver's foot on your thigh. Using your thumbs, press 6 points on the foot.

When you finish working on the 6 points on the one foot, place it gently on the mat, and repeat this technique on the other foot as well.

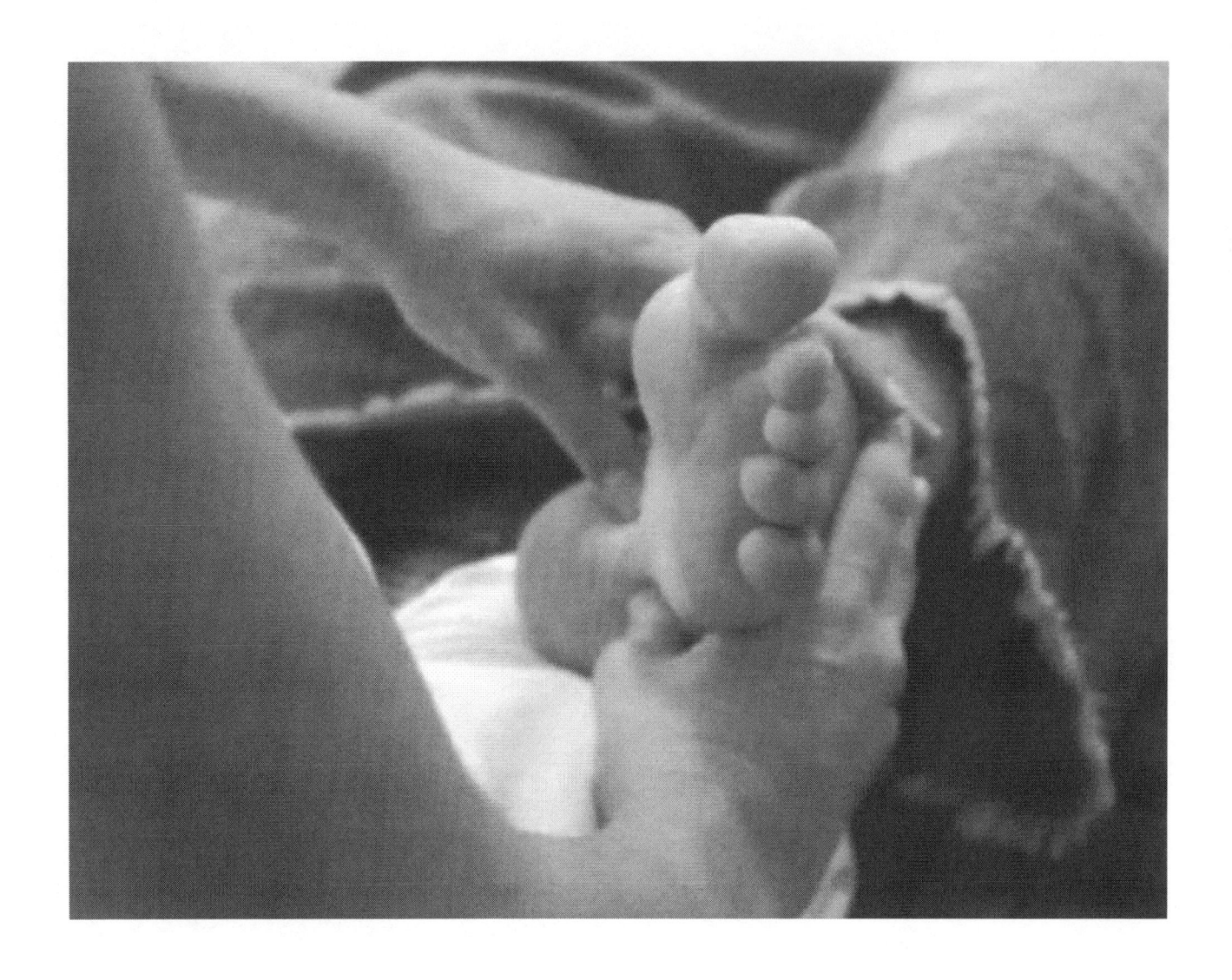

And this is Technique 8, just shot from a different angle.

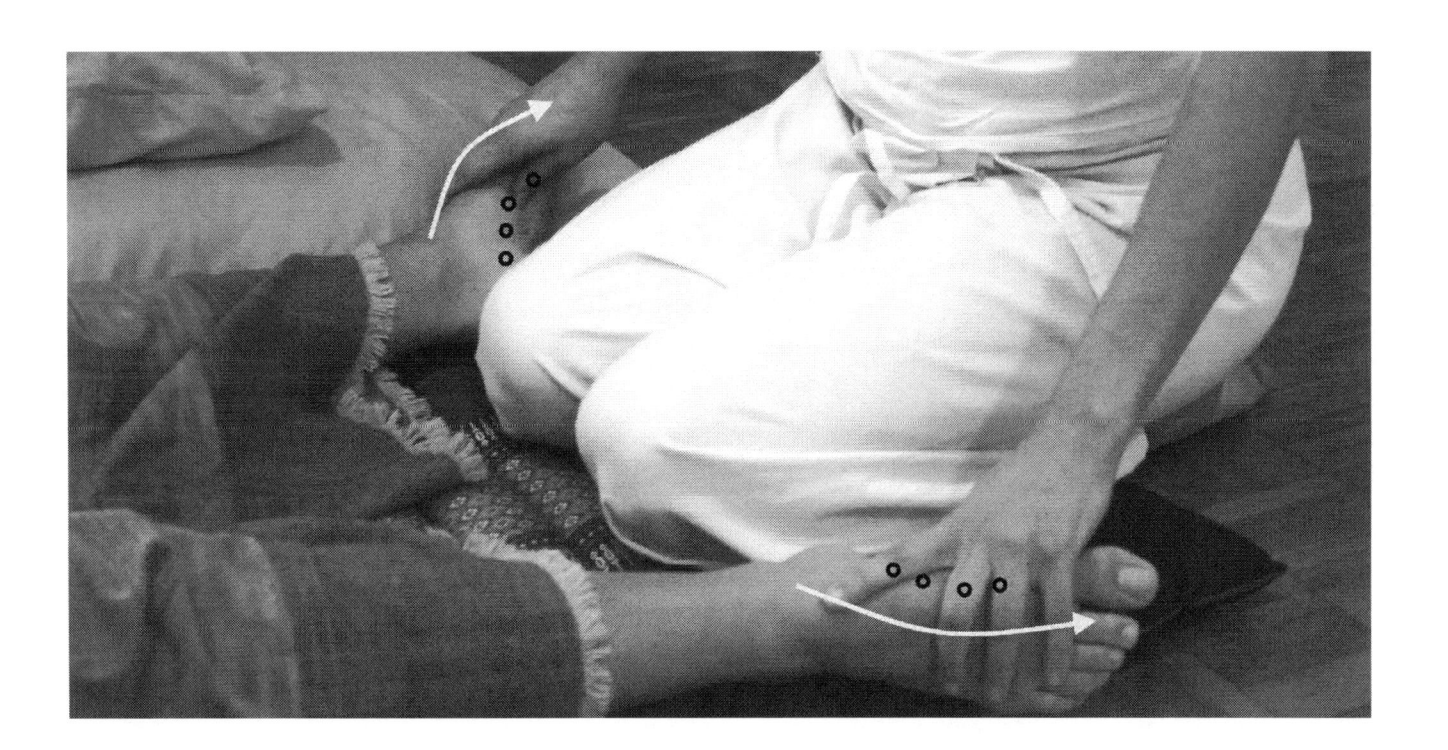

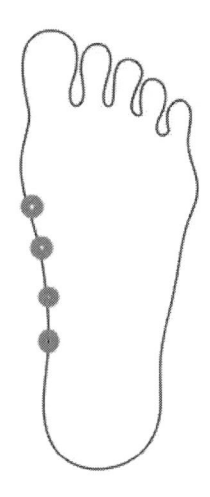

Using your thumbs, press the inner arch of both feet simultaneously. Do not apply pressure on the metatarsophalangeal joint.

what lies underneath

I am presenting some anatomical plates for your reference. They demonstrate some of the anatomy terms mentioned in the text.

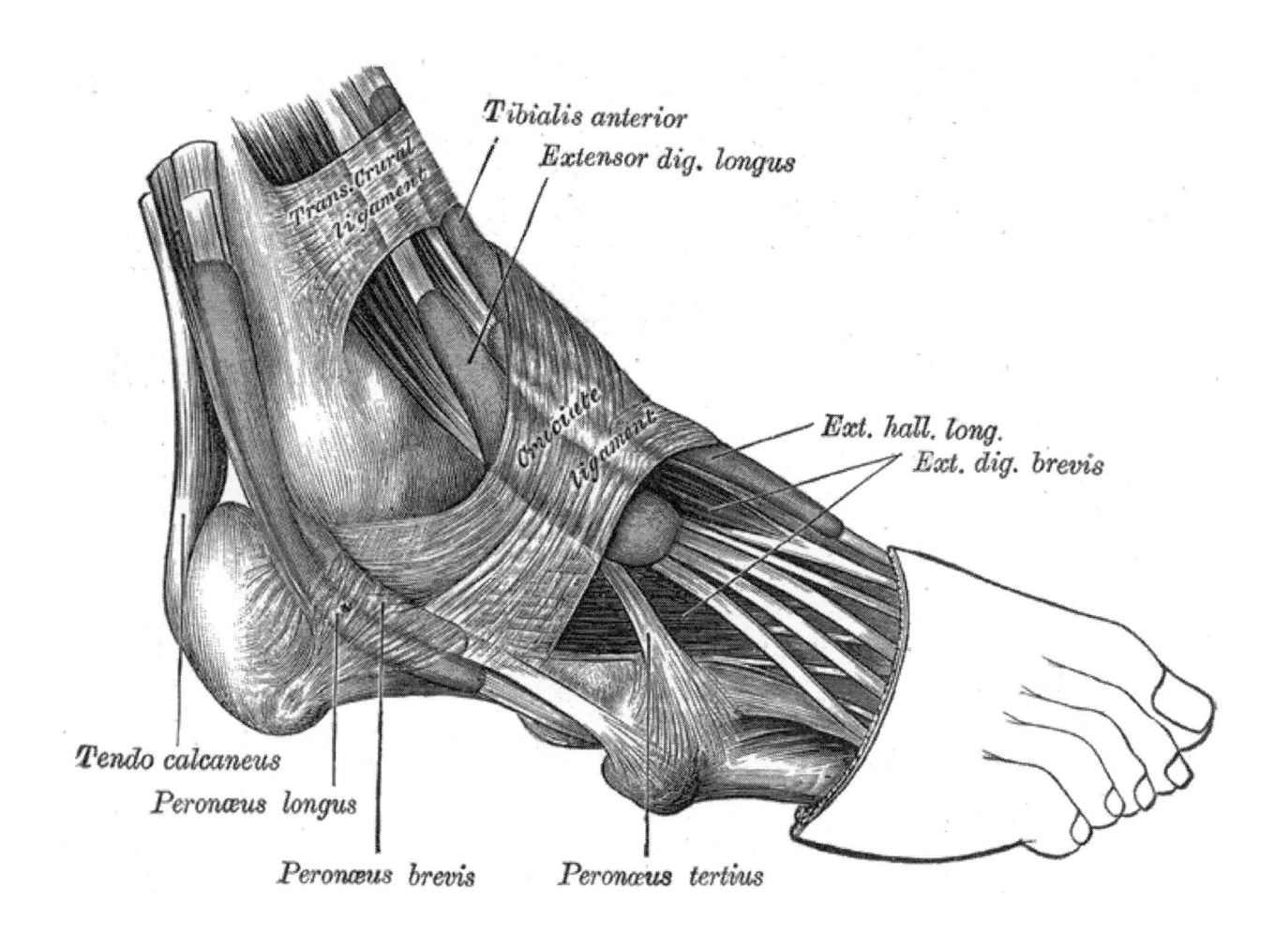

This plate shows the ligaments of the foot.

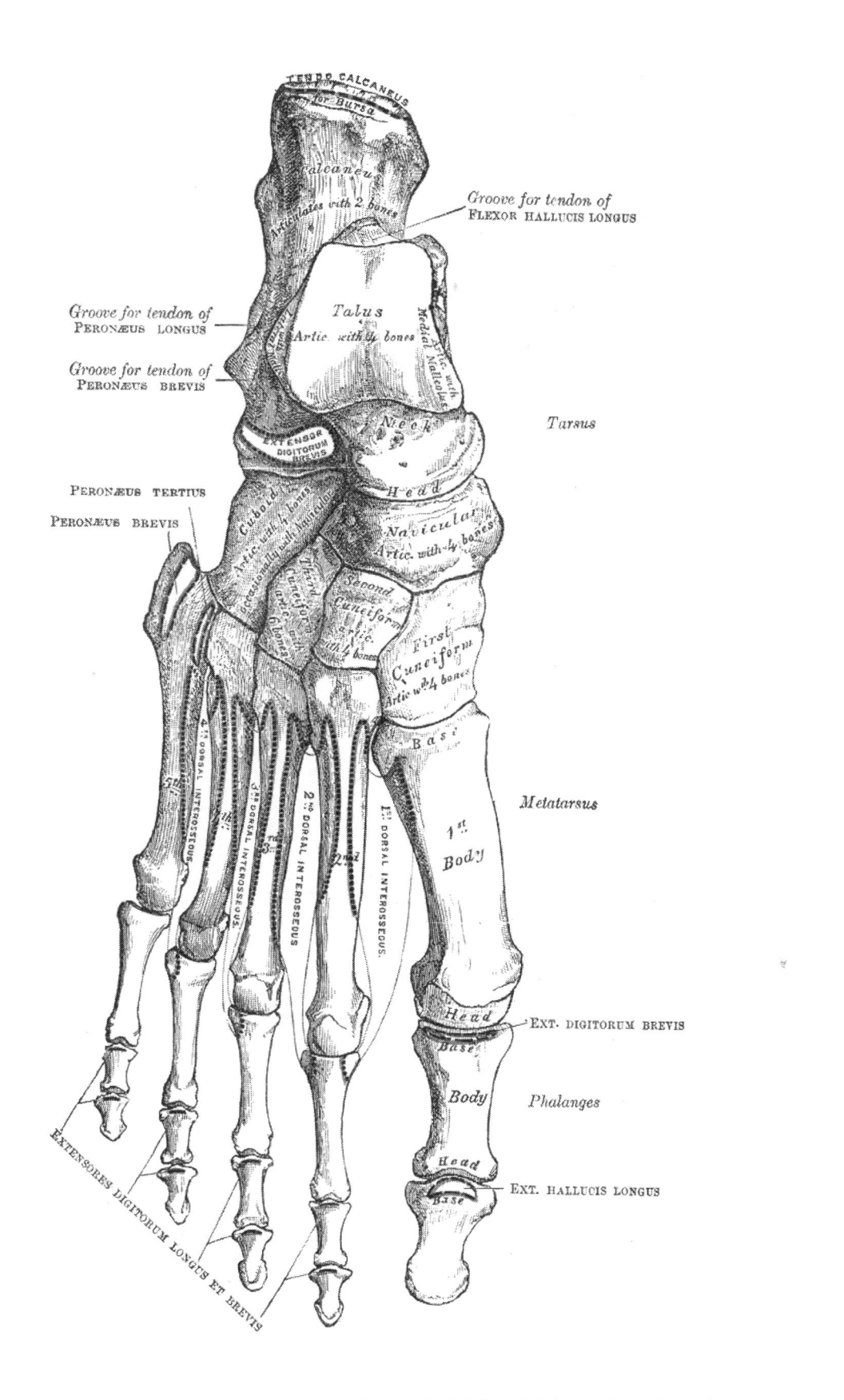

This plate shows the bones of the right foot (dorsal surface).

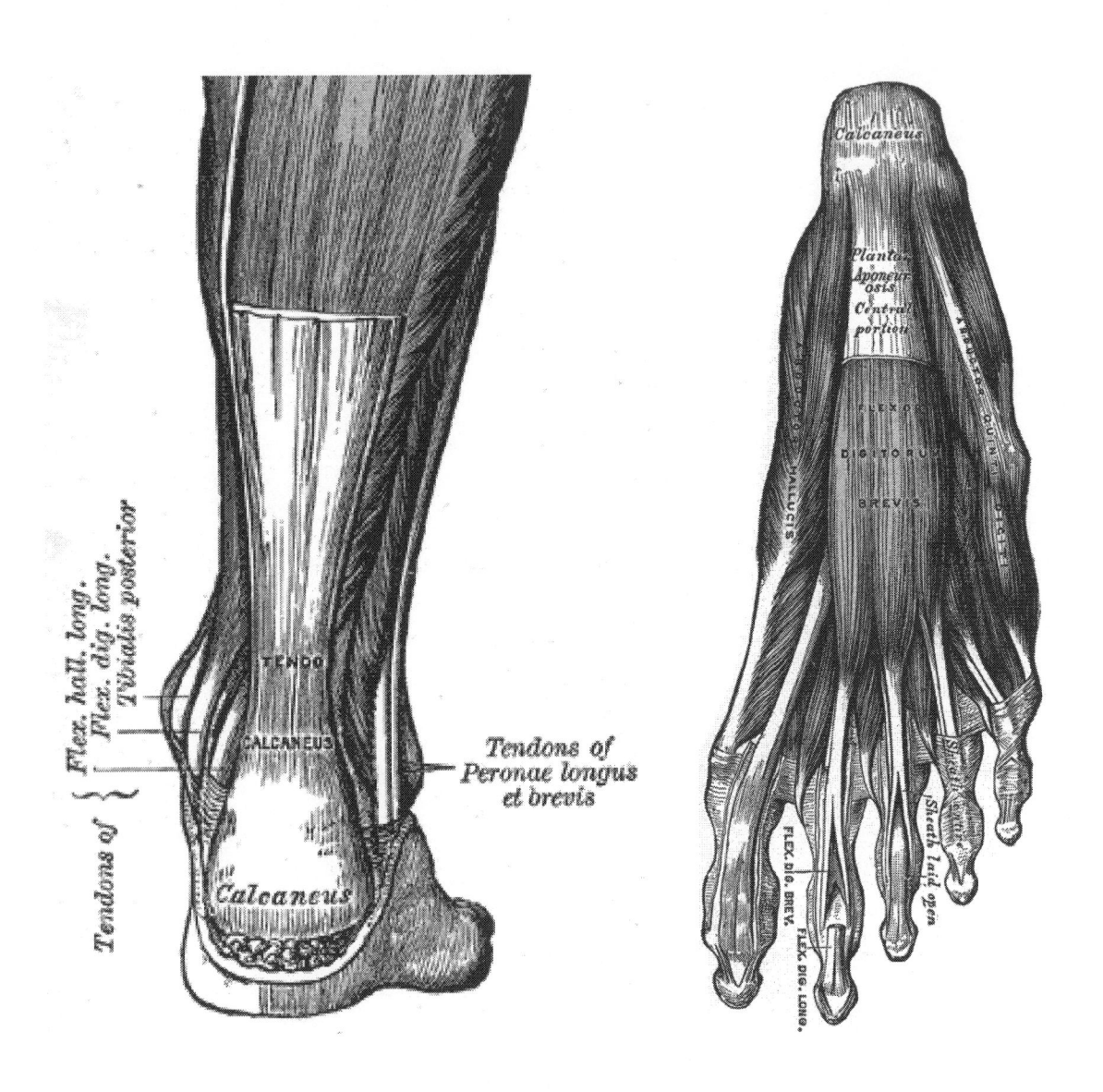

Achilles tendon (left) and muscles of the foot (right).

Thus end the Thai Massage feet techniques.

These techniques are considered suitable for the treatment of plantar fasciitis (during the chronic phase). Other traditional indications include painful, tired feet, headaches and stress.

According to Thai medicine, acupressure on the feet brings the energy down, thus removing the tension away from the body. For this reason, they are especially indicated for headaches.

leg techniques

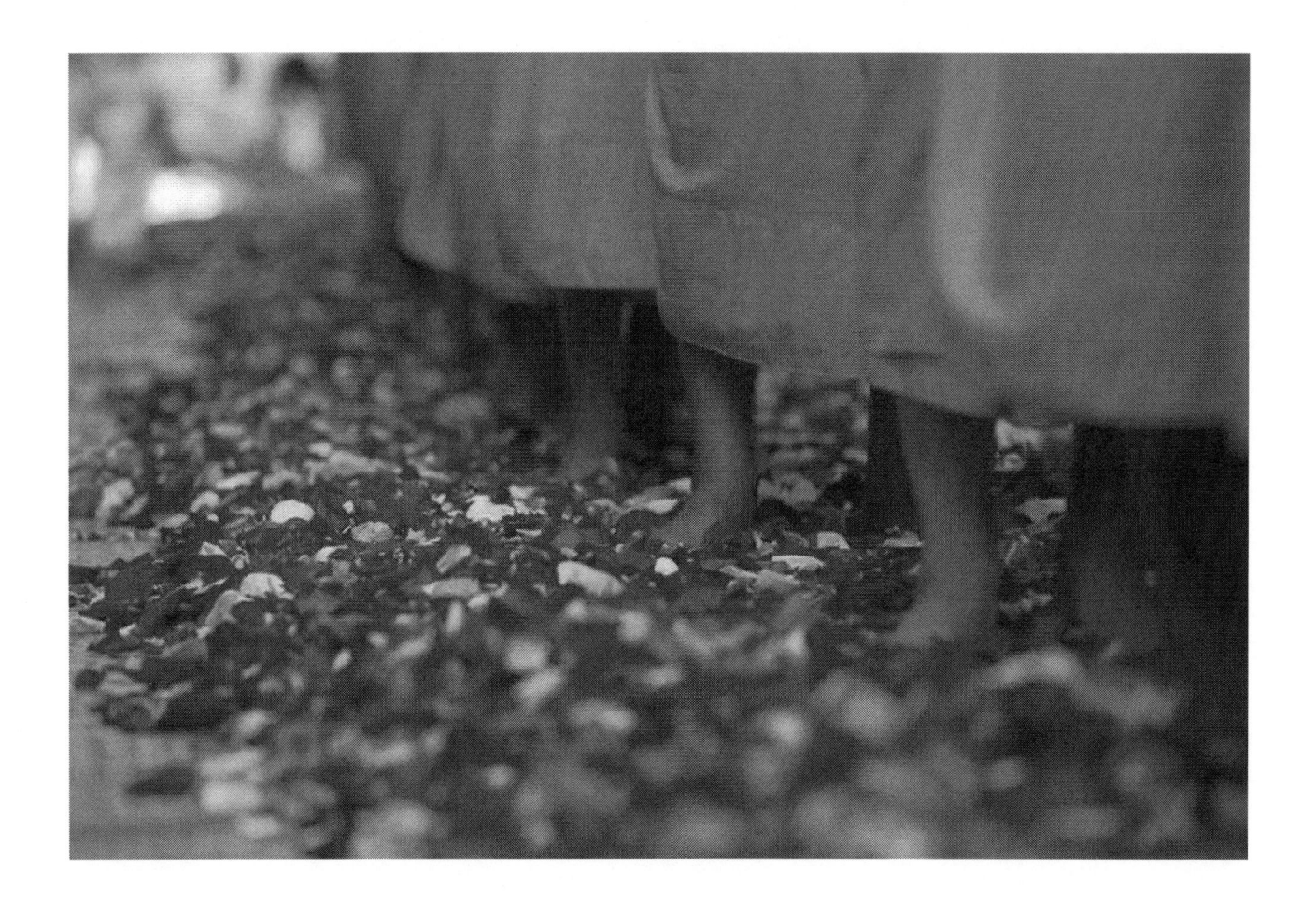

We can say that these techniques are the most representative feature of Thai Massage. Some of them are gentle and may be applied even to the elderly. However, some of them are unsuitable for older clients. Some techniques should never be applied to those who suffer from osteoarthritis of the hip.

If applied properly, these techniques can be effective not only for disorders of the legs, but also for lower back pain and sciatica. During their application, the therapist should respect the receiver's flexibility and boundaries. Clearly, you should never push the body beyond its limits.

The experienced therapist may use various props (pillows, yoga bricks, etc.), in order to support properly the receiver's body. This may be necessary especially if the receiver is an elderly person, a person with limited mobility or simply a person with limited flexibility.

single leg techniques

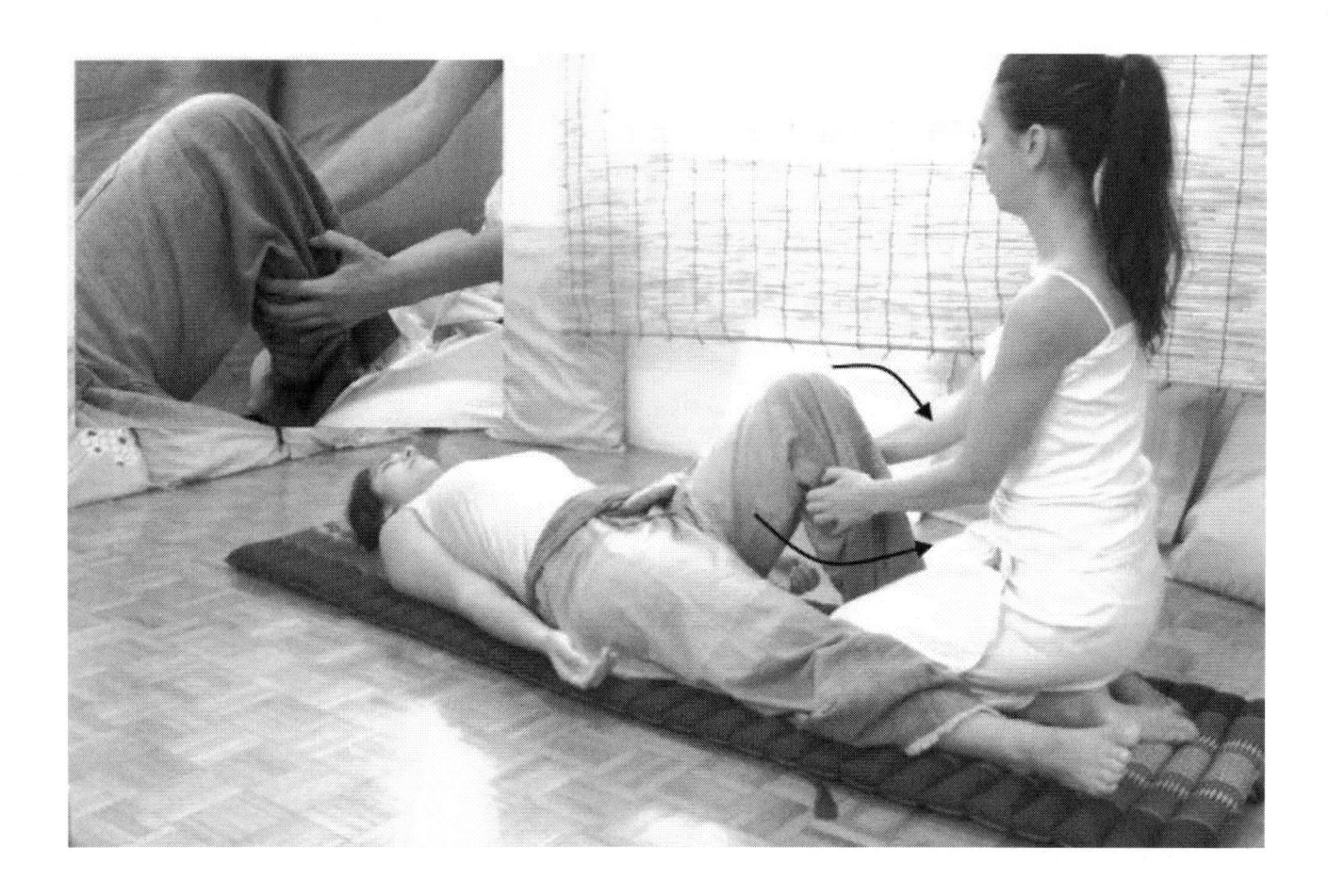

1. Stabilize the receiver's lower leg between your thighs. Using your fingers, try to separate the heads of the gastrocnemius muscle. Be careful not to continue this technique below the muscle – that is, on the Achilles tendon – because this would be painful.

With your hands in the same position, you can also let your body weight fall back, applying traction to the hip.

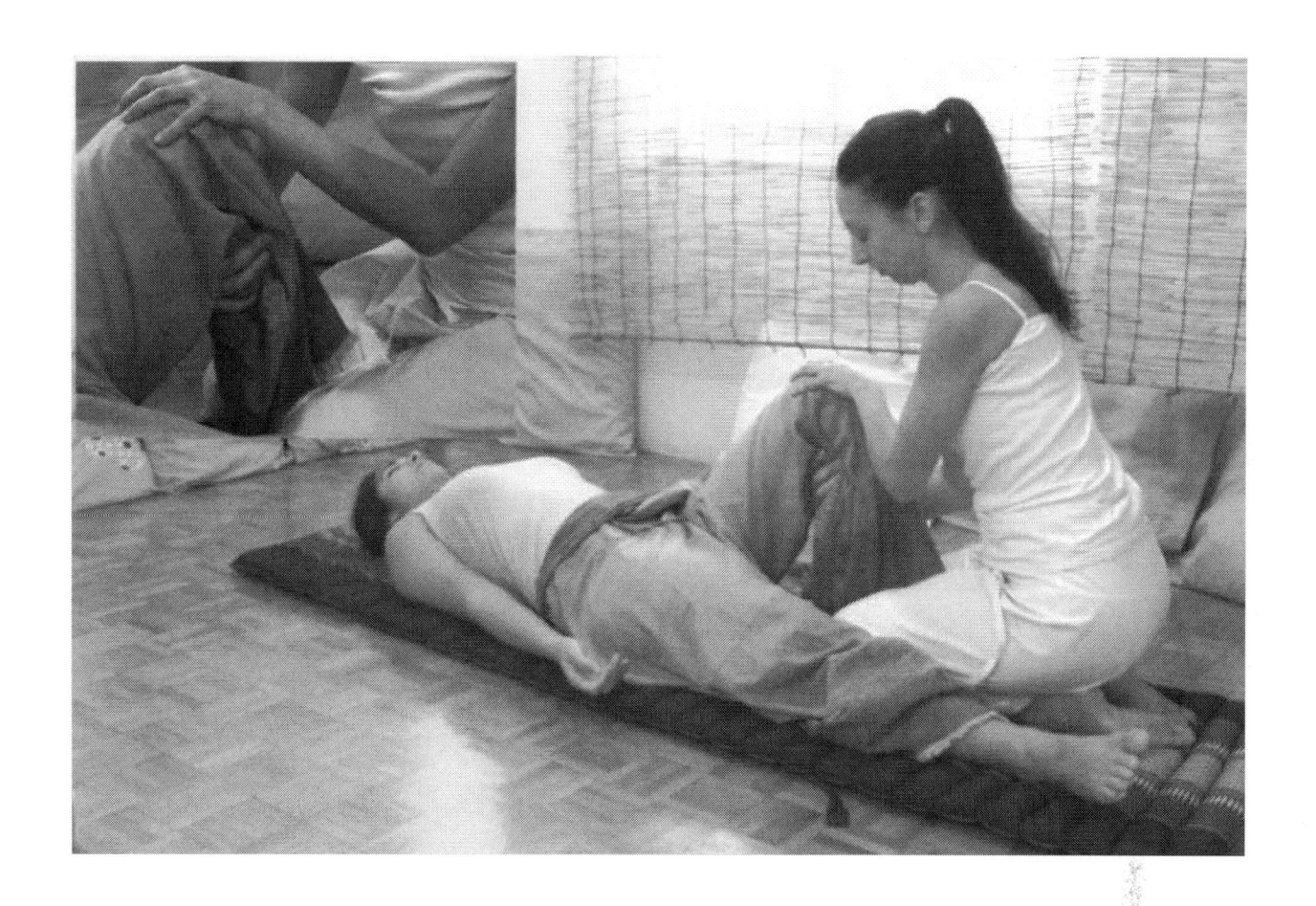

2. Then, place one palm on the receiver's patella. Using your other hand, knead the gastrocnemius muscle.

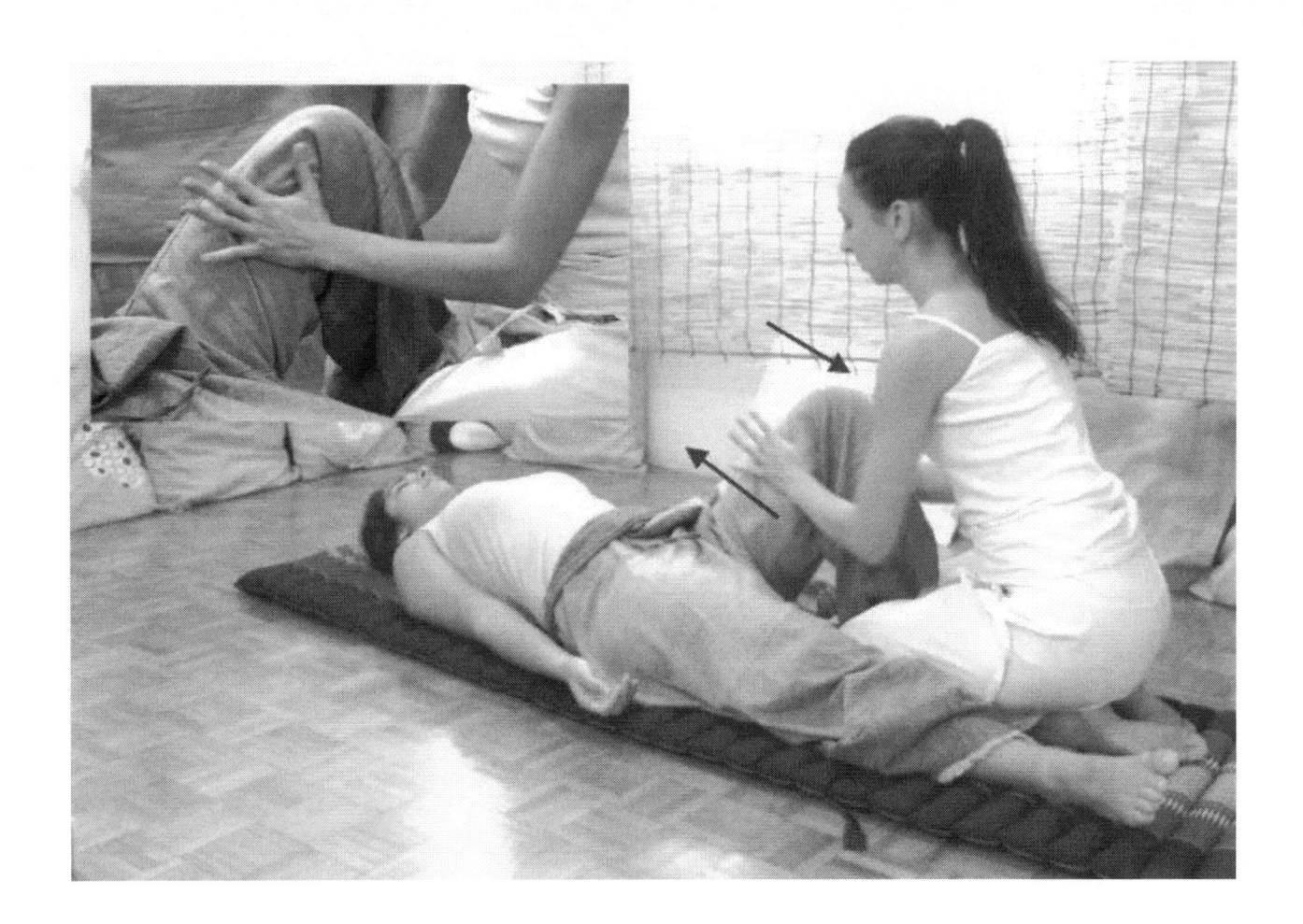

3. Maintaining the former leg lock, mobilize the receiver's thigh. Cover the entire thigh, as this technique is a sort of warm-up for the next steps.

Repeat 5-10 times, depending on how tight the muscles are.

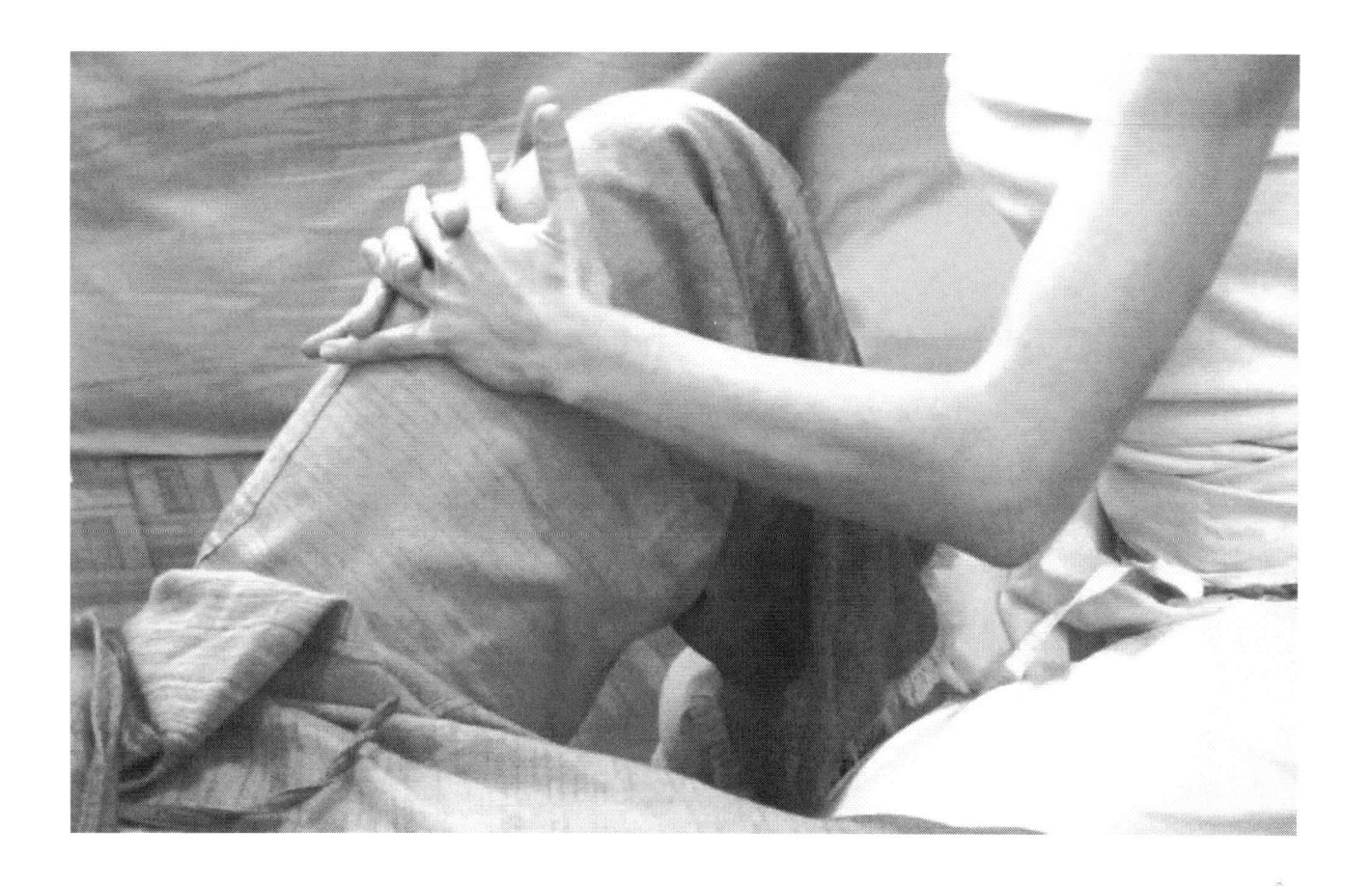

4. Interlock your fingers and perform circular massage, trying to separate the quadriceps muscle from the surrounding tissues.

You should actually try to lift the quadriceps muscle, not to squeeze it.

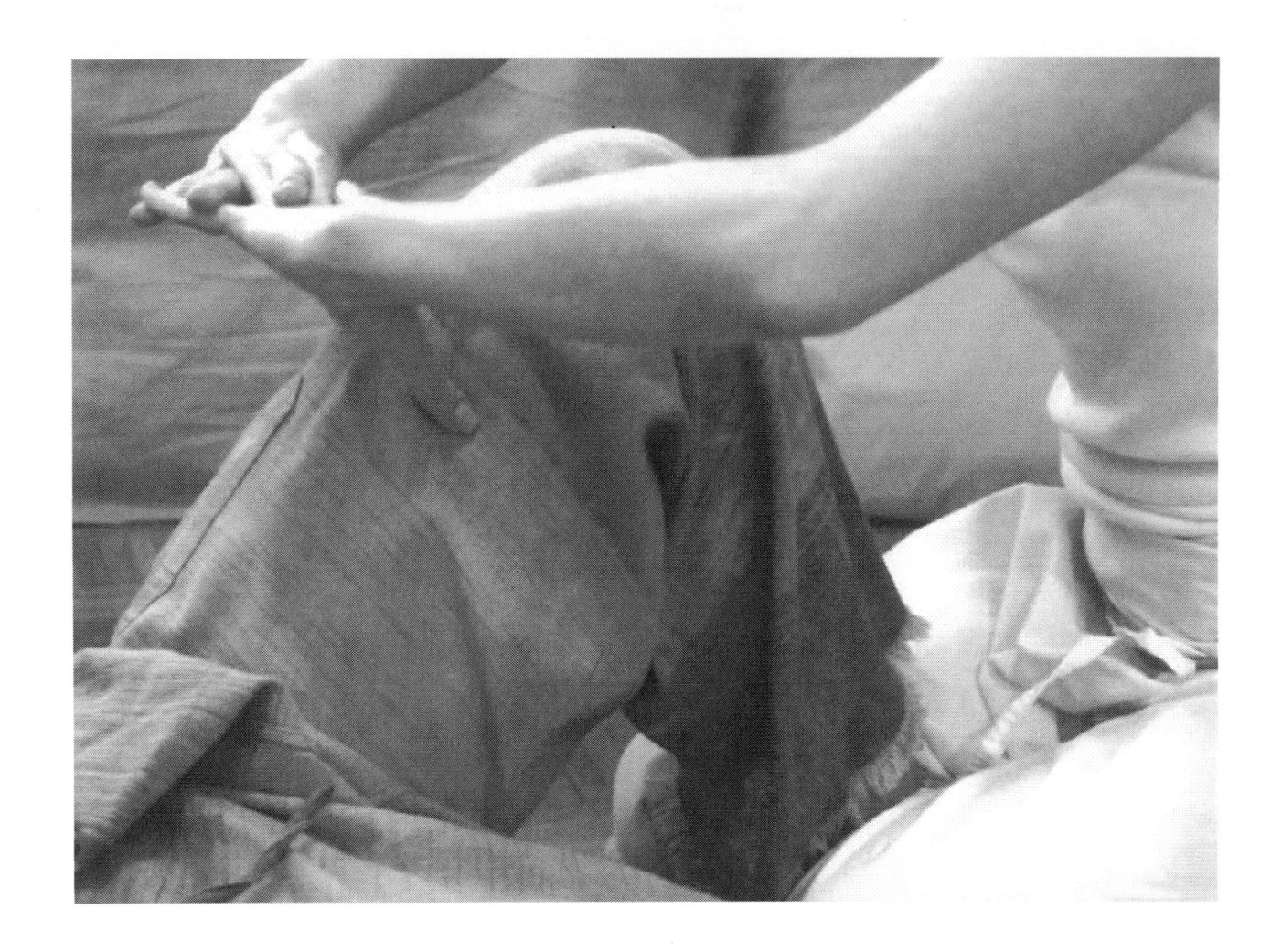

5. Then, interlock your fingers as shown in the photo, and using your thumbs, apply pressure on the 1st inner and 1st outer sen lines.

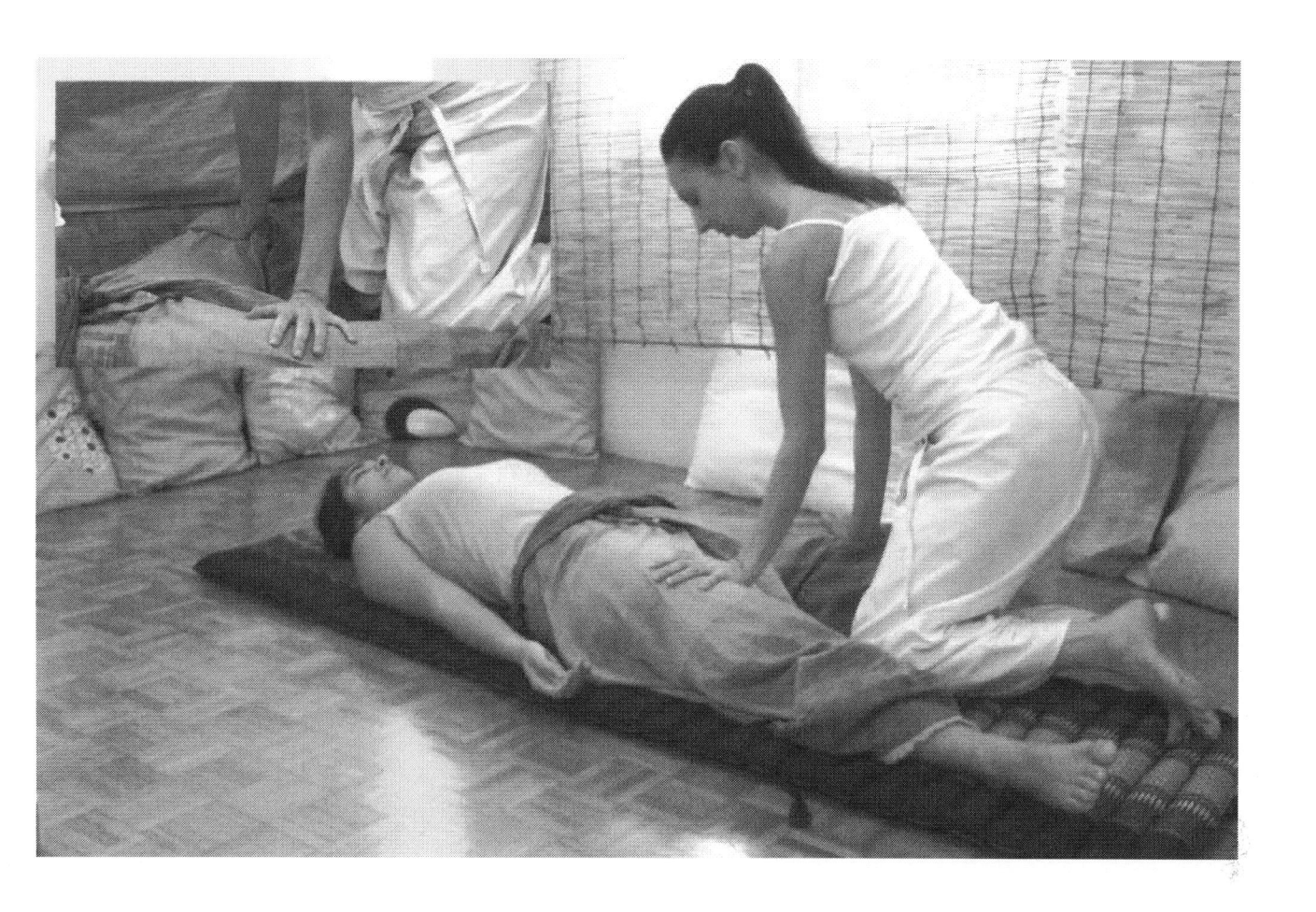

6. Now release the previous leg lock. Bend the receiver's foot and stabilize it with your knee. The transverse arch of the receiver's foot should face her knee joint. Then start walking with your palms on the receiver's thighs. Press the thighs alternatively.

Always go very gently with this technique, and observe carefully the receiver's facial expressions. Never go beyond the limits in this one, and whenever you apply it, be sure that you have warmed the muscles properly with the previous techniques.

This technique has some similarities with Patrick's test. Thus, any pain elicited during its application, may suggest hip joint disorders and / or sacroiliac joint dysfunction.

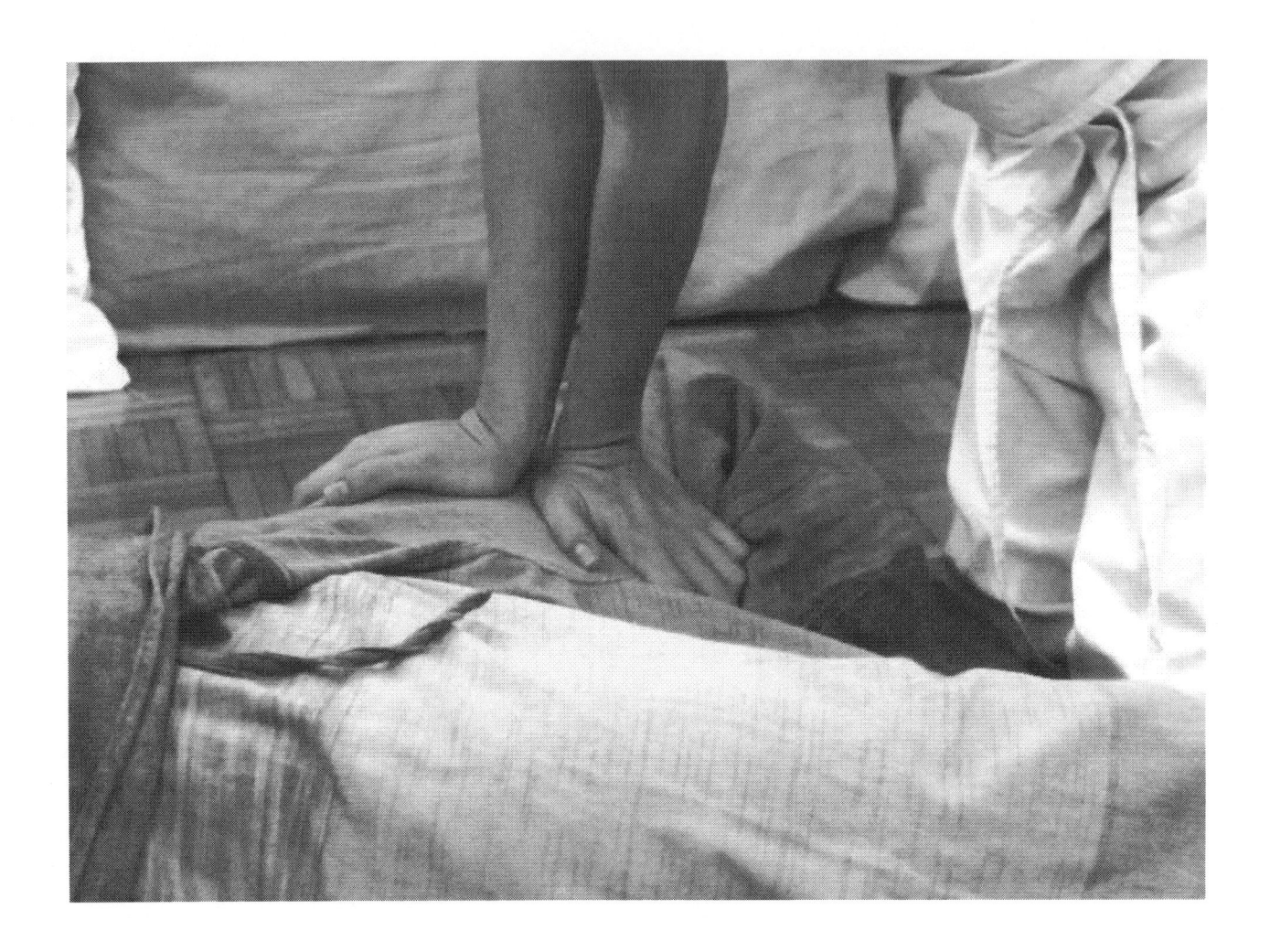

7. Also, in the same lock do "butterfly" walking with your palms.

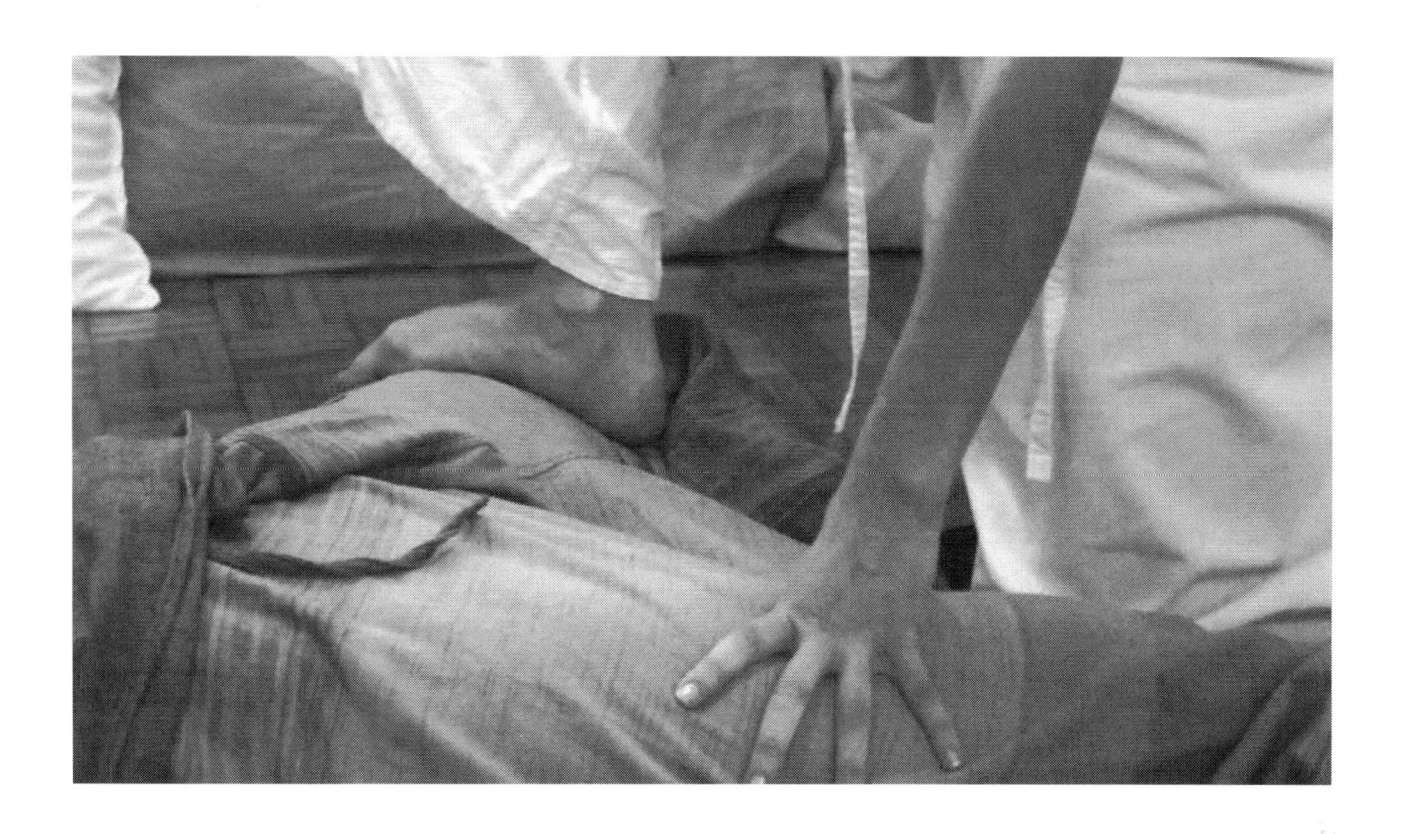

8. You can also press the thigh with your foot.

Place the transverse arch of your foot on the receiver's thigh, and let your body weight do the rest.

Never apply pressure from your leg – this may be painful and even dangerous.

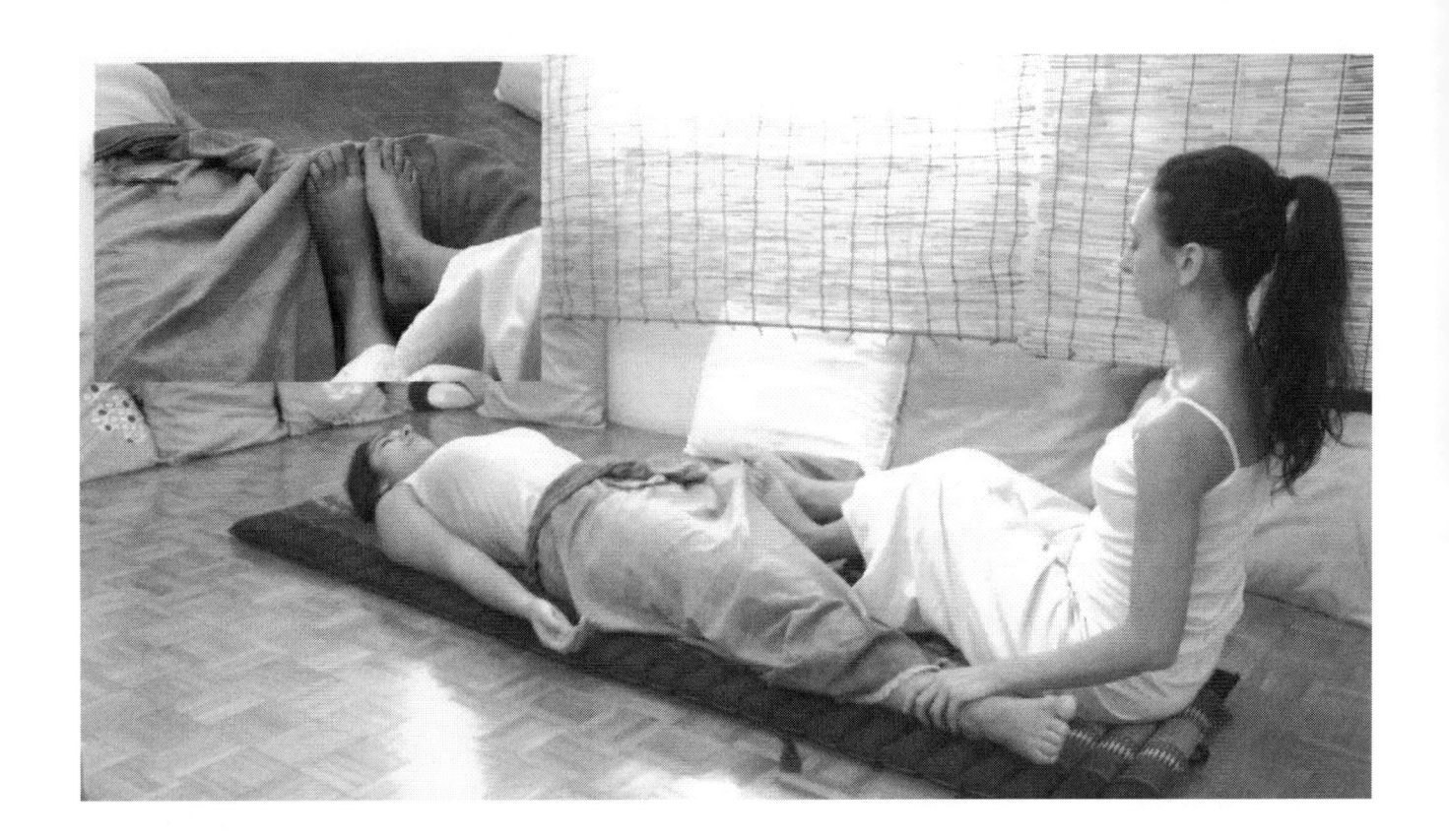

9. Release the previous lock and sit between the receiver's legs. Start pressing the adductors with your feet alternatively. Pressure should be applied with the transverse arch of the foot.

Do not push the thigh above the level of the hip joint, even if the receiver is flexible.

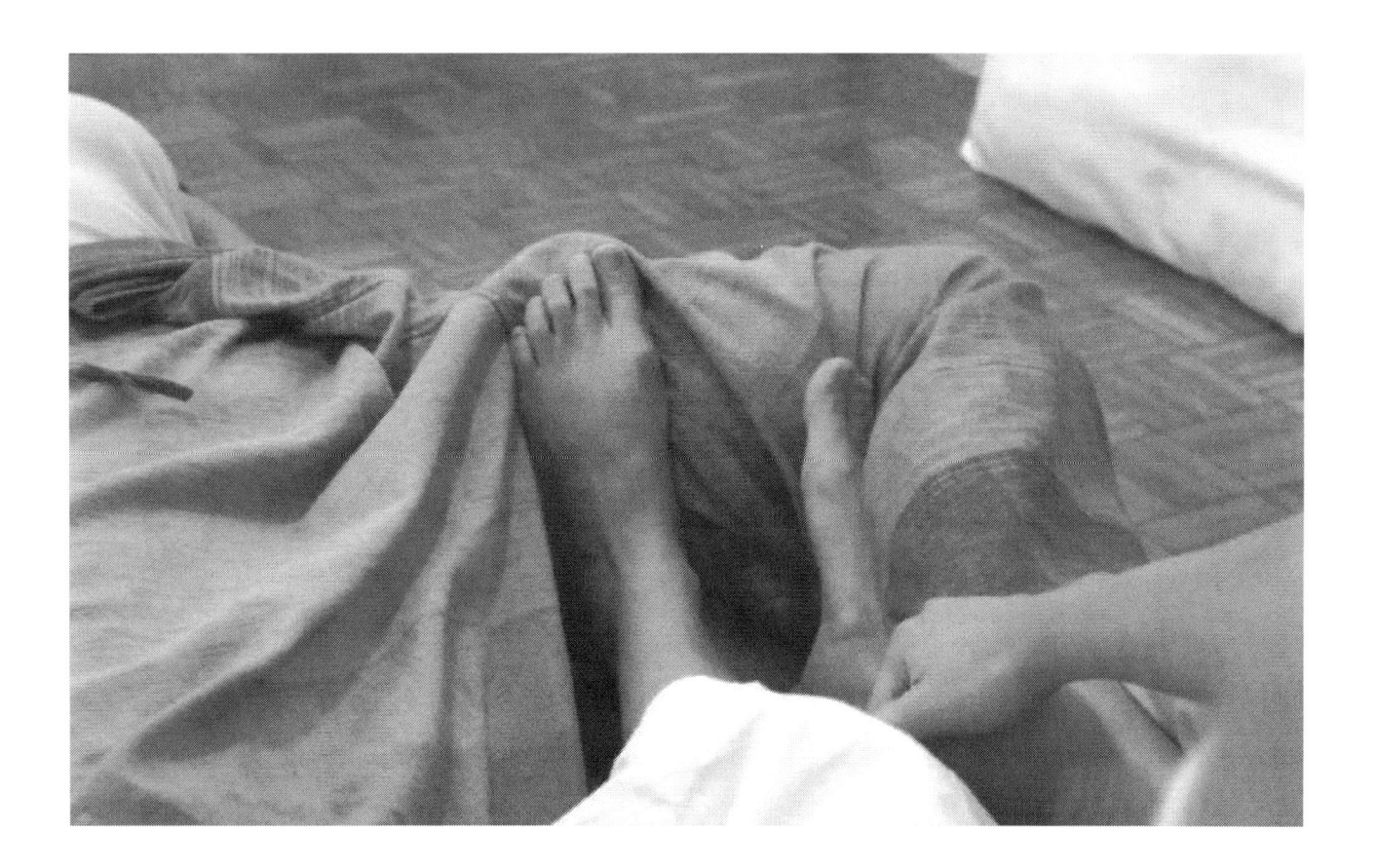

10. Still seated between the receiver's legs, lock the receiver's foot in your knee joint. Grasp her heel and other leg, and repeat the previous foot presses, with one foot. Simultaneously, pull the other leg of the receiver.

This technique targets the pelvis. It is recommended for people with anterior pelvic tilt, leg length discrepancies and generally poor alignment of the pelvis, as well as for lower back pain.

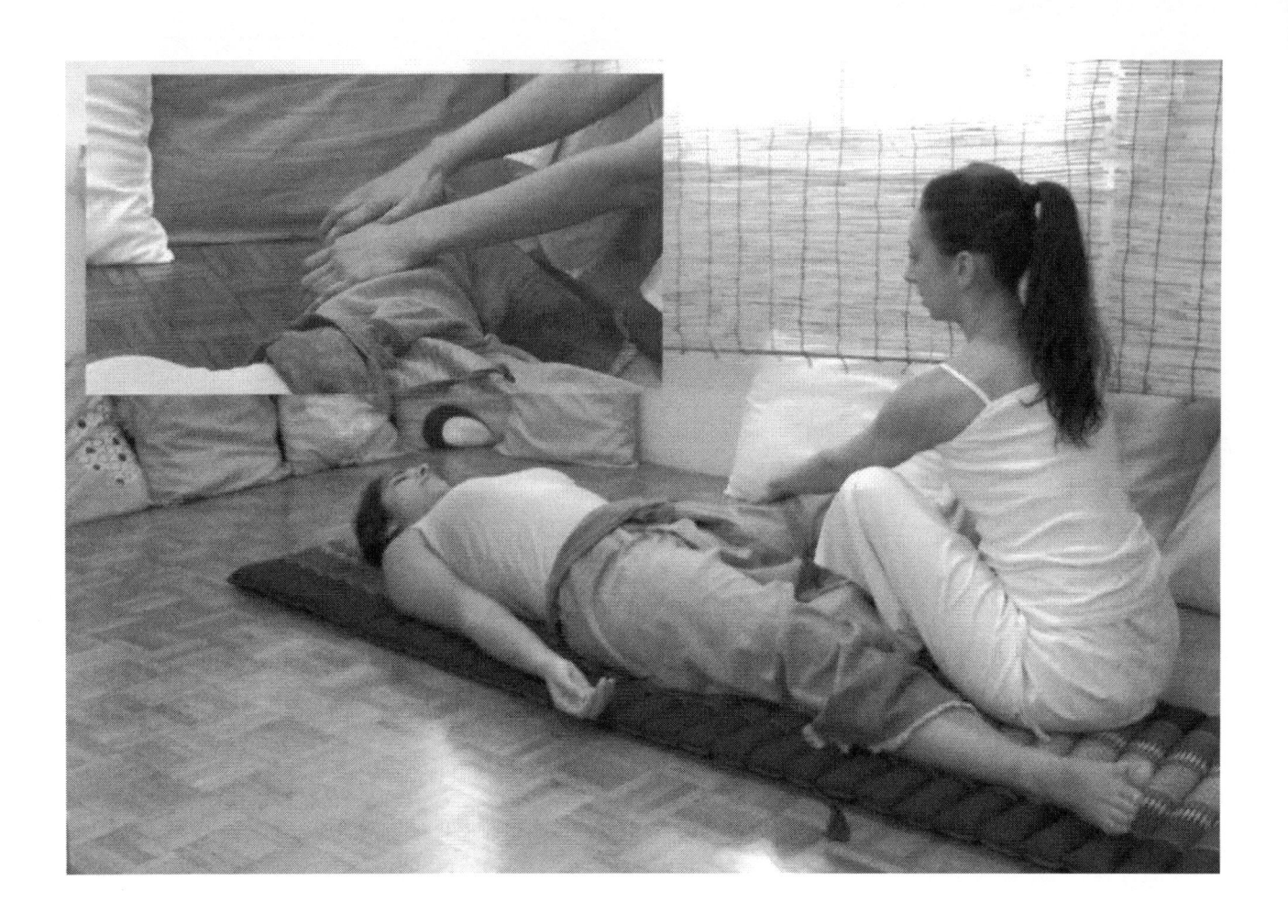

11. Now bring the receiver's leg in front of your feet, and work on the quadriceps muscle.

You can do deep tissue work on the rectus femoris muscle from this position: Just try to "separate" the muscle from the surrounding tissues, by doing transverse friction massage around it.

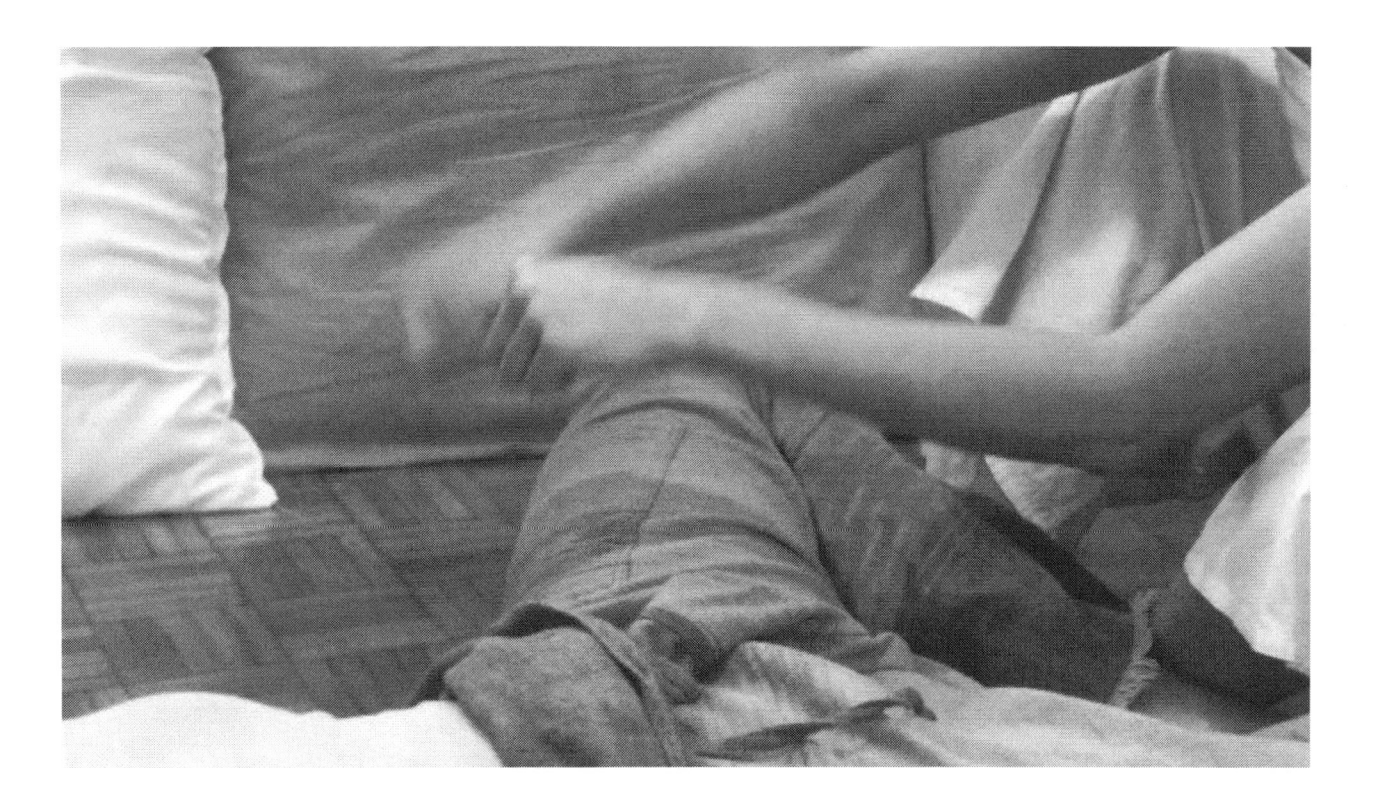

12. Then gently punch the quadriceps muscle.

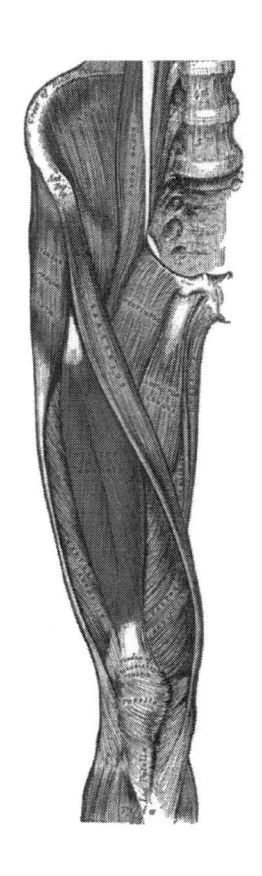

Quadriceps muscle – the rectus femoris muscle is highlighted in red color.

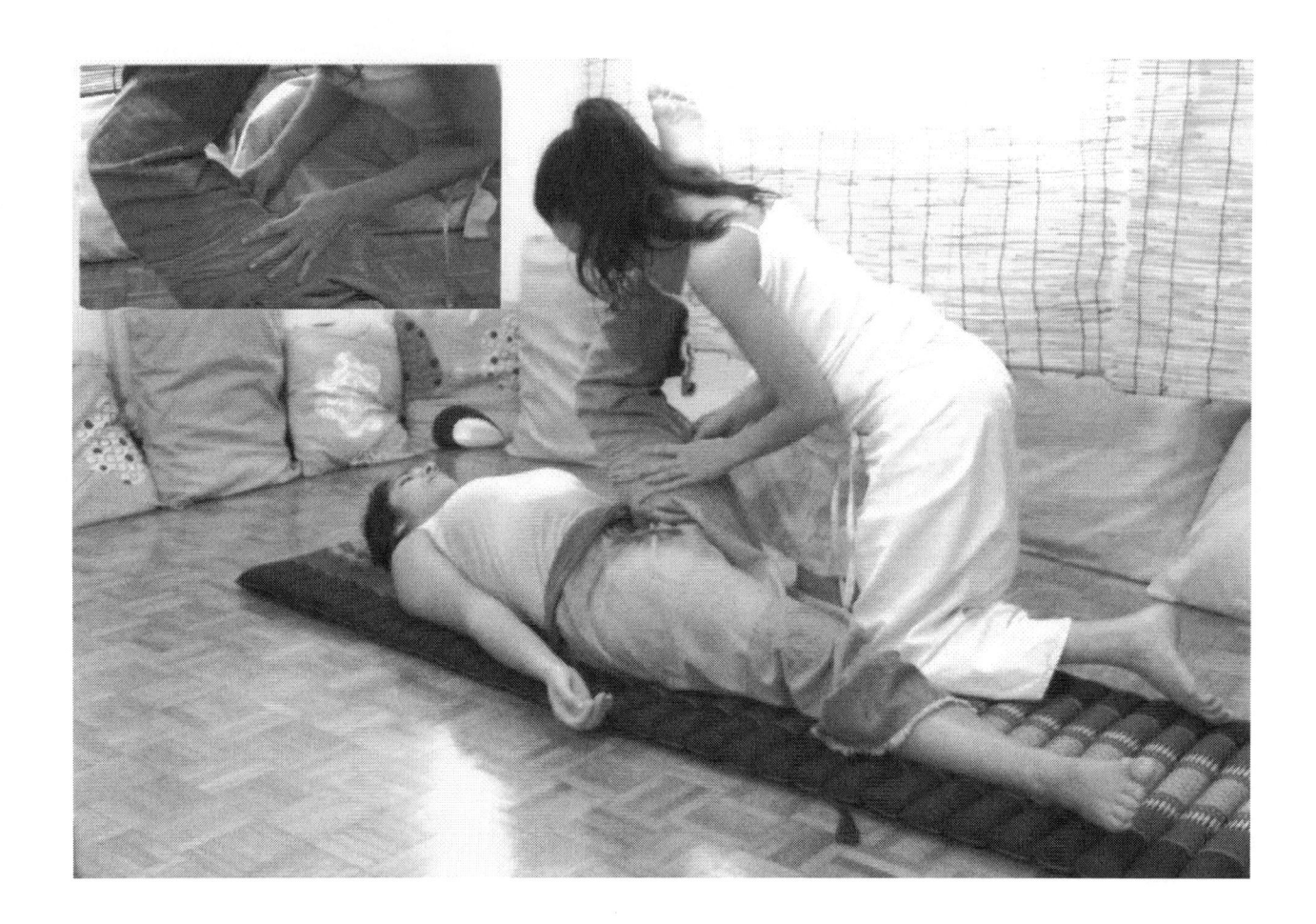

13. Release the previous lock, and place the receiver's leg on your shoulder. Do thumb presses on the biceps femoris muscle, on the 3rd inner line (*Itha & Pingkala Sen*). Cover the entire muscle.

Repeat 2-3 times.

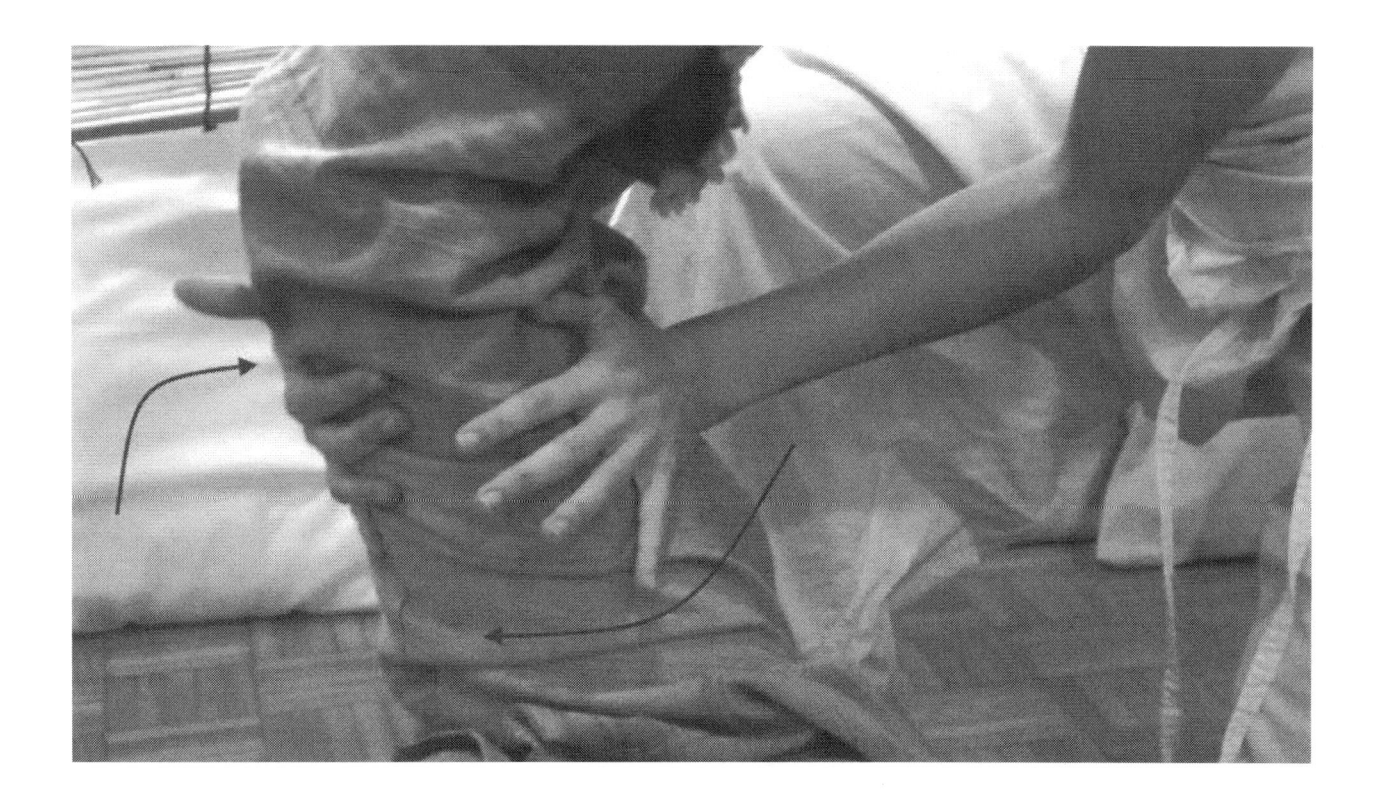

14. Now place one hand on the biceps femoris muscle and the other hand on the quadriceps muscle, and squeeze the leg by moving your hands at opposite directions.

This technique is recommended for sciatica.

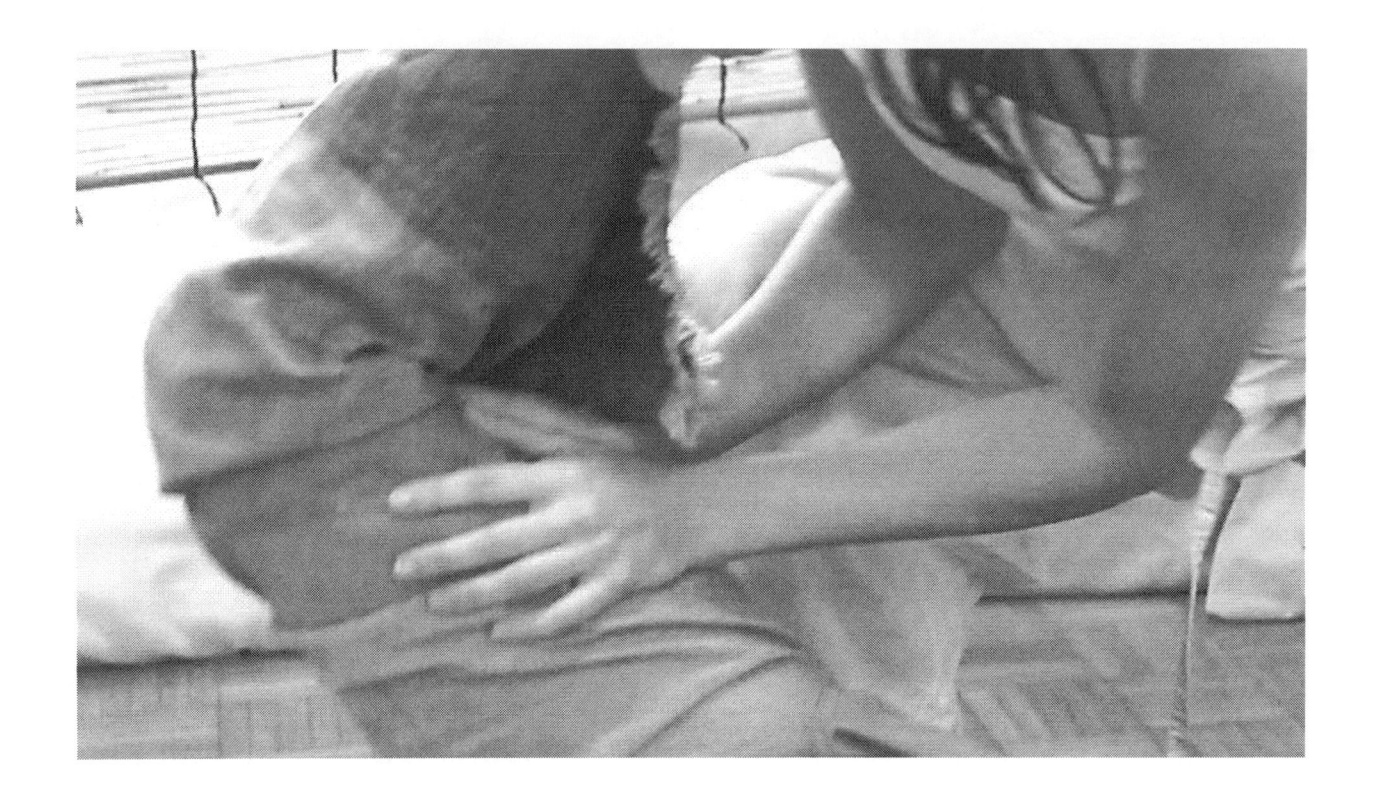

15. From this position, you can also do a good palm press to the biceps femoris muscle. Each time you press, bring your pelvis forward – in this way, you work with your body weight and put less strain on your wrists.

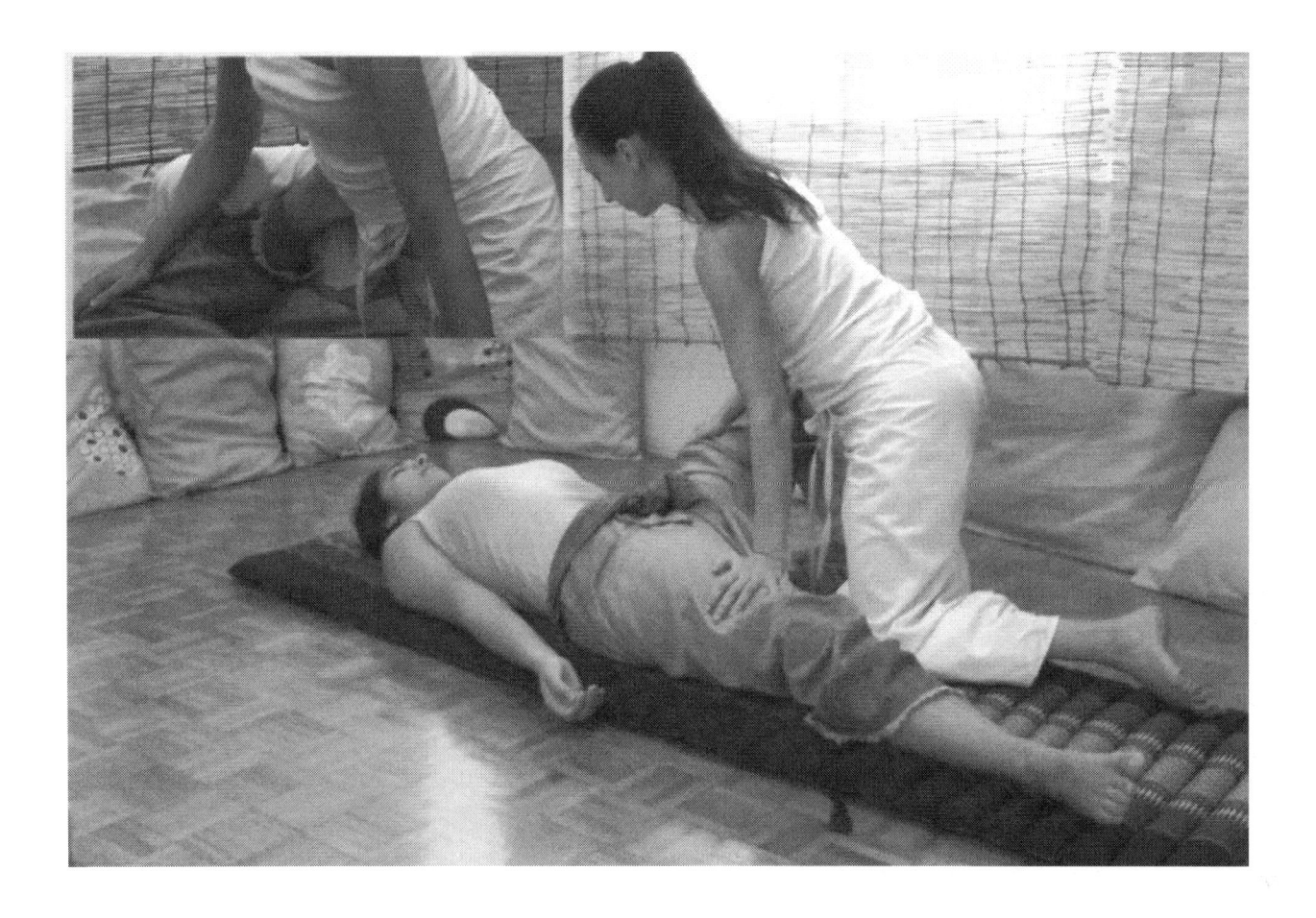

16. Place the receiver's foot on the upper part of your quadriceps muscle, and start stretching gently her adductors. One palm should be places on the receiver's bent leg, and one on the other leg. Each time you apply the technique, bring your pelvis forward.

It is best to apply the stretch as the receiver exhales. Also, go for it very slowly and observe the body's structural limitations. Repeat 4-5 times.

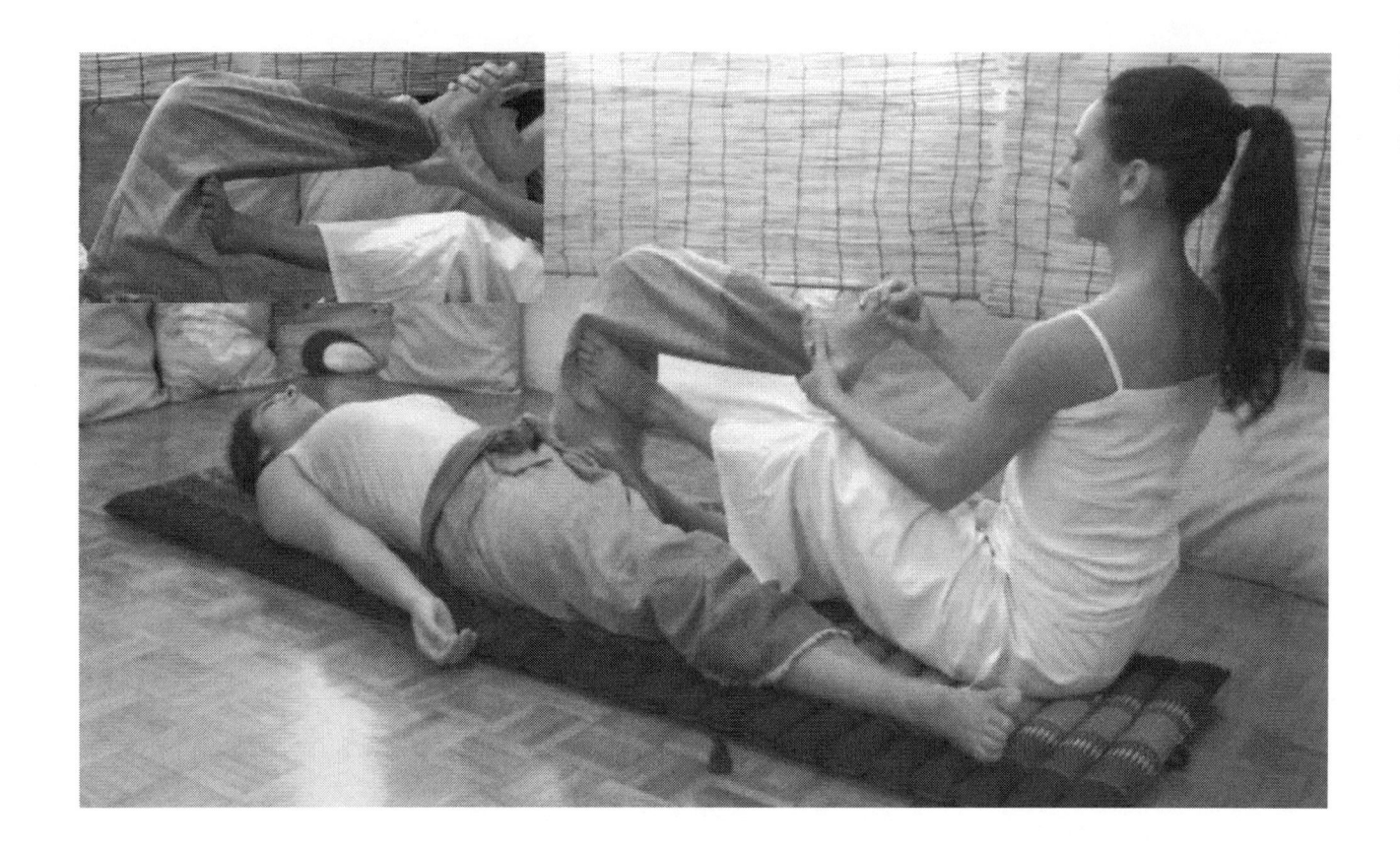

17. Now sit down, grasp the receiver's foot, and do leg presses on the biceps femoris muscle. Simultaneously, pull gently the foot.

Do not perform this technique if the receiver has loose ligaments of the foot (you will hear the typical sounds in the joint, in that case).

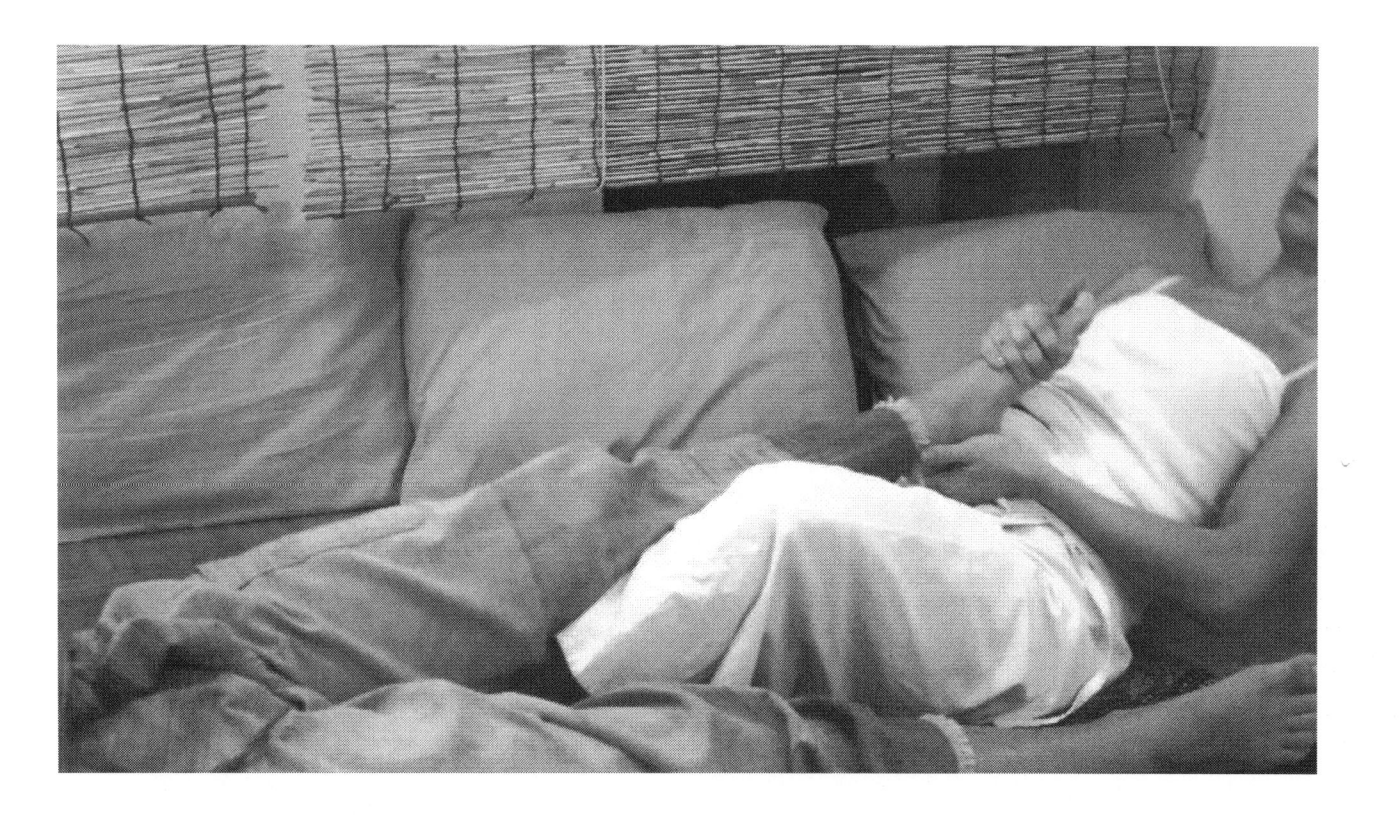

18. Then, place your flexed foot under the receiver's gluteus muscle. Grasp her foot and fall back. This technique is indicated for the decompression of the hip joint. It is great for lower back pain.

Again, as this technique involves a pull of the foot joint, avoid it if the receiver has loose ligaments of the foot.

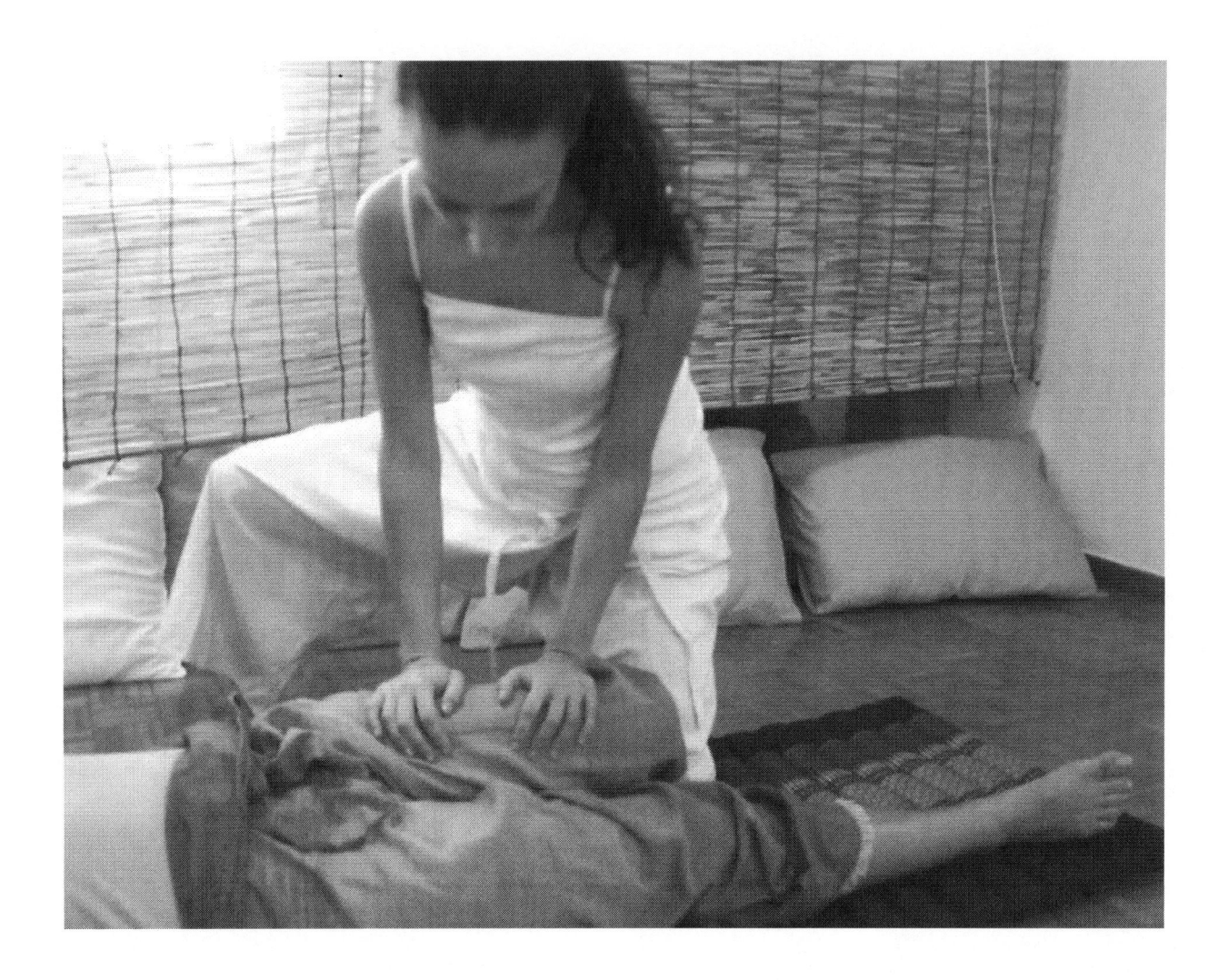

19. Flex the receiver's knee inwards, and do palm presses on the iliotibial band.

You may have to place a pillow (or a yoga brick) under the receiver's knee, if the receiver is not flexible enough in order to bend his knee.

An excellent technique for iliotibial band syndrome (not during the acute phase, but highly recommended for the chronic phase).

Skip this technique if the receiver suffers from any knee disorders (like cartilage damage, injuries etc.).

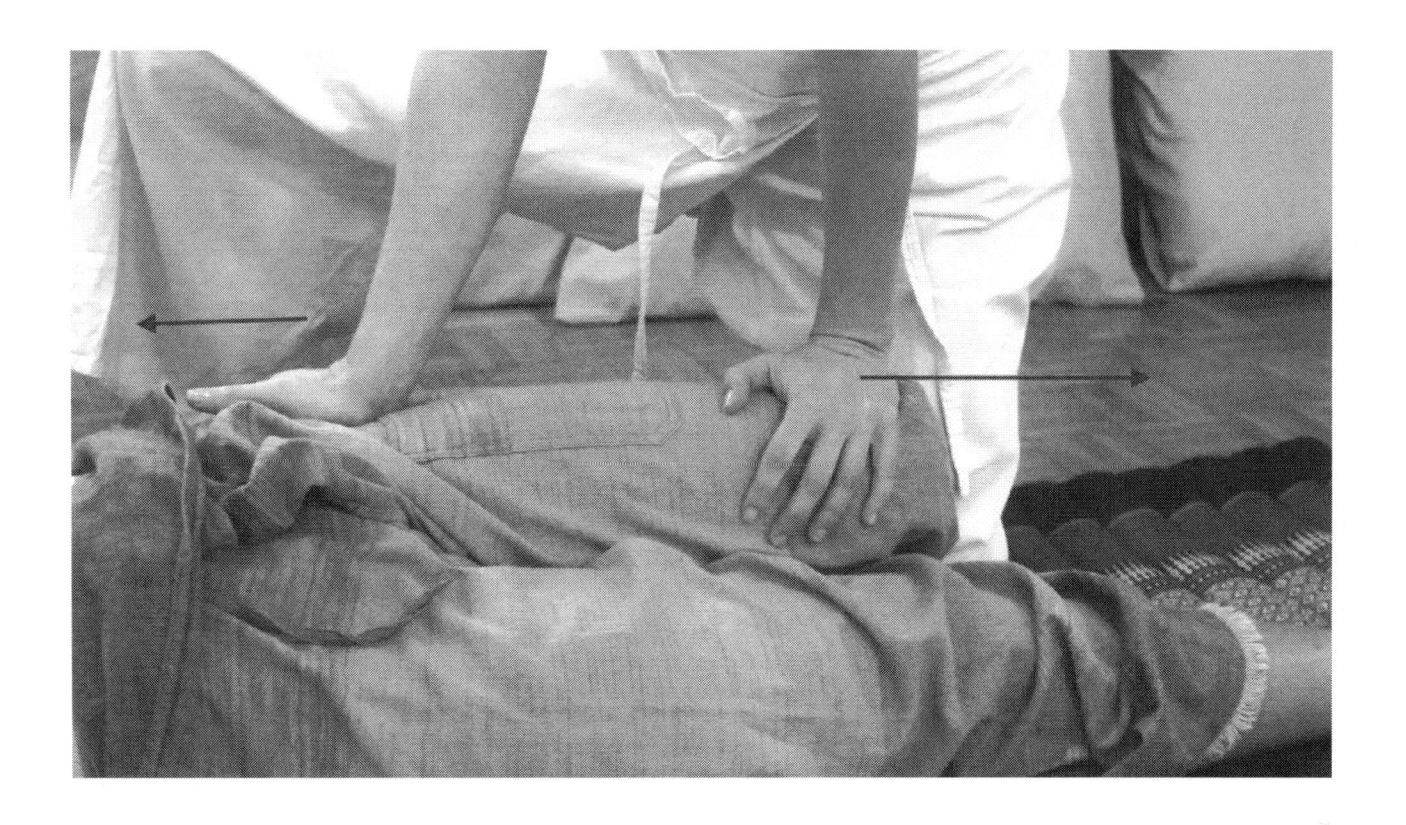

From this position, you can also stretch the abductors and / or focus on the iliotibial band.

In order to apply this technique, place one hand under the hip joint, and one hand above the receiver's knee. As she exhales, transfer your body weight forward, and push your hands in opposite directions (the "arrows" are parallel to the ground), thus applying the stretch.

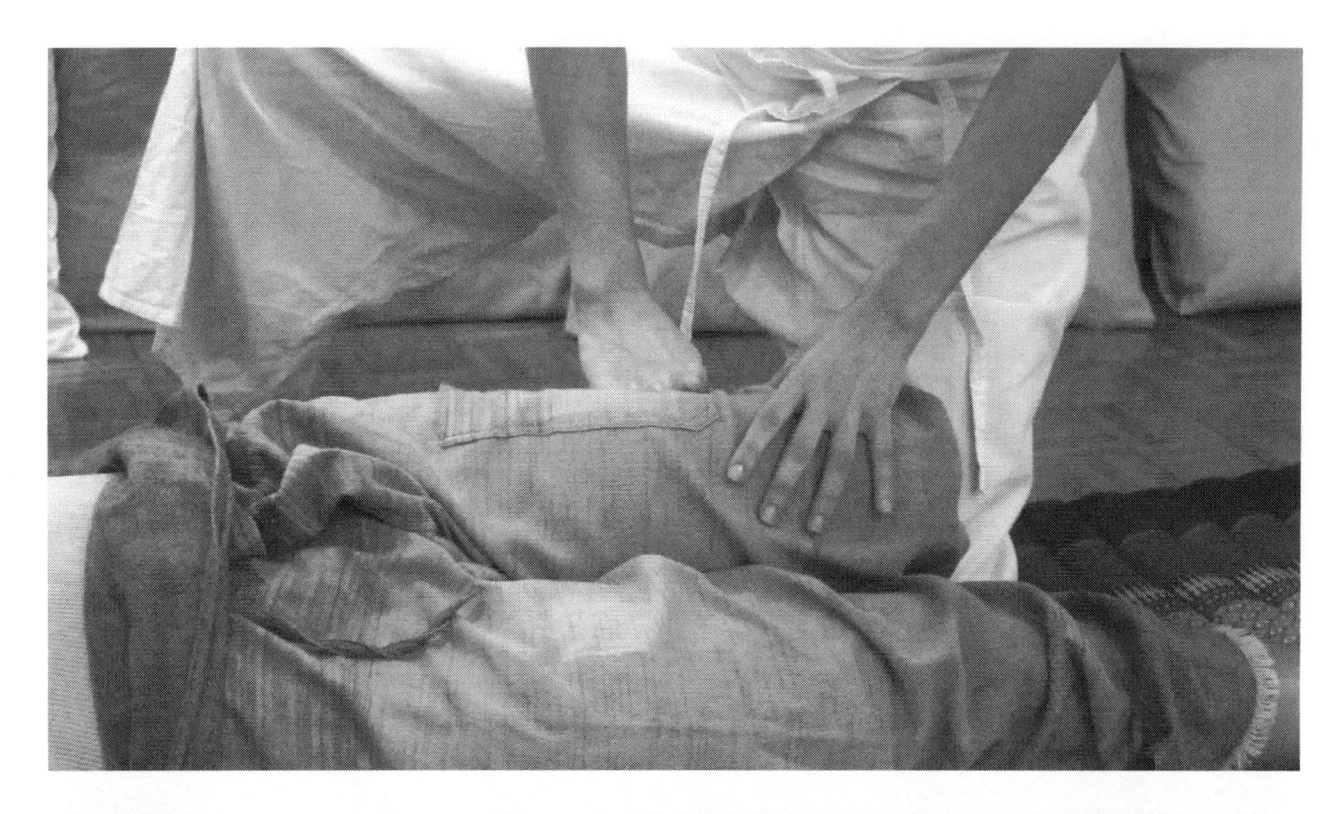

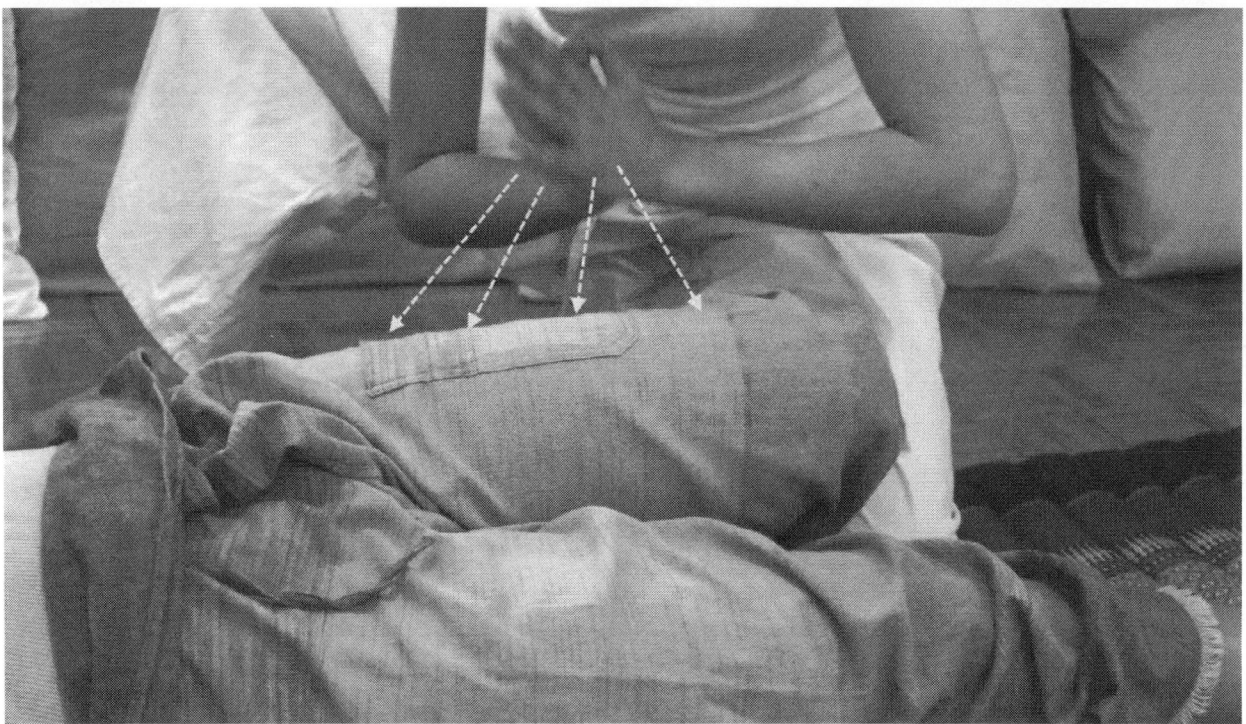

You can also do transverse friction massage and tapotement techniques.

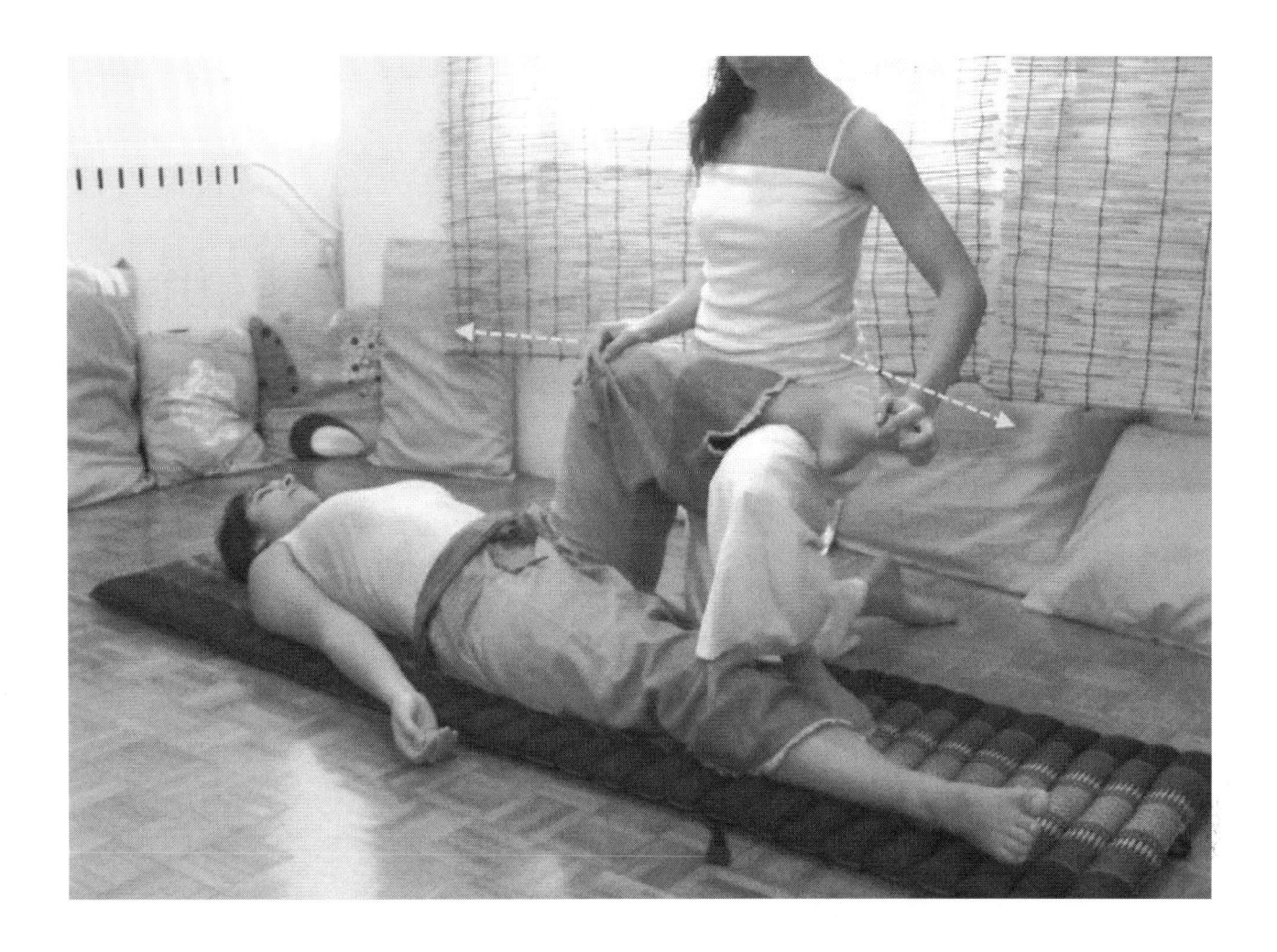

20. Place the receiver's lower leg on your thigh, and stretch the anterior muscles of the lower leg.

In order to apply the technique, place one hand on the receiver's patella, and one hand on her foot. Perform the stretch as the receiver exhales.

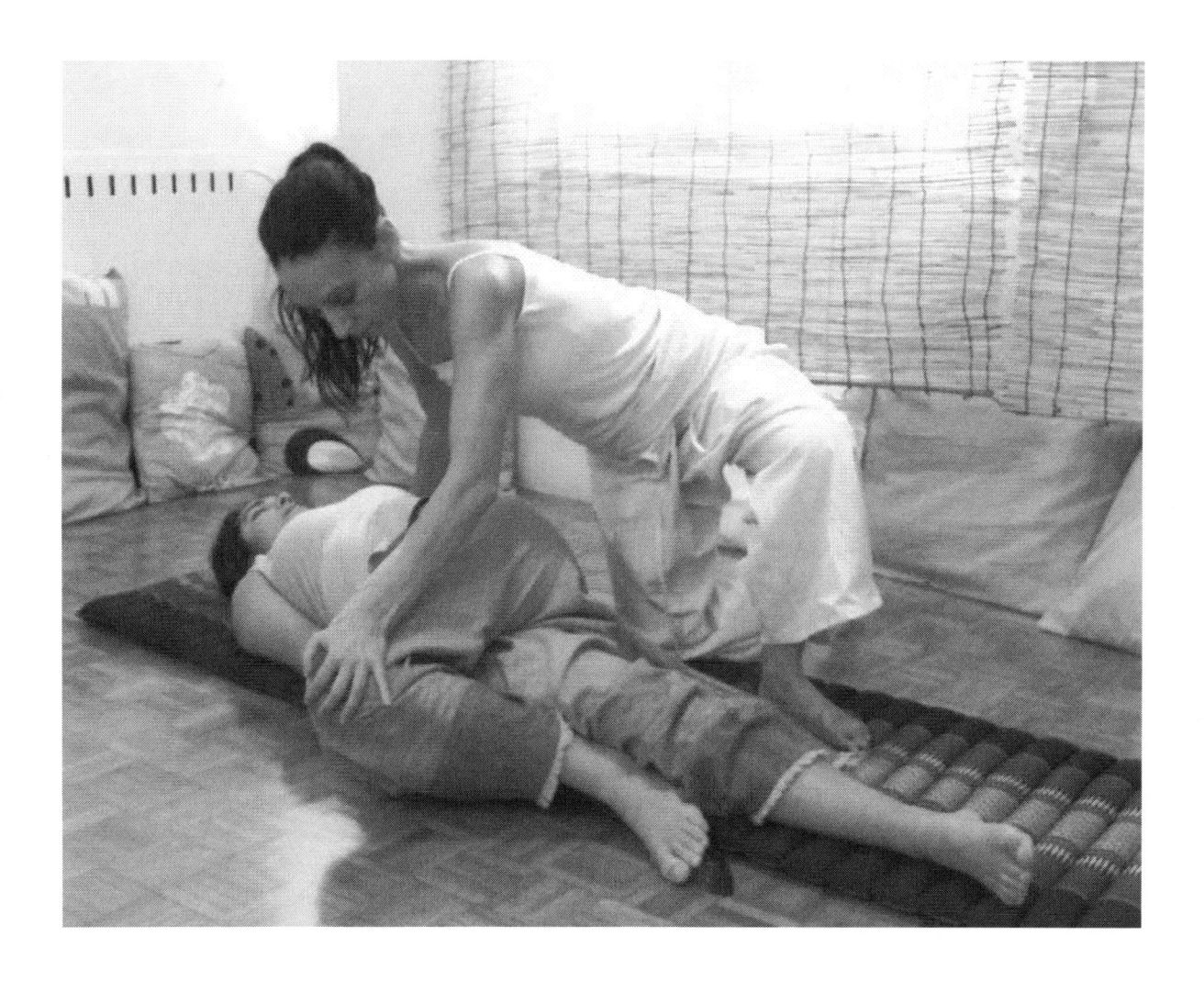

21. Now place one hand on the receiver's shoulder, and one hand on her knee, in order to apply this spinal twist.

It is important not to apply any pressure on the receiver's shoulder. Apply the technique as the receiver exhales, and respect the body limits. Stay on the stretch at least for 10 seconds, allowing the receiver to breathe.

Then place the receiver gently back to the initial supine position.

This technique is a passive application of the yogic asana Supta Matsyendrasana.

Be very careful when applying the technique to people with degenerated discs on the lumbar spine.

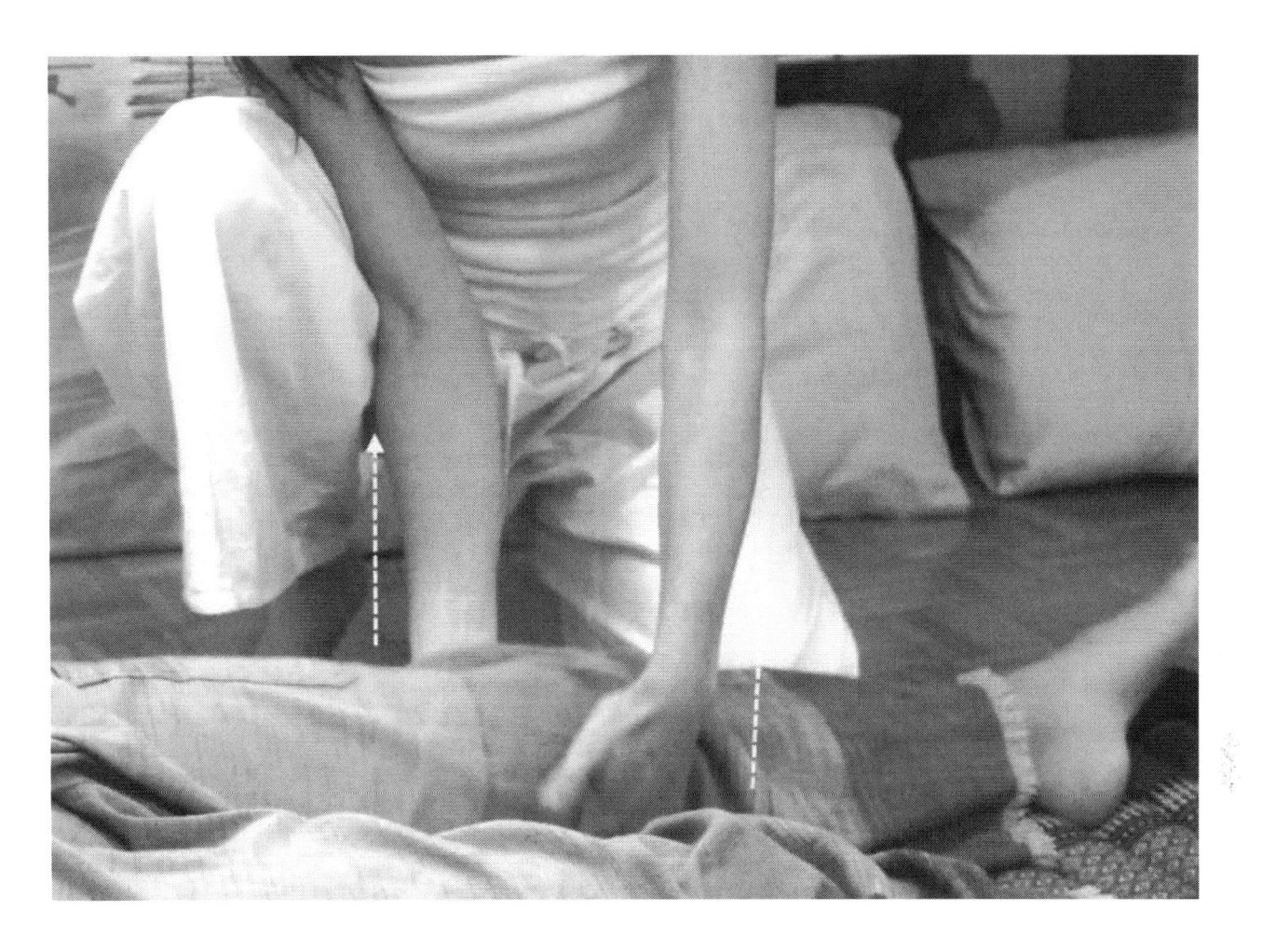

22. In order to relax the leg, place your hands under the knee joint, and shake it gently upwards and downwards. Repeat 8-10 times.

When you complete all the techniques on one leg, apply them on the other leg too. In the next section, you will see the techniques that involve both legs simultaneously.

two legs techniques

These techniques are very interactive and very dynamic. They should be applied only after the receiver's muscles have been properly warmed.

Many of them are not suitable for the elderly. Have in mind that clients who are not familiar with the Thai bodywork may feel quite uncomfortable with some of these techniques.

The following techniques are excellent for sciatica and lower back pain. However, be gentle and careful with any back bend when treating people with degenerated discs and spinal stenosis.

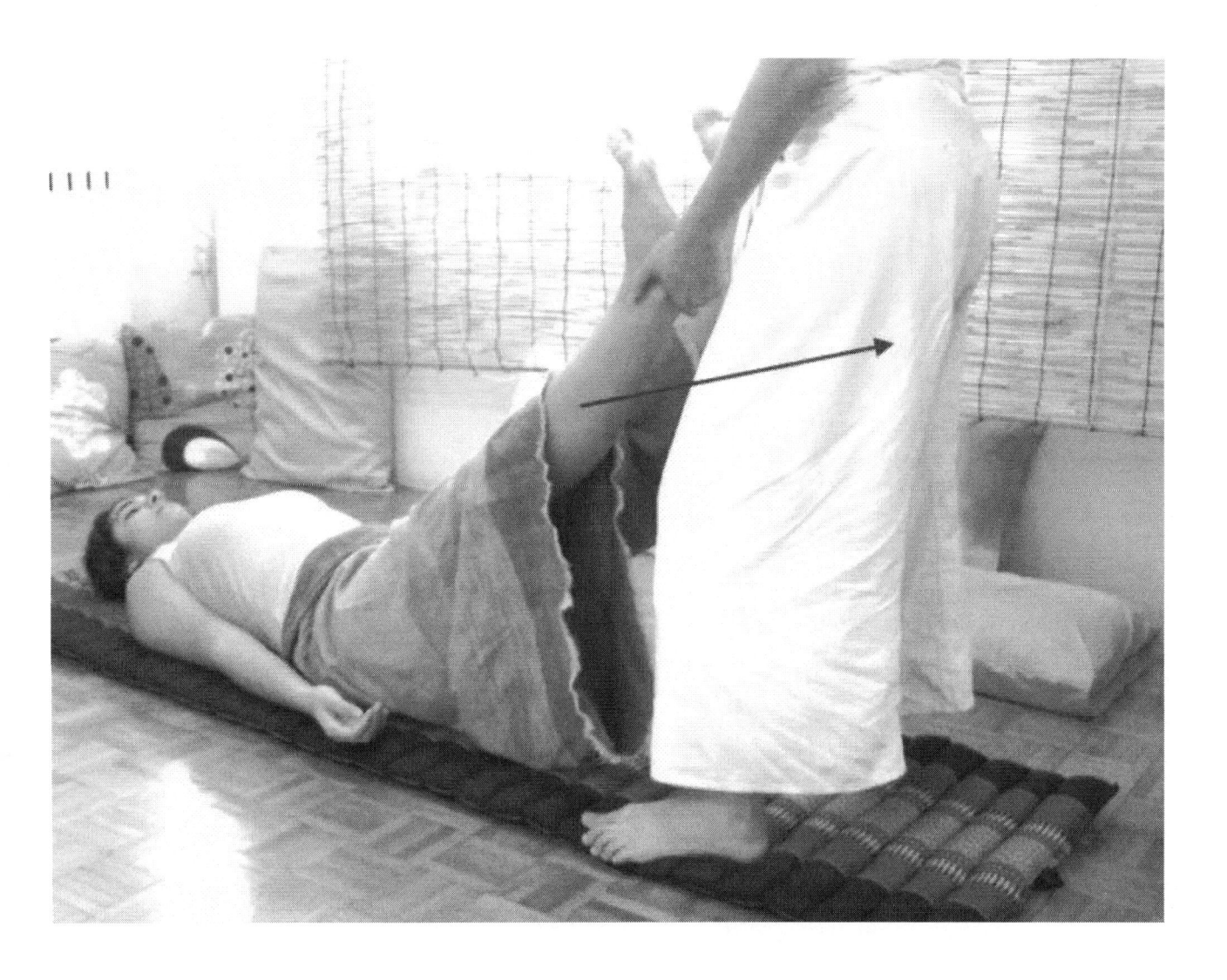

1. Grasp the receiver's feet from the heel, and pull them. This technique creates a gentle decompression of the lumbar spine.

The closer the receiver's legs are on the ground, the stronger the traction. Of course, this is more demanding for the therapist, especially if the client is heavier.

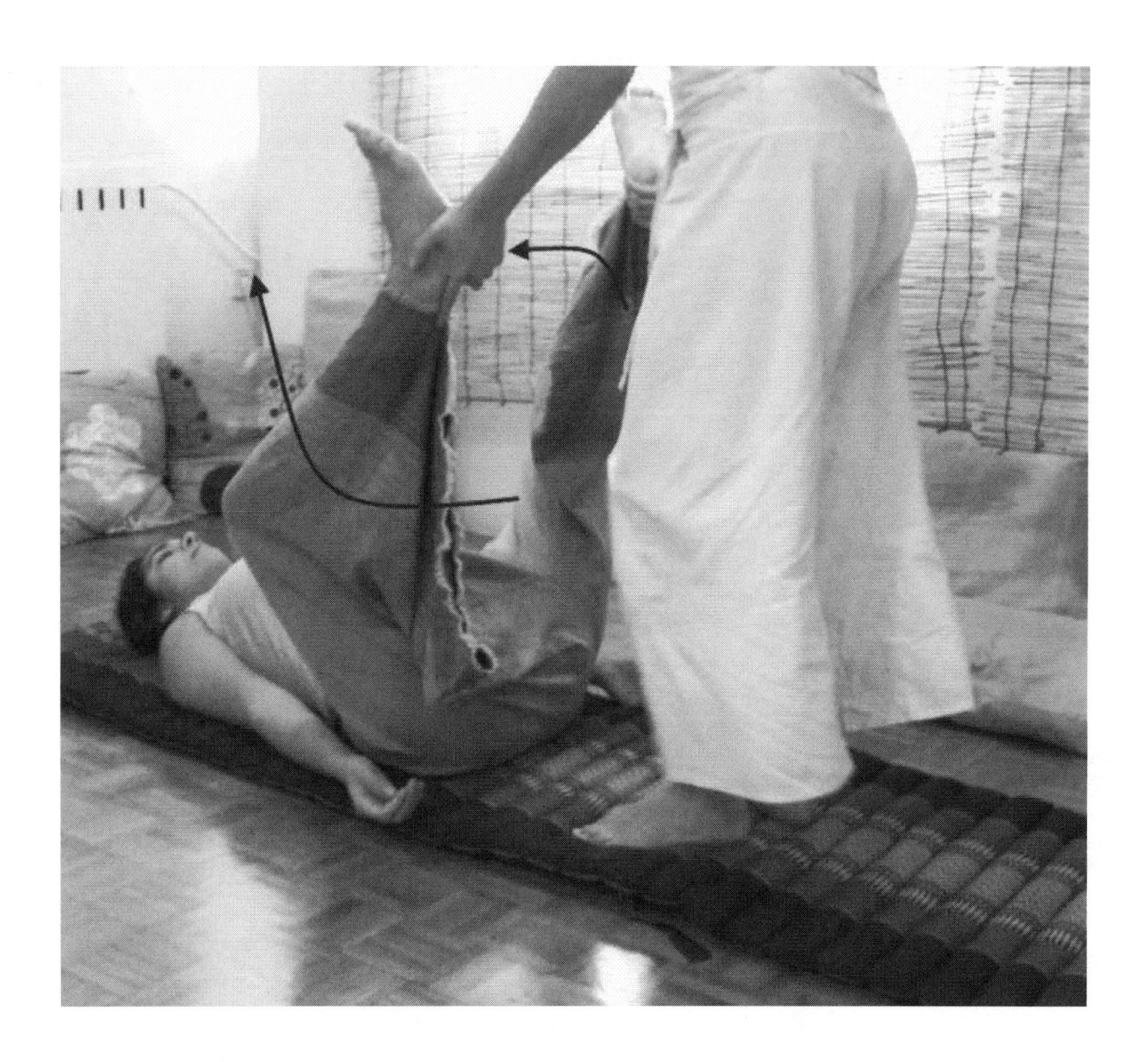

2. Then mobilize the receiver's legs, with slow and gentle movements. Still holding them from the heels, move them towards the left and towards the right.

This technique targets the pelvis, and if applied properly, can be very relaxing.

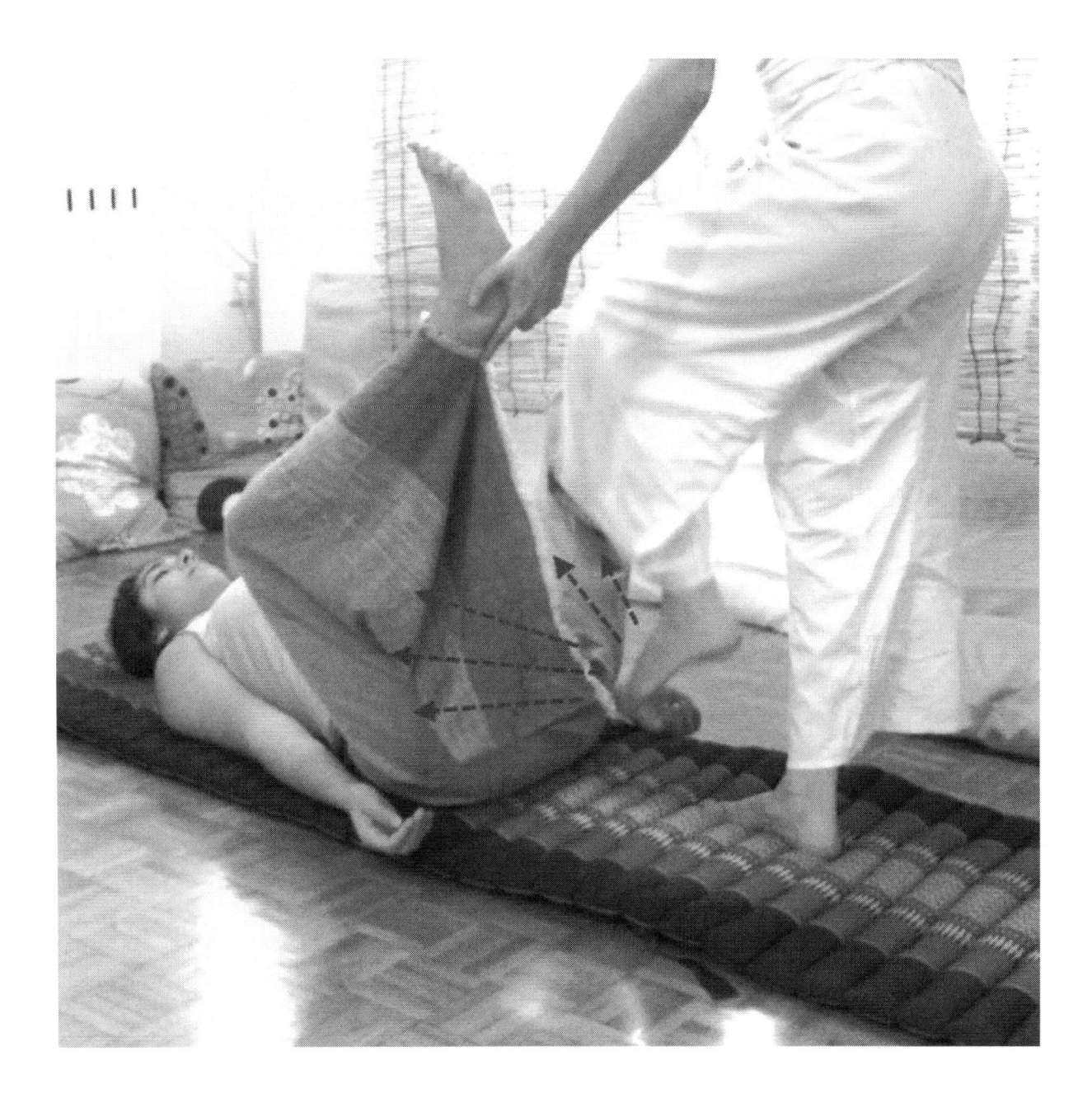

3. Hit gently the receiver's posterior thigh muscles with your feet. Your left foot should hit the receiver's left foot, and your right one her right thigh.

This warms the muscles. Do not be afraid to hit a bit harder – it is not at all painful;, and actually very pleasant!

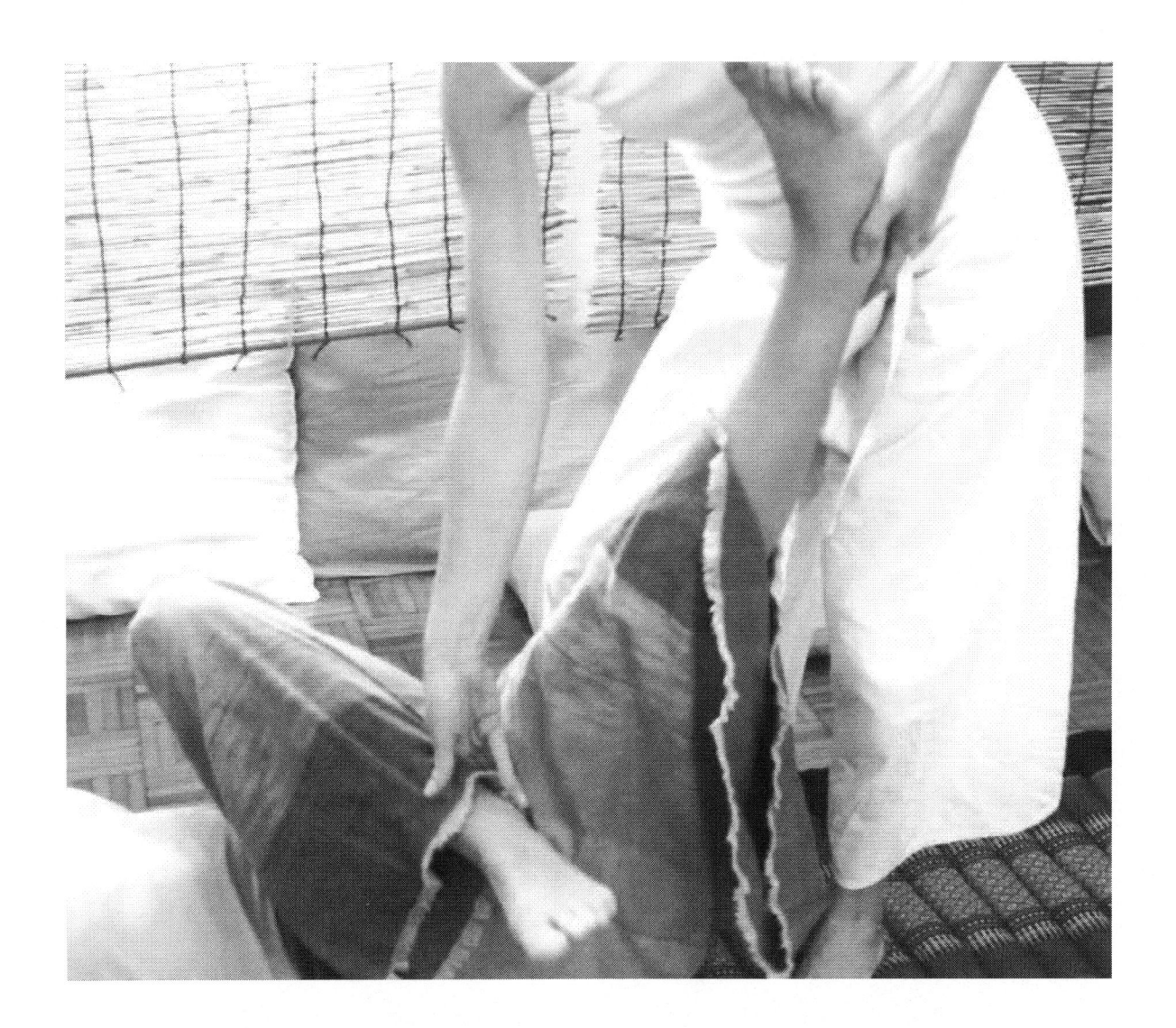

4. Bend the receiver's leg, and place it above the knee joint. Her ankle should be placed outside of her thigh. Actually, this lock suffices for the application of the following techniques, if the receiver is not flexible enough for the next step of the lock. Now, if the receiver can do it, go on and perform the next step...

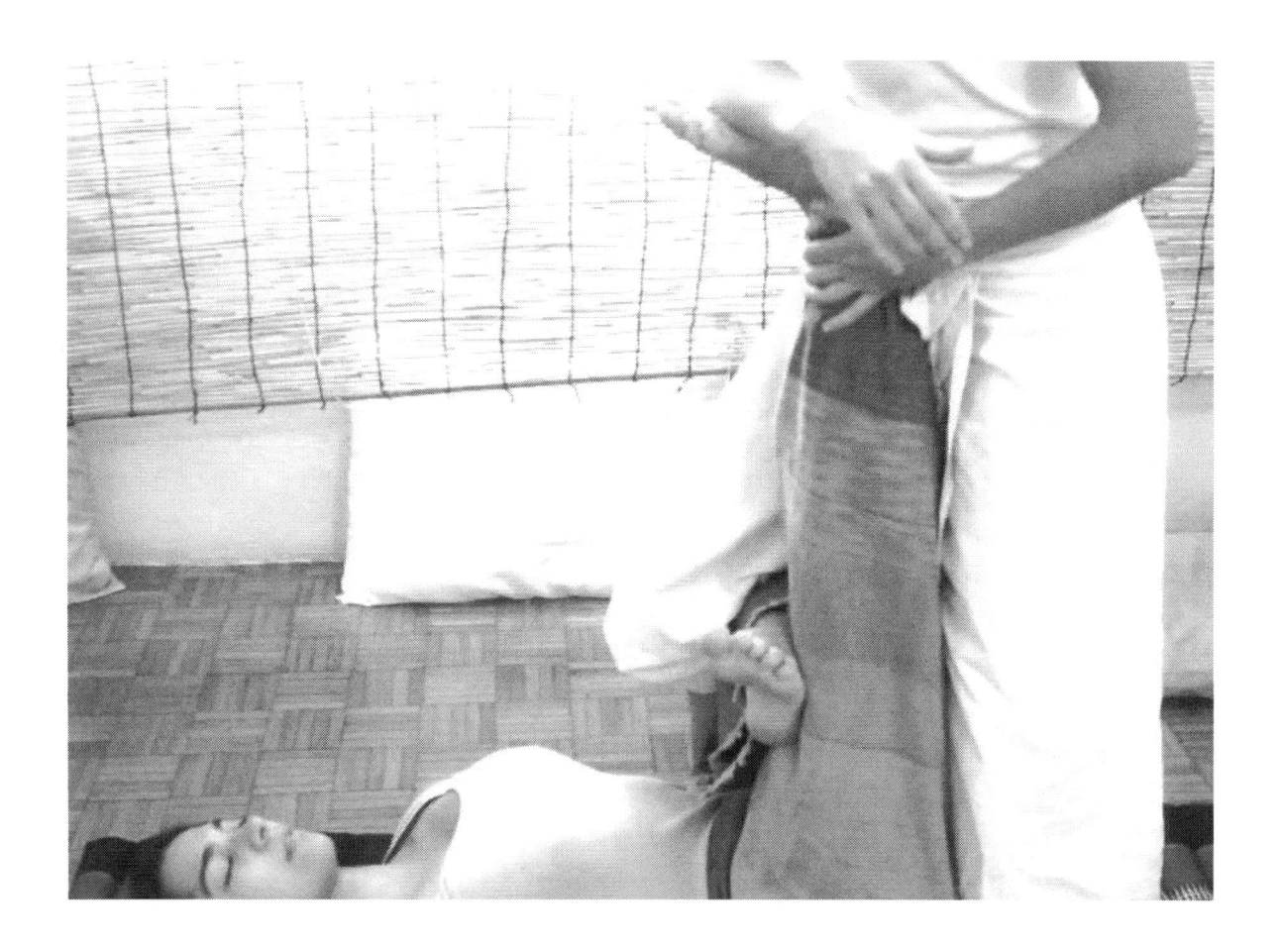

Bring your leg in front of the receiver's leg, in order to stabilize this lock perfectly. Then, press gently her foot with your forearm.

This technique targets the sciatic nerve and the popliteal tendon.

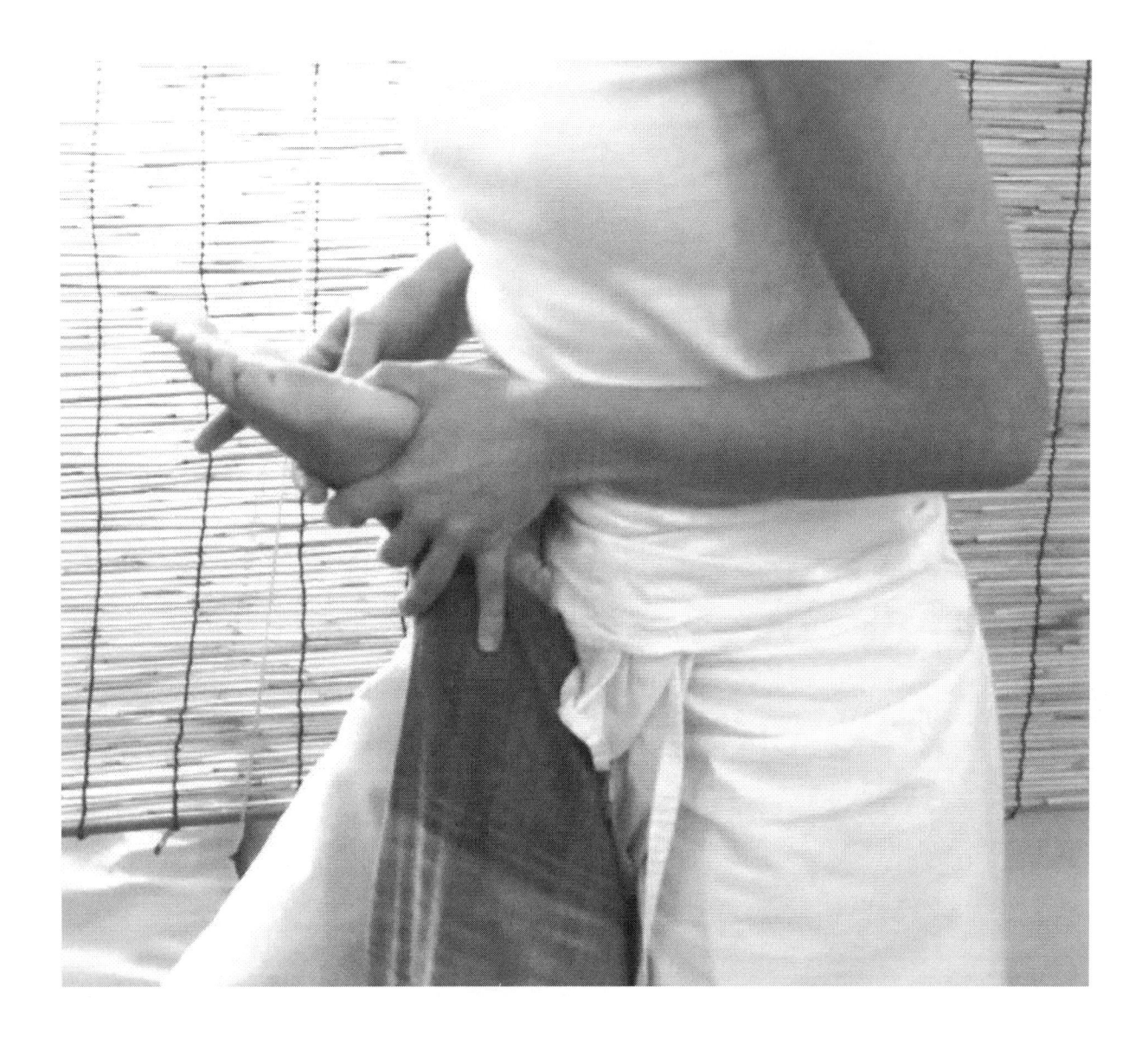

You can also press the 6 points on the feet with your thumbs. It is also possible to use your elbow for this.

Refer to the feet section for these points.

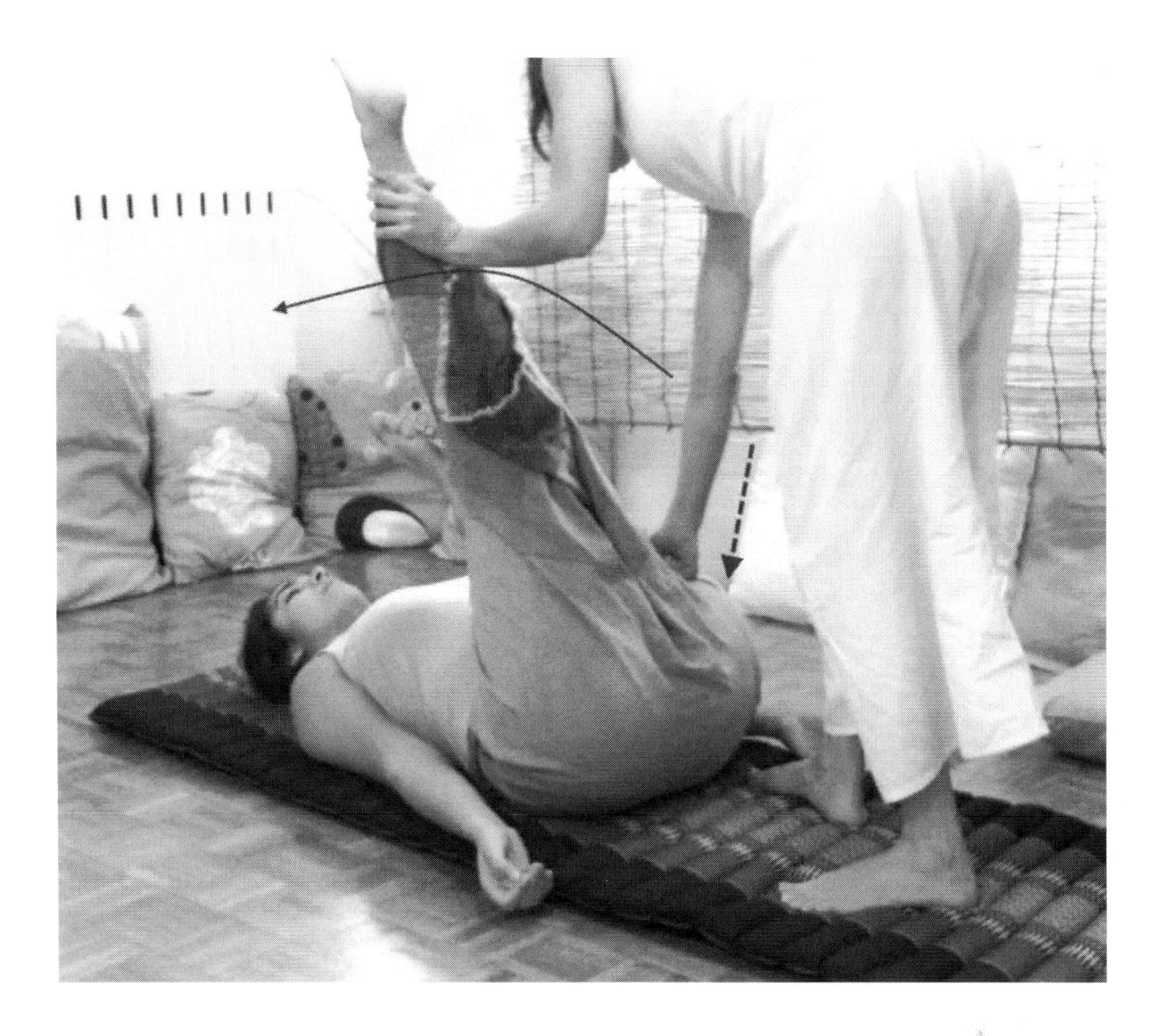

Now press the posterior thigh muscles with your fist, and simultaneously press the other leg towards the receiver's head.

These presses can also be done with your palm, and you can even do thumb pressing between the heads of the muscles of this area.

If you wish, you could also place your hand below the receiver's sacrum and push gently her leg towards her head. In that case, the technique becomes a passive application of the yogic asana *Sarvangasana*.

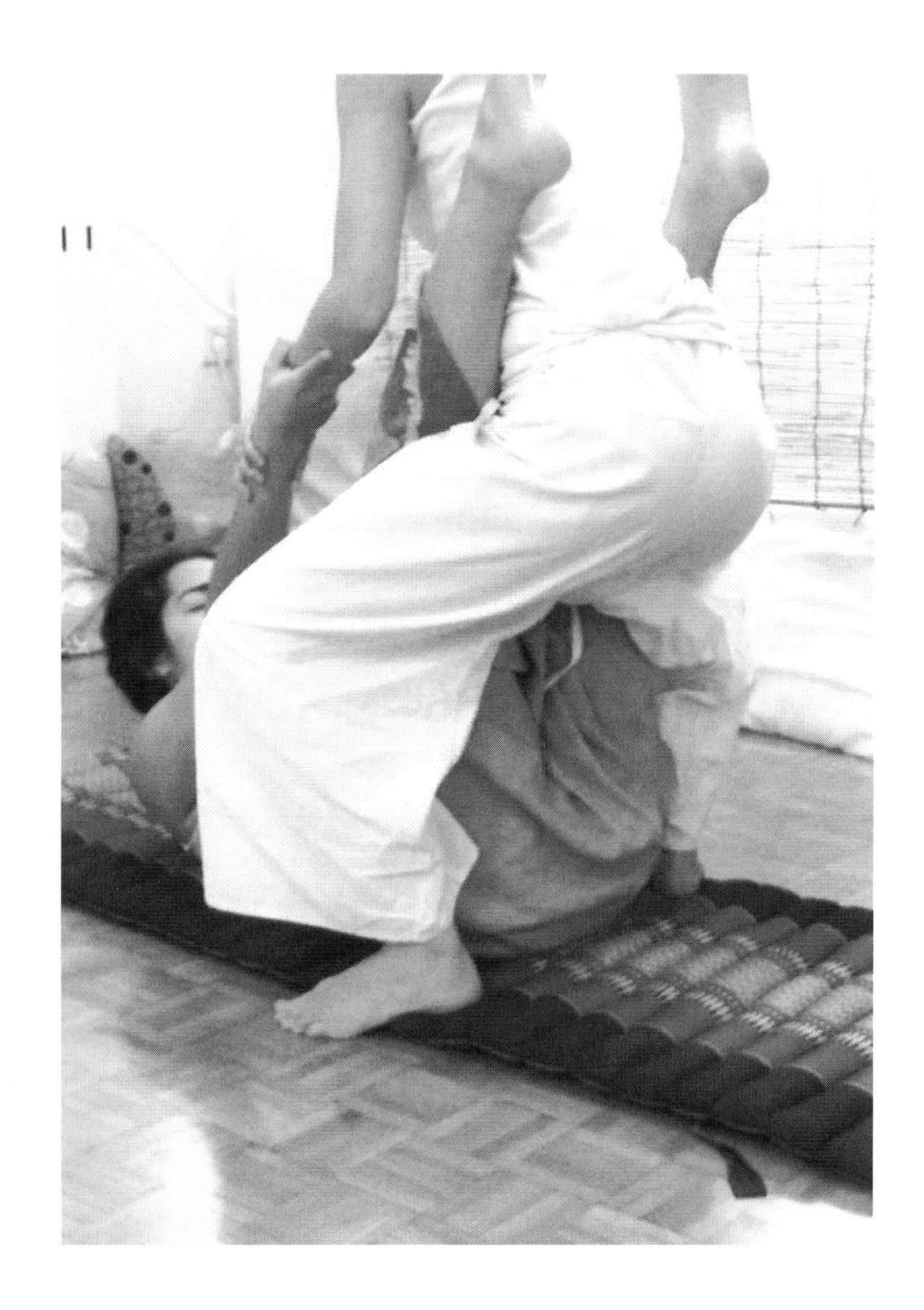

5. Then lift and stabilize the receiver's legs on your quadriceps muscle, and lift her arms. Do the lift as the receiver exhales.

This is a good technique for scoliosis and slight kyphosis.

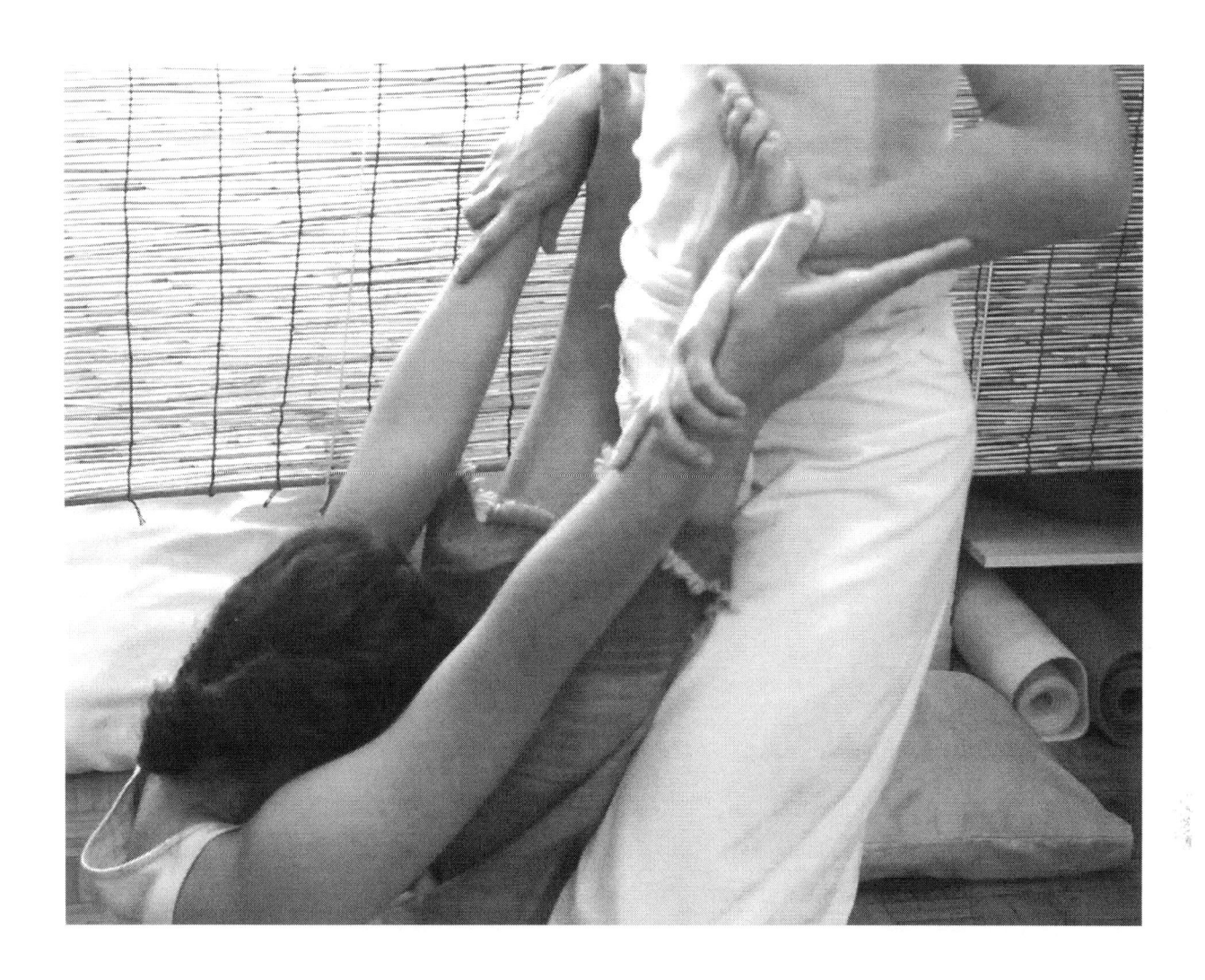

How to grasp hands

It is important to grasp the receiver's arms from the forearm – never from the wrists. Always ask the receiver to grasp your arms as well.

It goes without saying that the skin should be completely dry. If there is any oil, the arms could slip, and that could be dangerous.

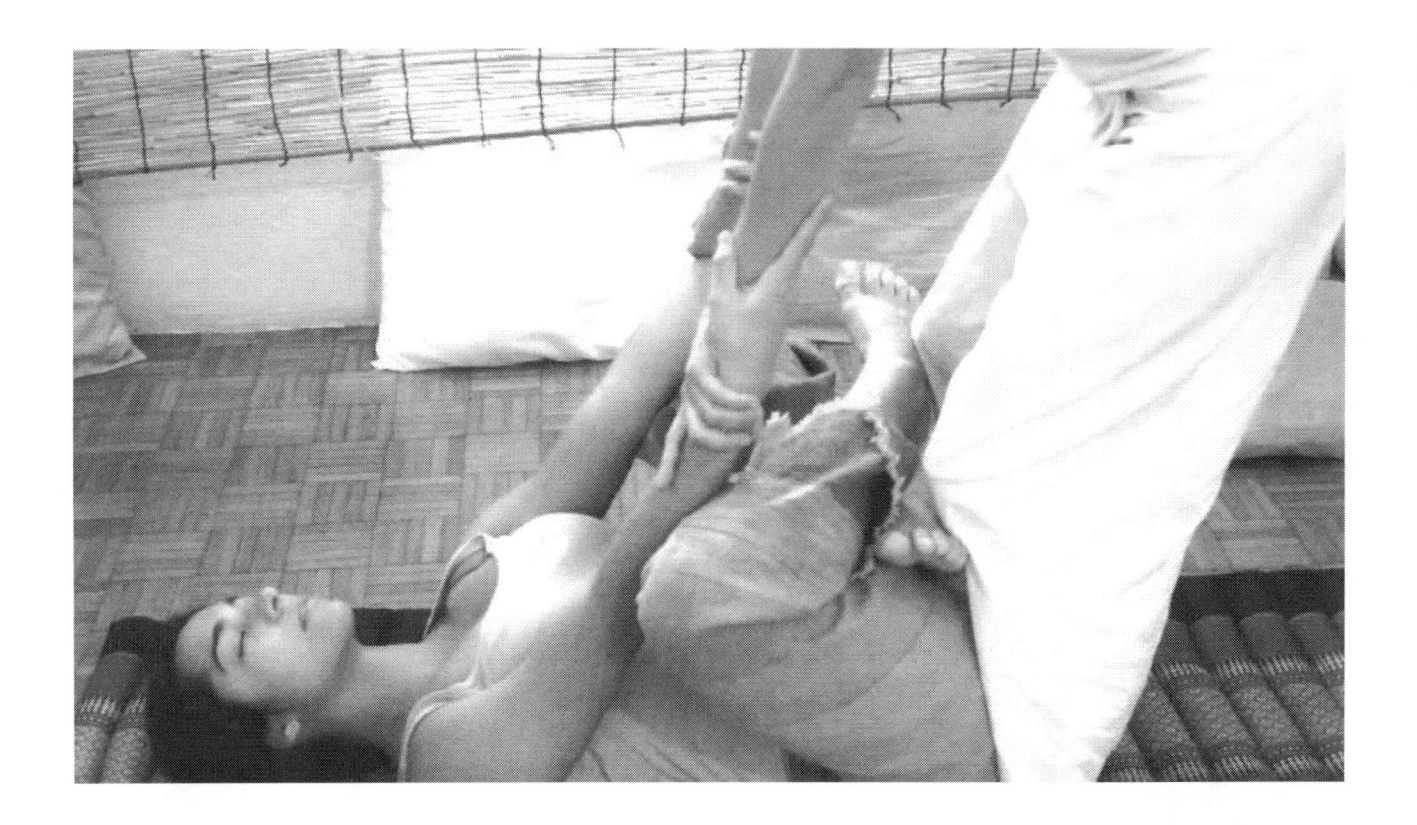

6. Repeat the previous technique – only this time, with crossed legs.

In order to achieve the lock, place the receiver's legs below your knees. The patella works as a "barrier" and stabilizes the legs.

How to lift clients
Always bend your legs and keep your back straight, when lifting the client in Thai Massage. Let the muscles of your legs do the work, not the back muscles.

> ### *How to lift clients*
>
> *Always bend your legs and keep your back straight, when lifting the client in Thai Massage. Let the muscles of your legs do the work, not the back muscles.*

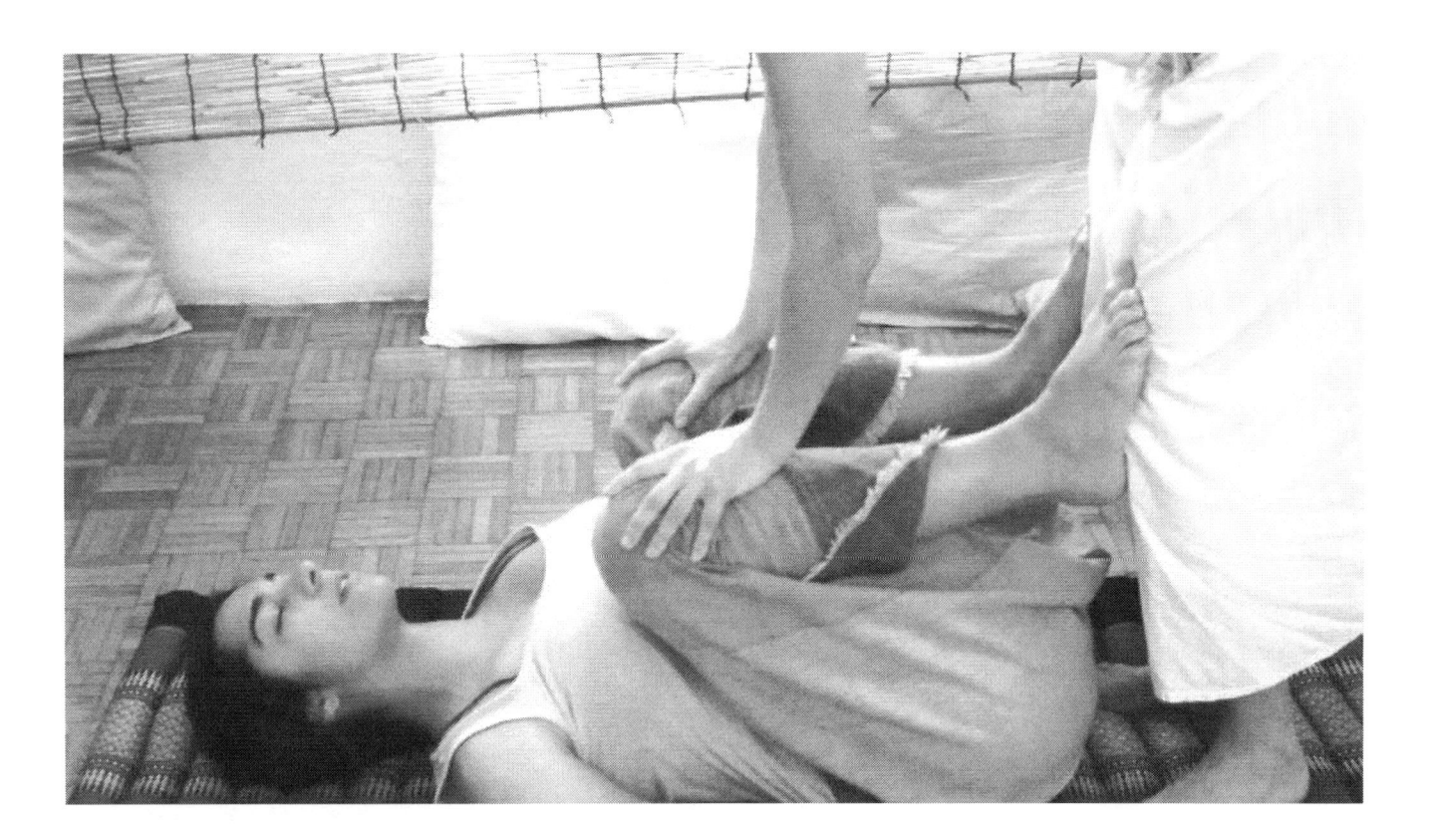

7. Stabilize the receiver's feet on your patella, and grasp her knees. When she exhales, push her legs towards her chest. It is helpful if you synchronize your breath with the receiver's breath – that is, you can exhale as she exhales.

This technique is a passive application of the yogic asana *Pawanmuktasana*.

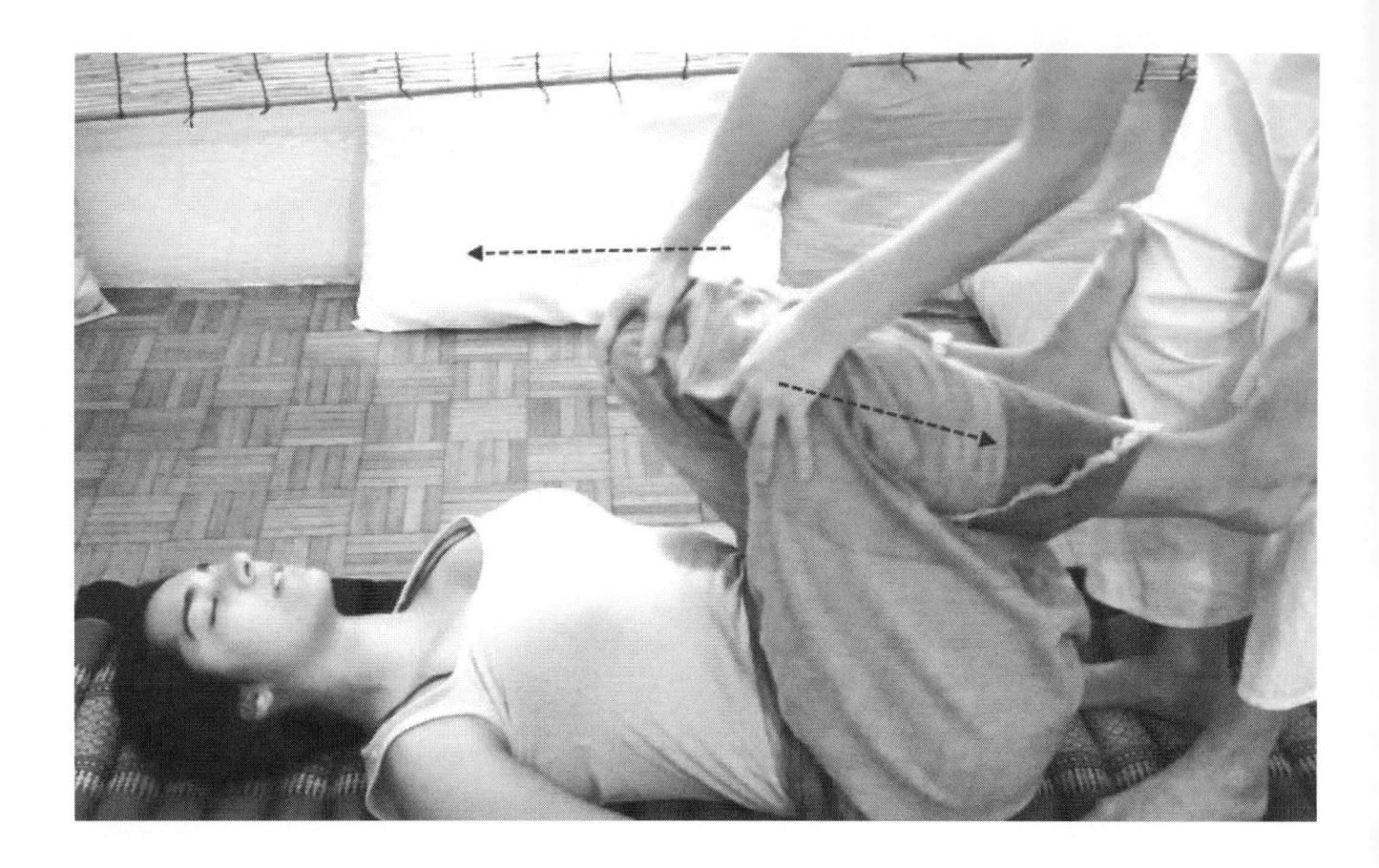

8. Then bring your knees forwards alternatively. This technique is very relaxing for the pelvis.

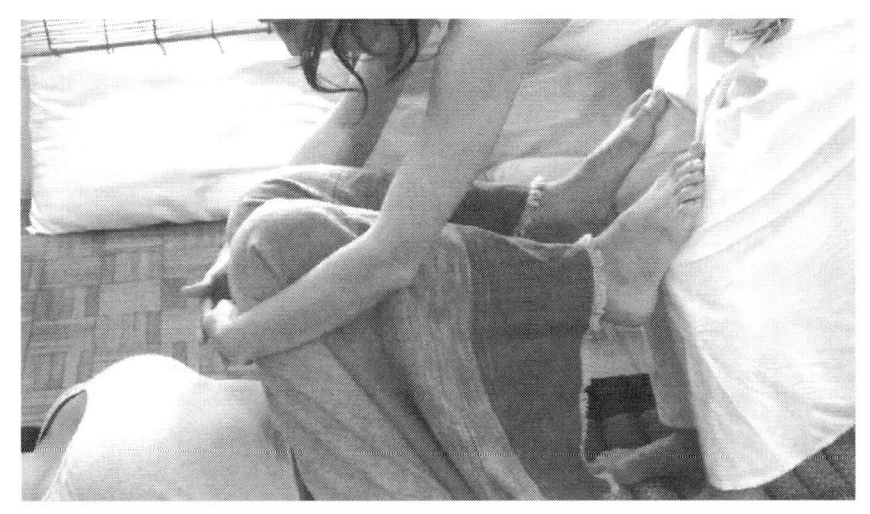

9. Now interlock your fingers and grasp the receiver's thighs...

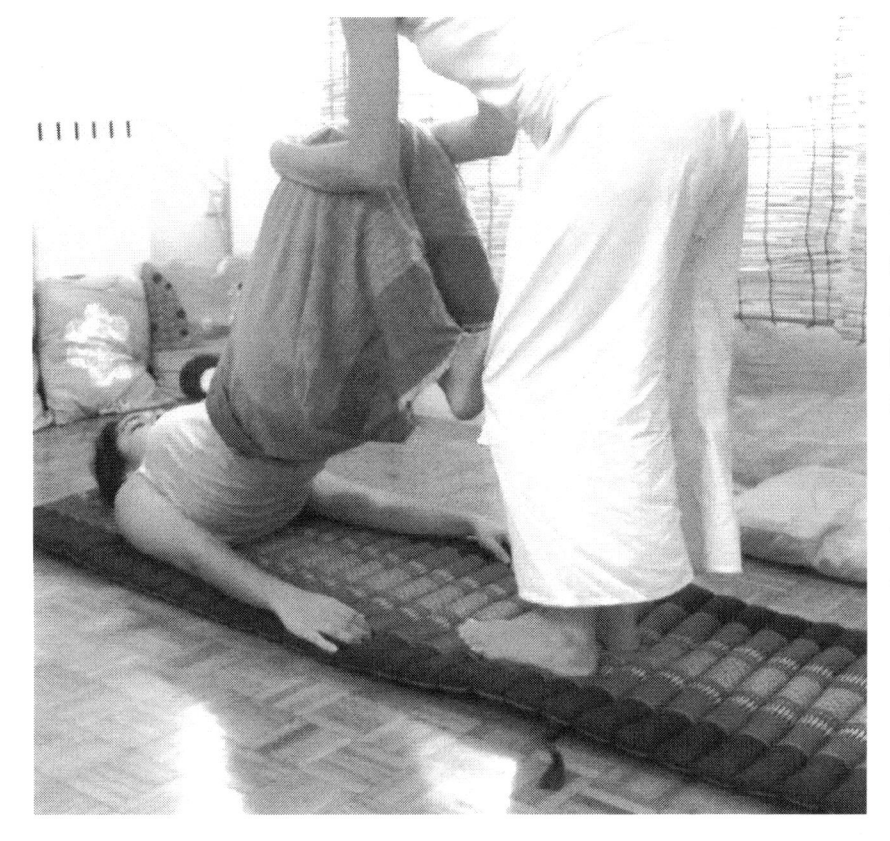

... and lift her torso from the ground. Hold the stretch for 5-10 seconds, and bring the receiver back to the ground gently.

Do not perform this technique on heavier clients.

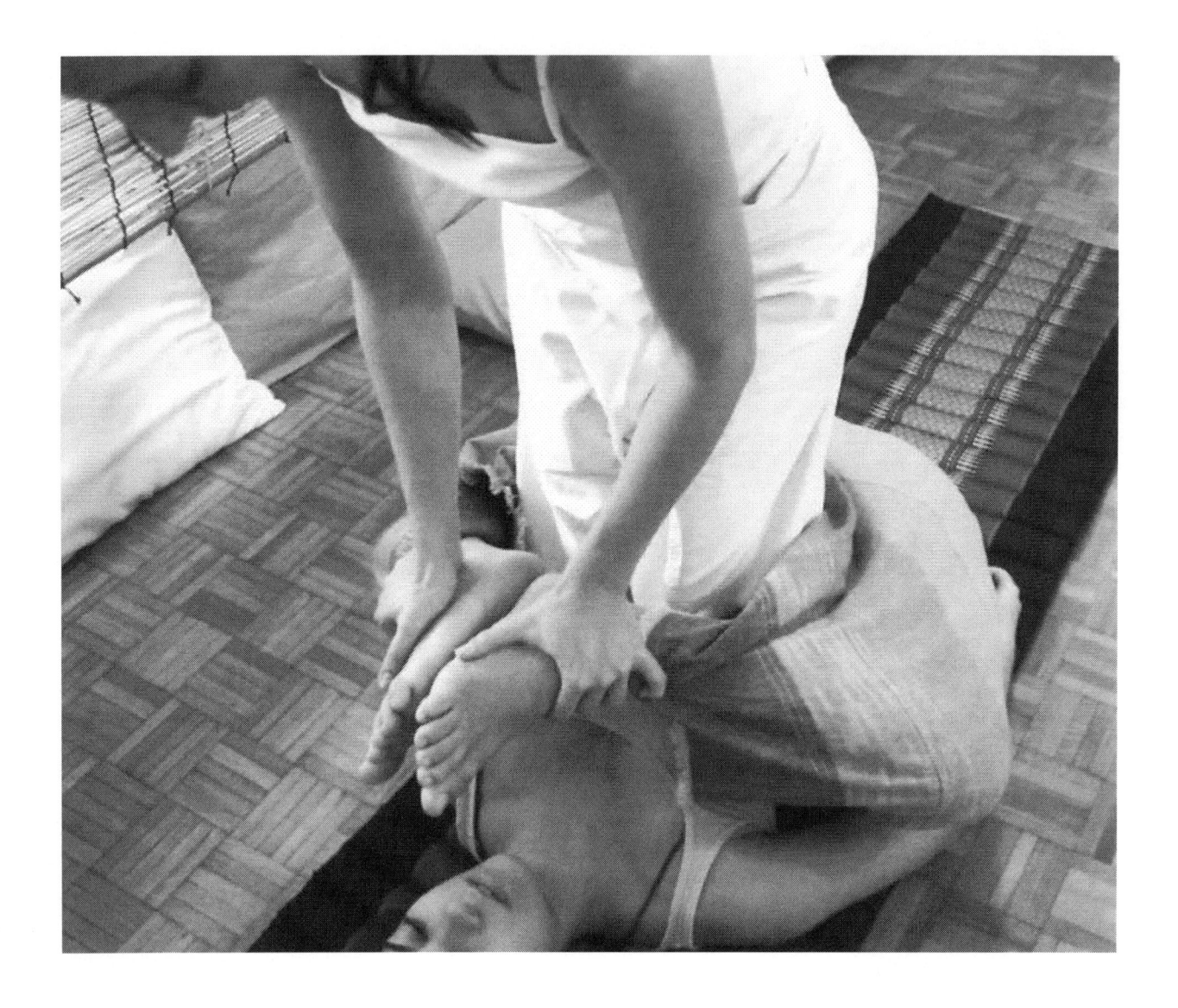

10. Bring your feet next to the receiver's hip joints, passing them through her thighs. Lift the receiver's legs and try to bring her feet together, in front of your knees.

Then push them downwards, as the receiver exhales. The "goal" is to bring them behind her head. However, you should never push the body beyond its limits.

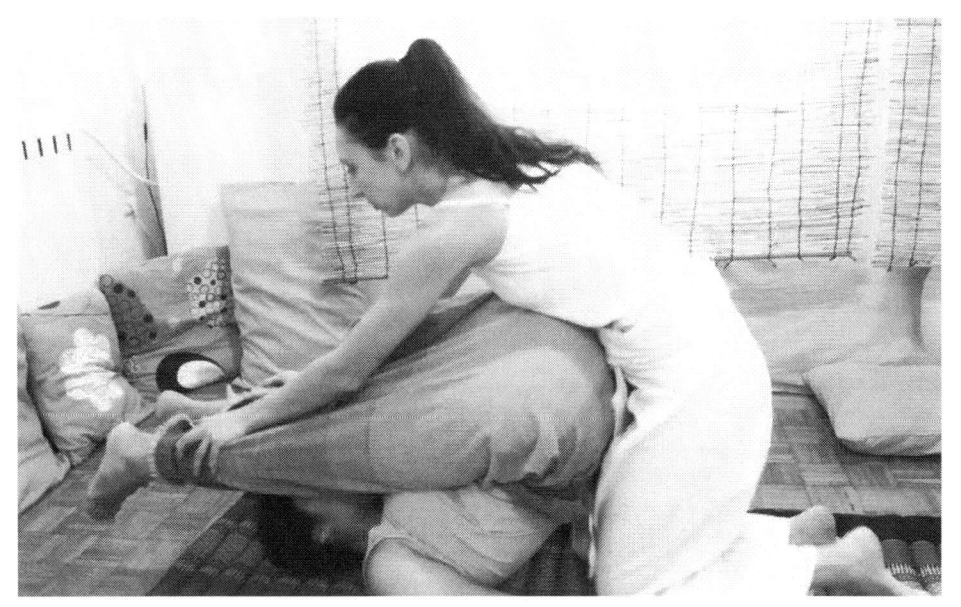

11. Lift the receiver's legs. Walk on your knees, until you reach the scapula.

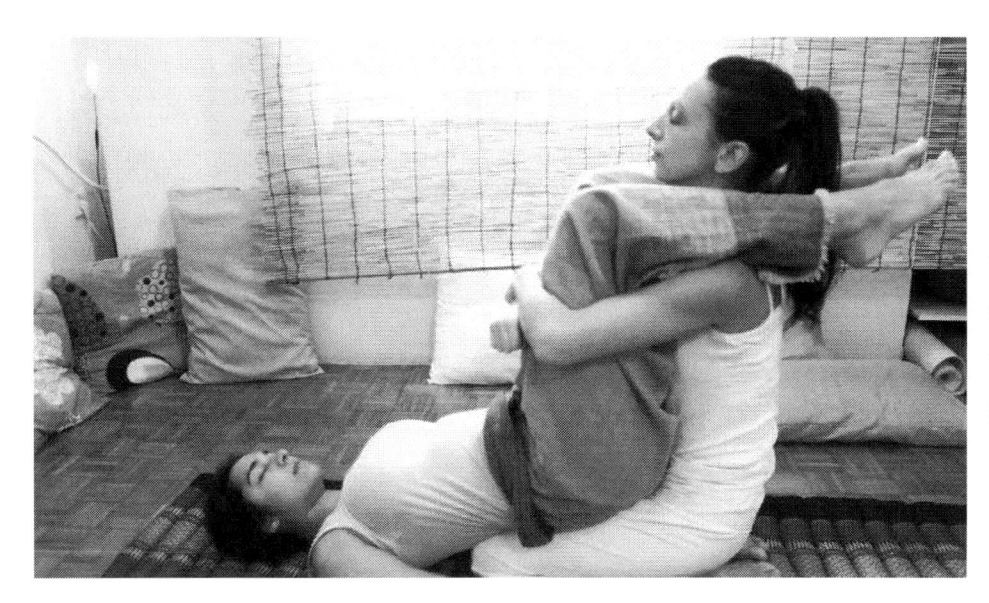

Then place the receiver's legs on your shoulders, and grasp her thighs.

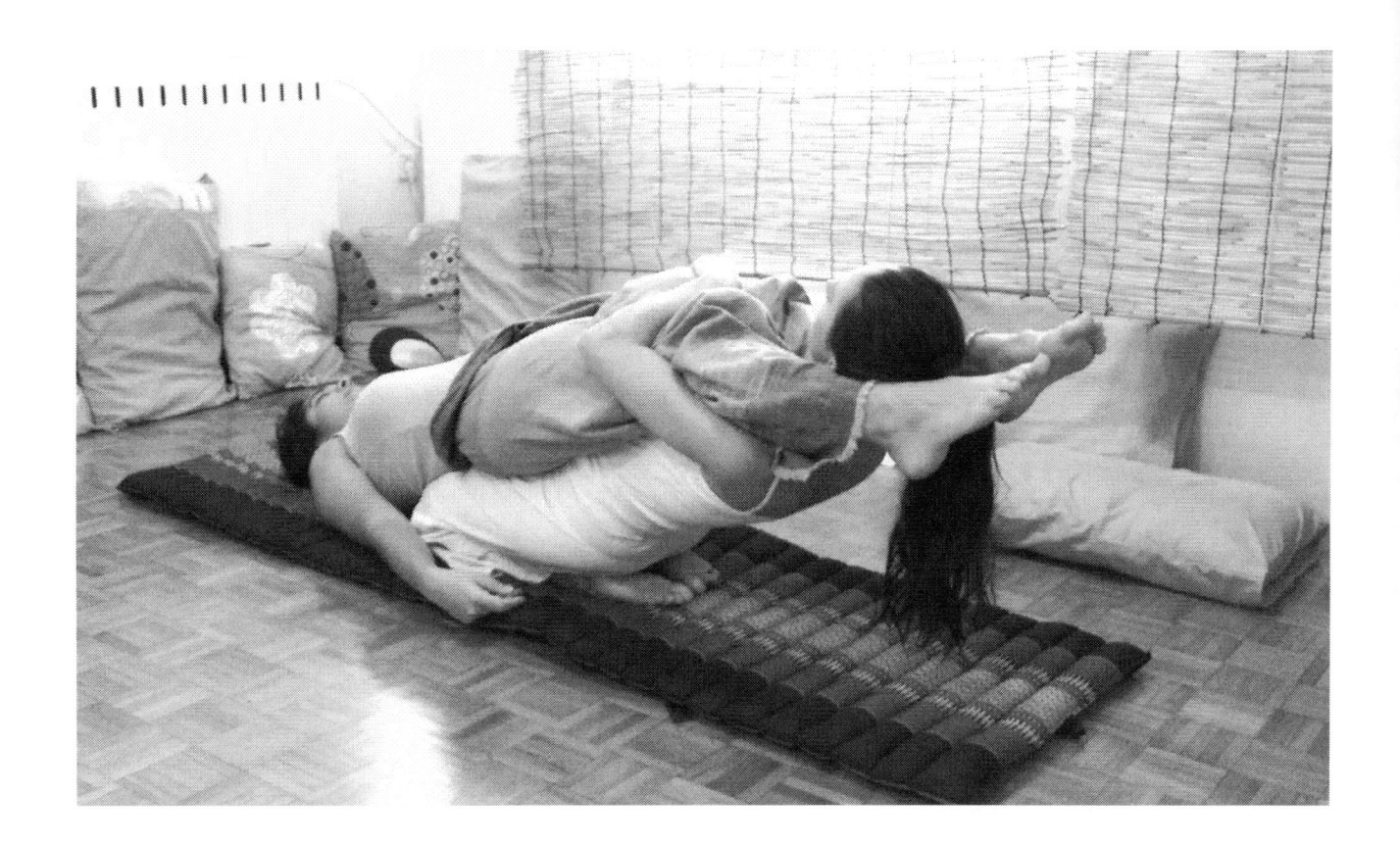

Then fall back, in order to decompress the receiver's lumbar spine. Stay in this position for at least 10 seconds.

In order to return the receiver's body to the supine position, lift her legs and walk slowly back on your knees.

Thus end the techniques that involve both legs.

The next section – that is, techniques for the abdominal and the thoracic cavity - includes far more gentle techniques.

what lies underneath

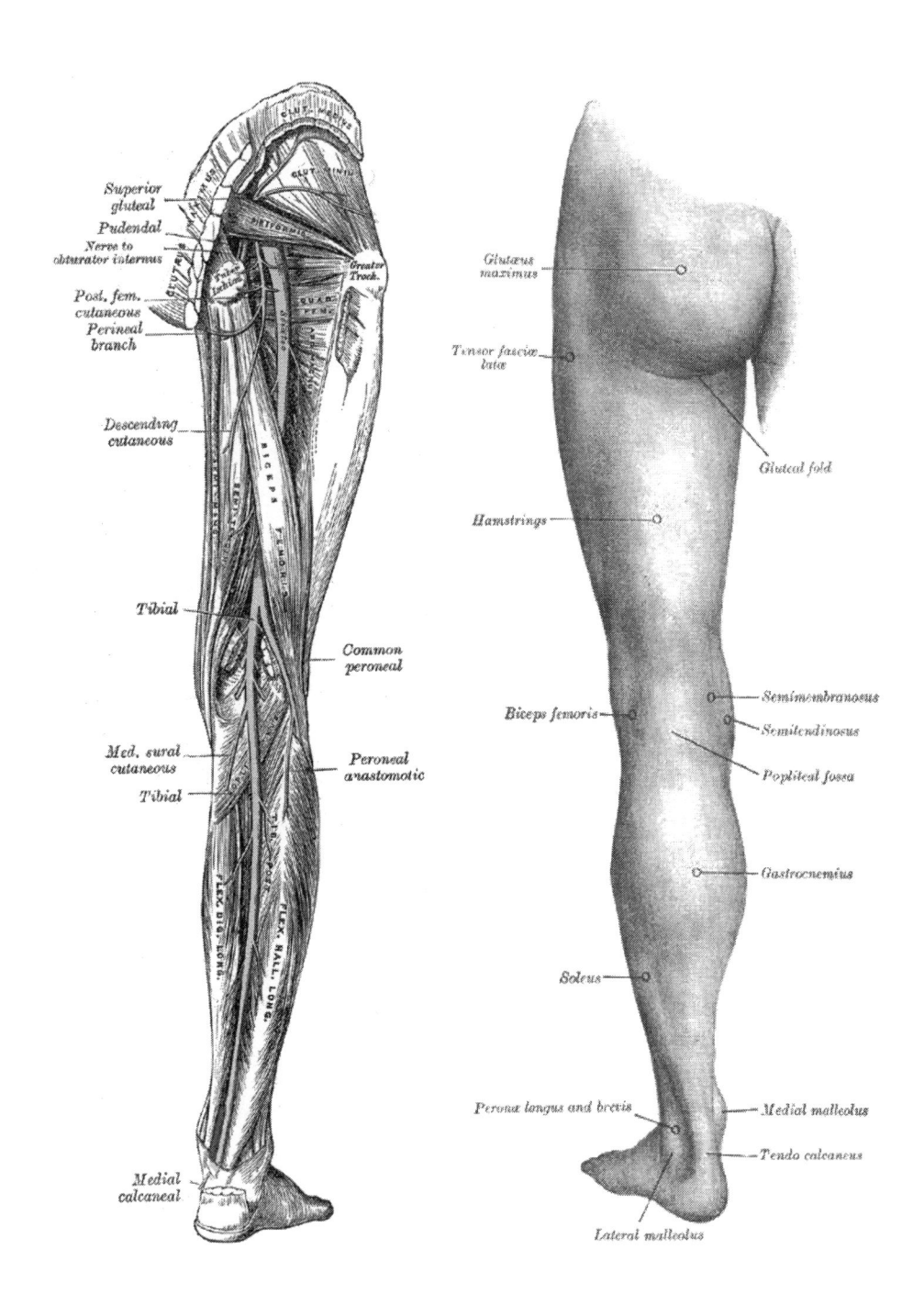

The sciatic nerve

Surface anatomy of the leg

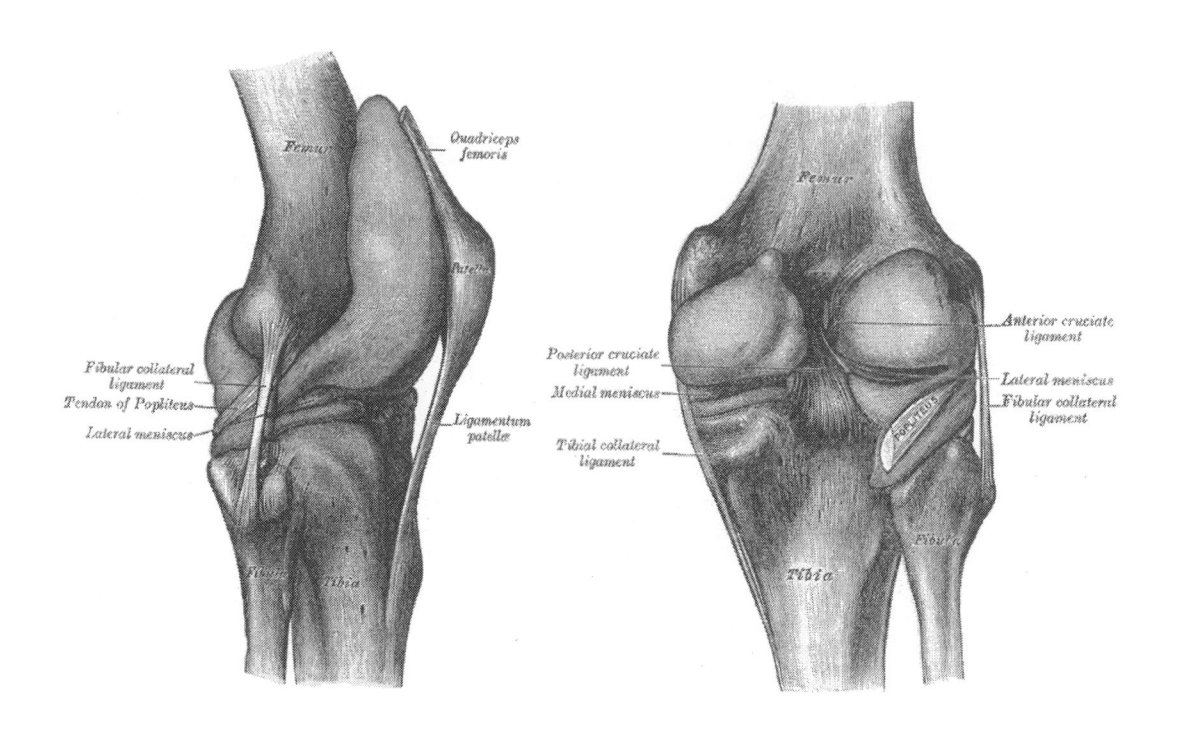

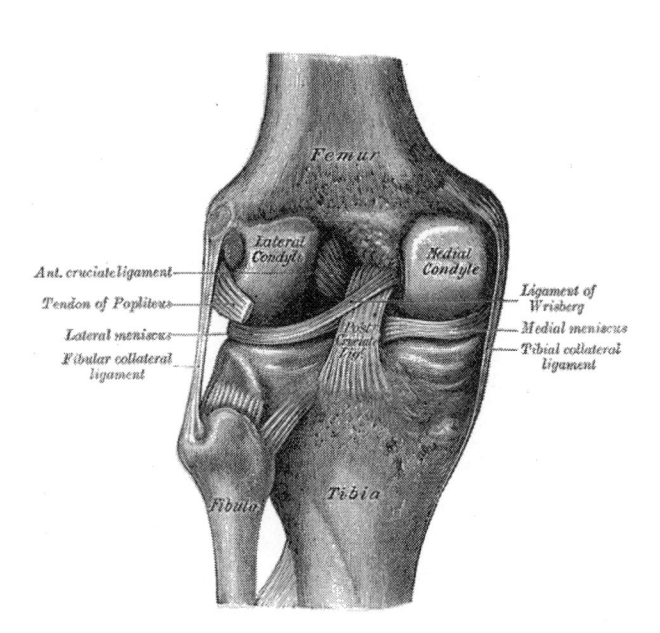

Anatomy of the knee

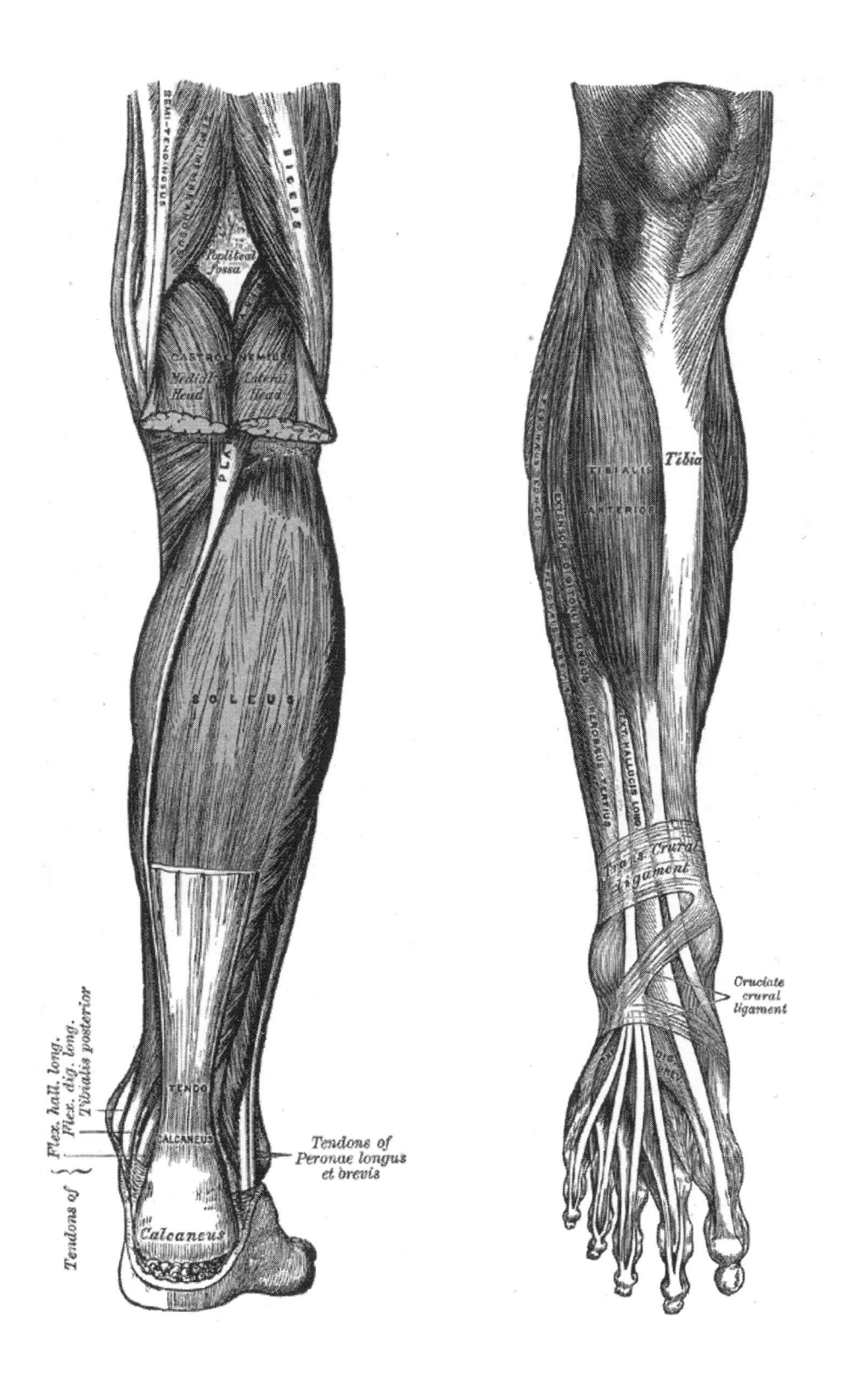

Posterior and anterior lower leg muscles

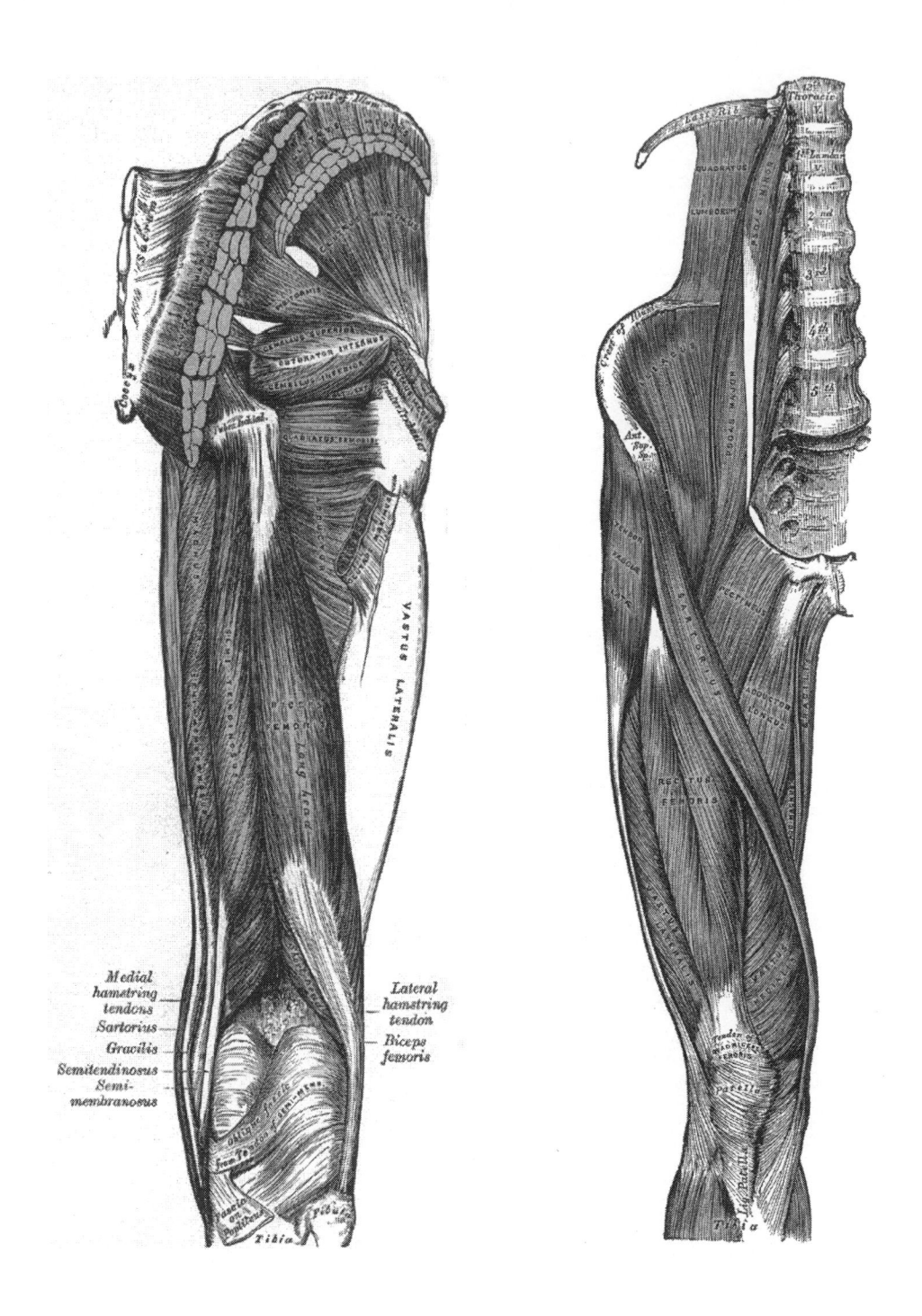

Posterior and anterior thigh muscles

trunk

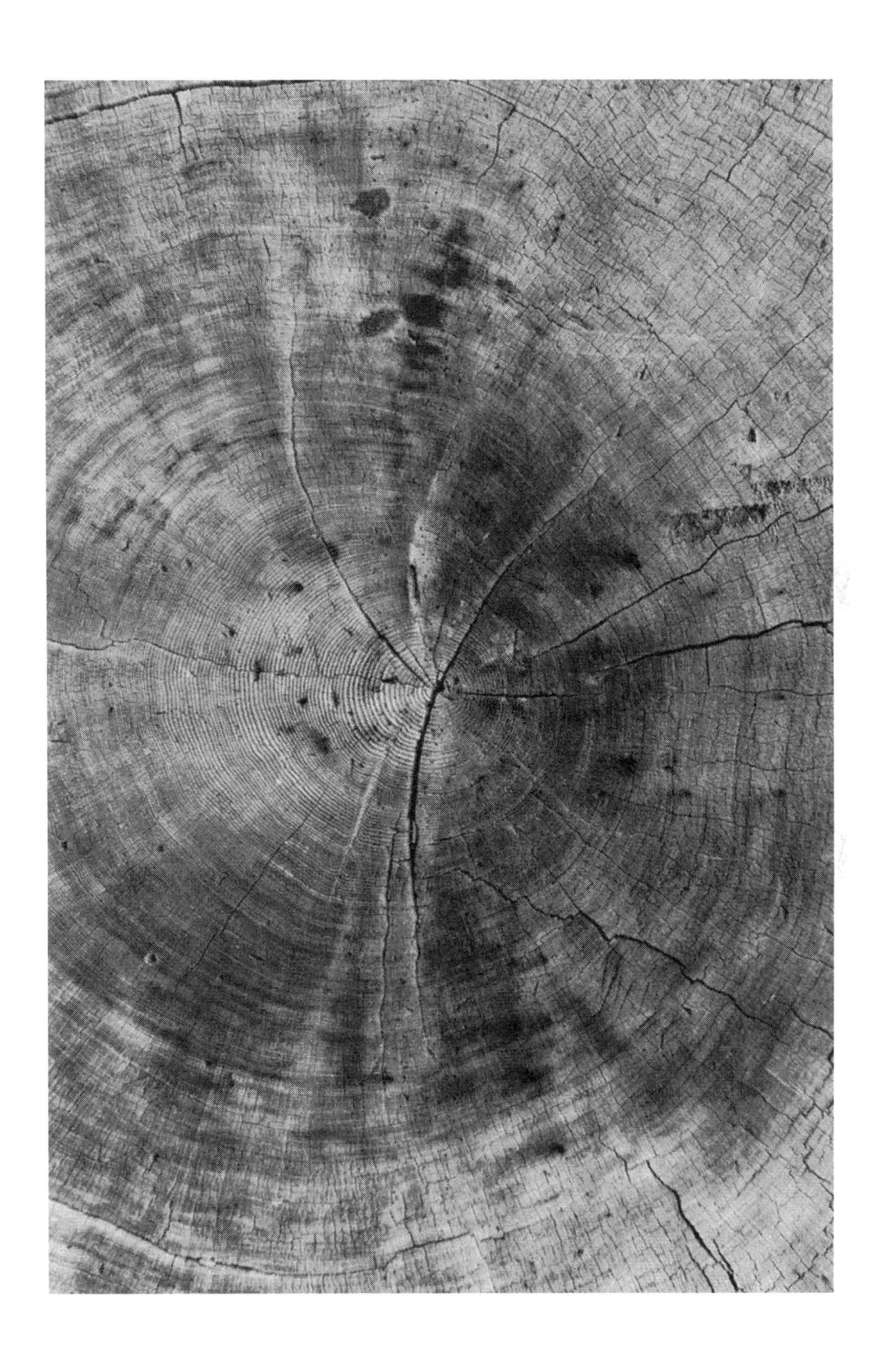

Now we will see the techniques for the torso – more specifically, for the abdomen and the thorax. Most of them are quite gentle and can be applied at any age group, as they do not involve too dynamic mobilizations.

They are especially indicated for arrythmias, stress, nervous tension, and chronic digestive and breathing disorders. Moreover, some abdominal techniques can also be helpful for lower back pain.

If you intend to work for some time on the trunk, please place a pillow under the receiver's knees. This will help proper pelvis alignment.

The following techniques (especially the techniques for the thorax) are more effective when combined with hot herbal packs and heat rubs.

abdominal techniques

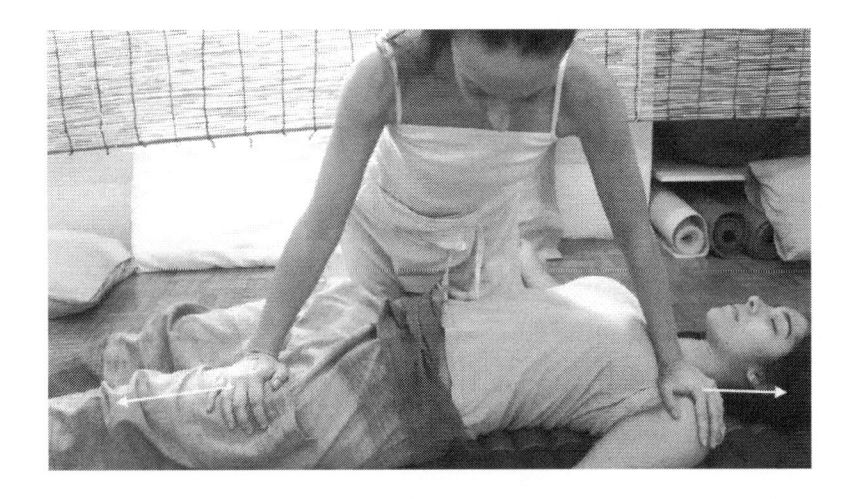

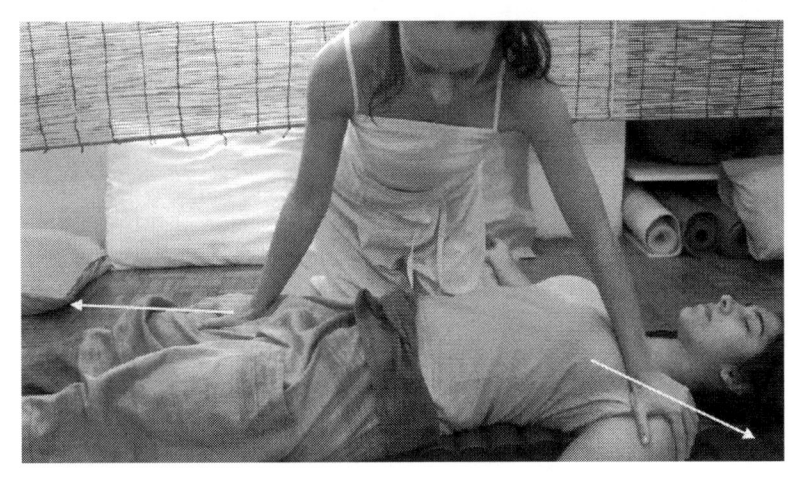

1. The session begins with 4 stretches on the torso. Place one palm on the receiver's shoulder, and one palm on the quadriceps muscle.

Apply two stretches with your palms on the same side of the receiver's body, and two stretches with your palms on opposite sides. It does not matter from which stretch or from which side you will start.

For best results, perform the stretch while exhaling – that applies for the therapist and the receiver.

This is an excellent technique. Not only it "opens" the torso, preparing the area for deeper work, but it is also helpful for lower back pain, as it decompresses the lumbar spine.

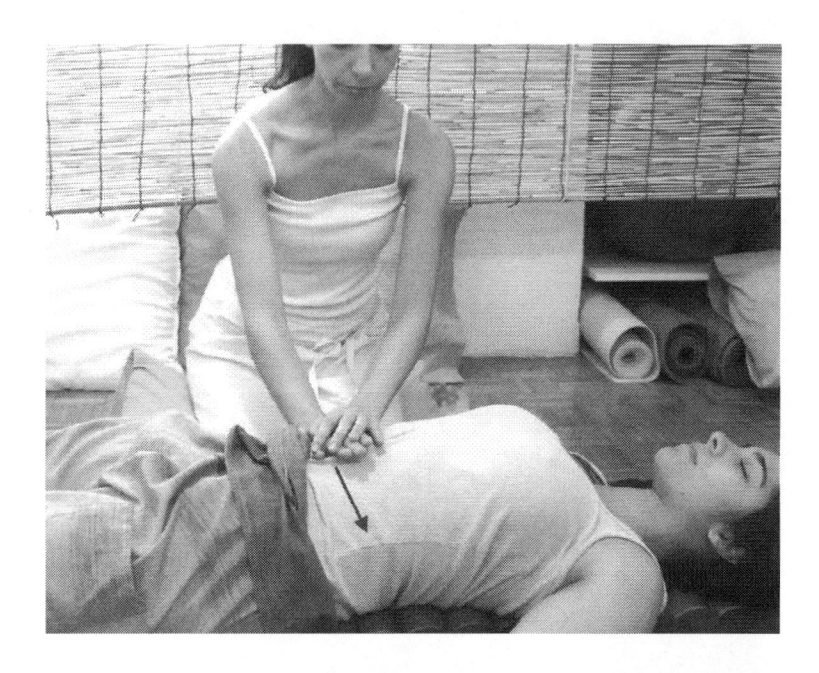

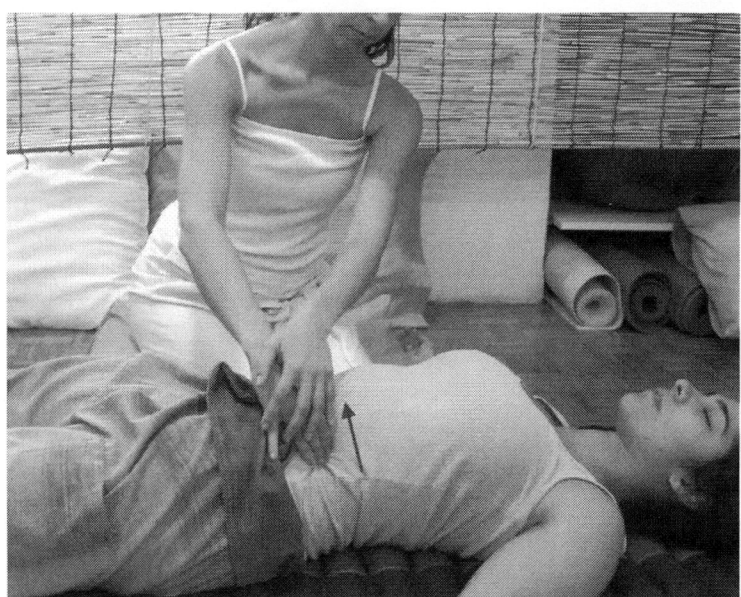

2. This technique is called the "wave". Massage the abdomen with your palms, in a wave-like pattern. This technique stimulates the intestinal peristalsis.

Push and pull the abdomen as shown in the photos. Your movement should be parallel to the ground. Pushing is done with thenar and hypothenar eminences, and pulling with your fingers.

Repeat 5-10 times, slowly and deeply.

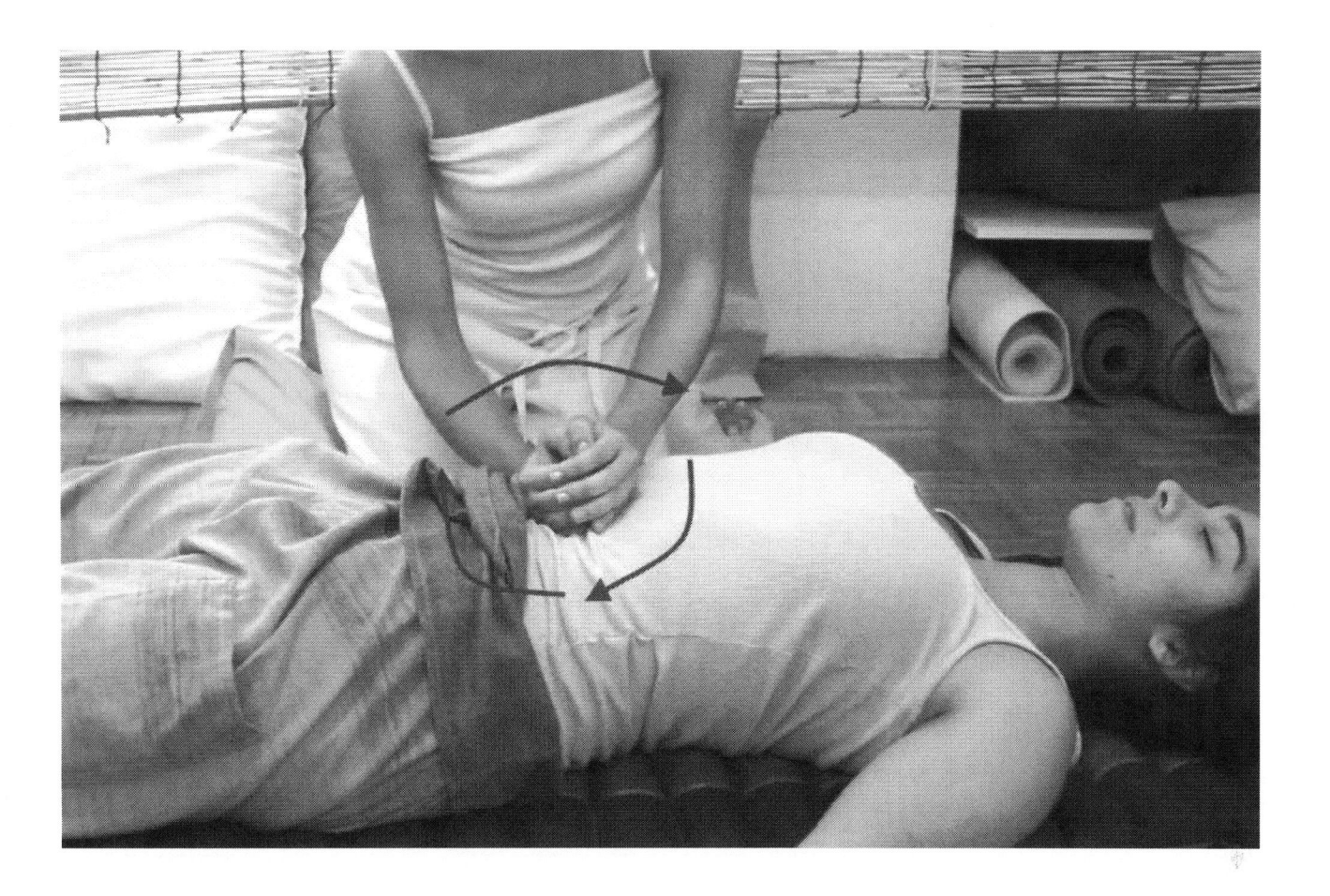

3. This technique is called "cup". Place your palms on the abdomen, and rotate the hypothenar eminence slowly around the umbilicus.

Use your body weight – do not apply direct pressure with your hands.

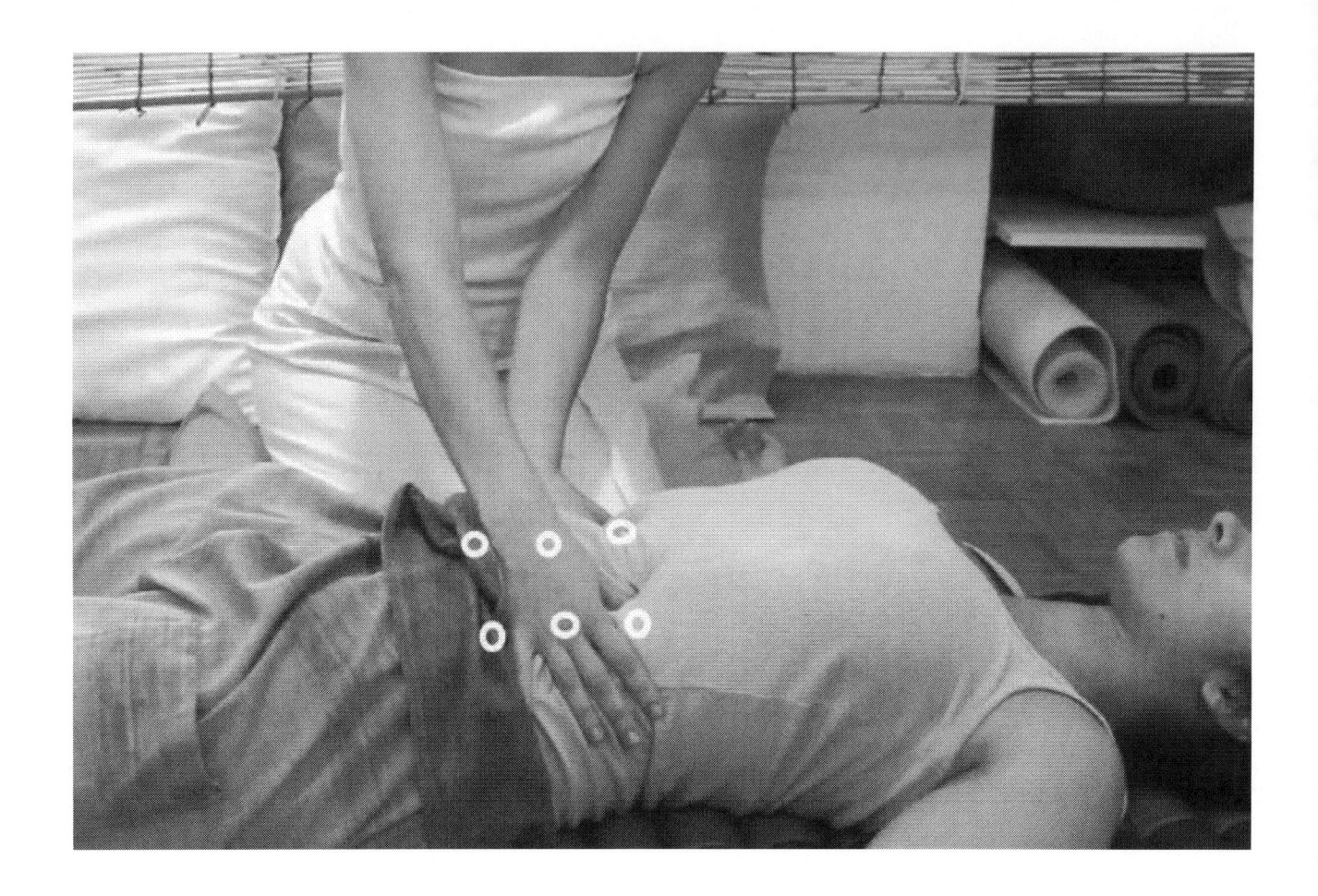

4. Now press 6 points next to the rectus abdominis muscle.

Points 1 and 2 are located two fingers beside the umbilicus, and two fingers above its level. Points 3 and 4 are also located two fingers beside the umbilicus, and at the same level with it. Points 5 and 6 are located two fingers beside the umbilicus, and two fingers below its level.

Begin by pressing 1 and 2 simultaneously, then 3 and 4, and finally 5 and 6. Always press when the receiver exhales.

Points are connected to *Itha & Pingkala Sen*.

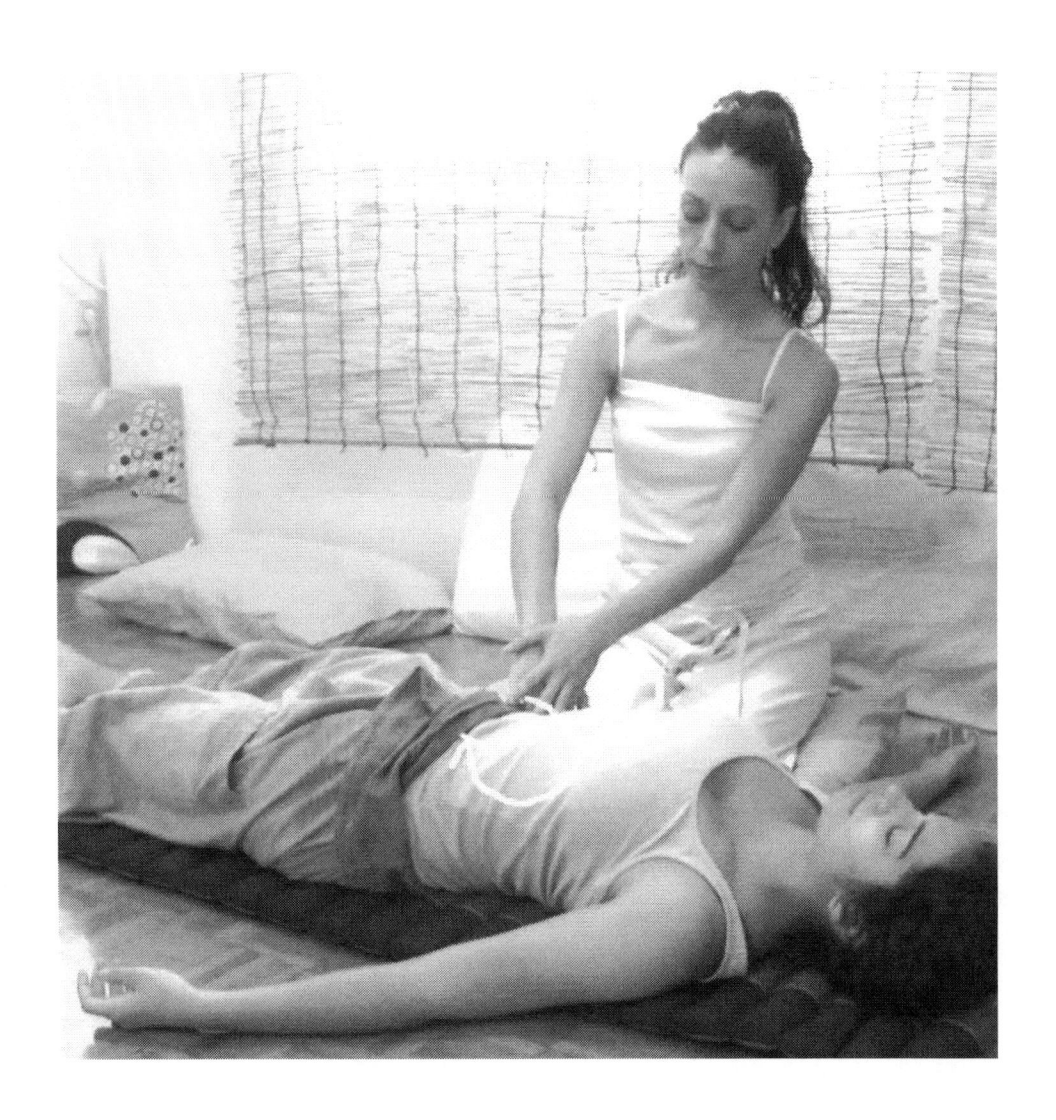

5. Then, press 9 points around the umbilicus, in a clockwise direction. Points 1 and 9 are located above the superior anterior iliac spine, while 5 is located below the xiphoid process. The other points are distributed evenly on this "circle", on the belly.

The 9 Points are connected to *Nantakawat Sen*. However, as Point 5 is specifically connected to *Sumana Sen*, it is used for breathing disorders, and problems pertaining to the heart and the mind. It is located on the diaphragm.

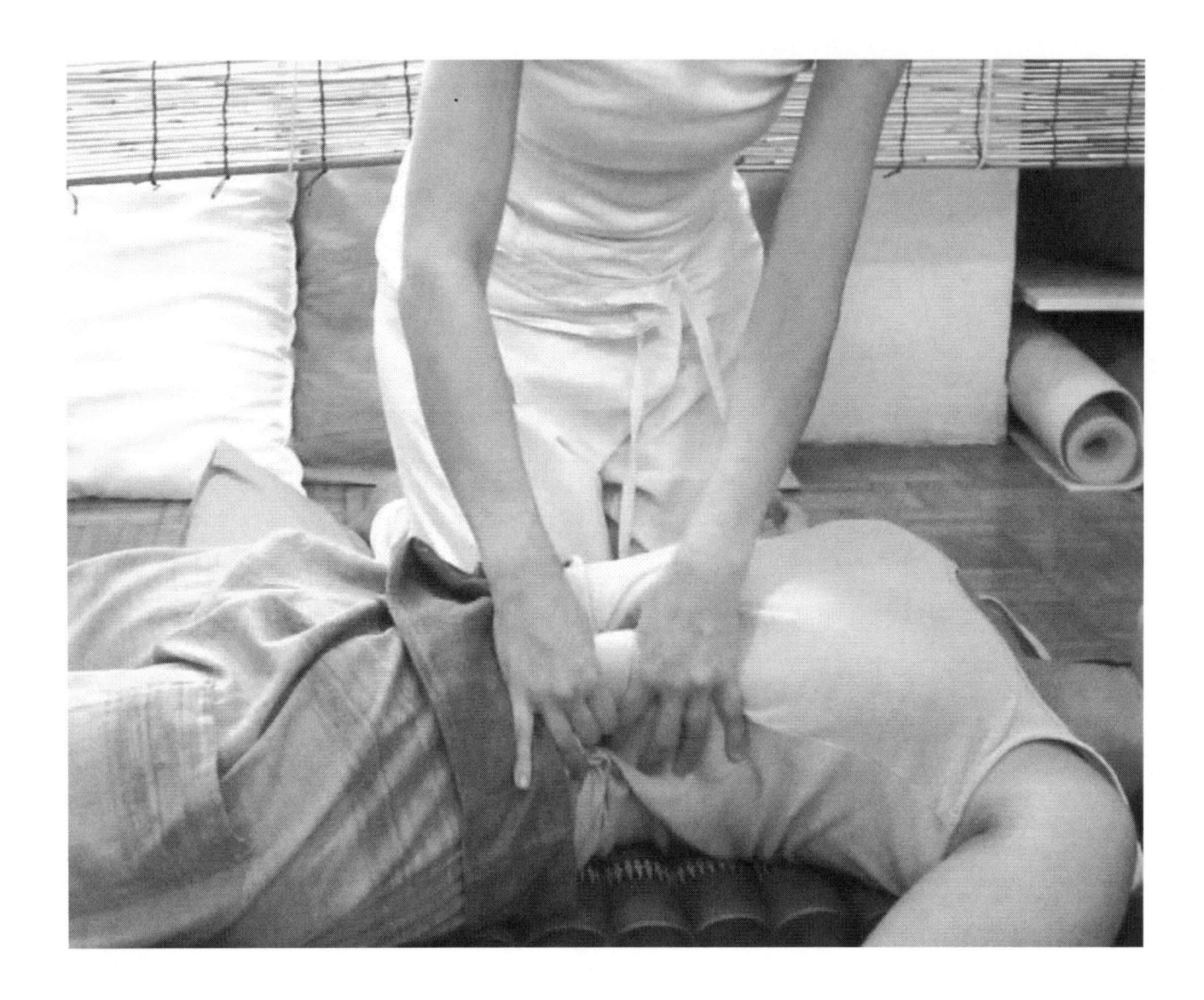

6. Follow with massage above the pelvis. Actually, thus technique is good for lower back pain.

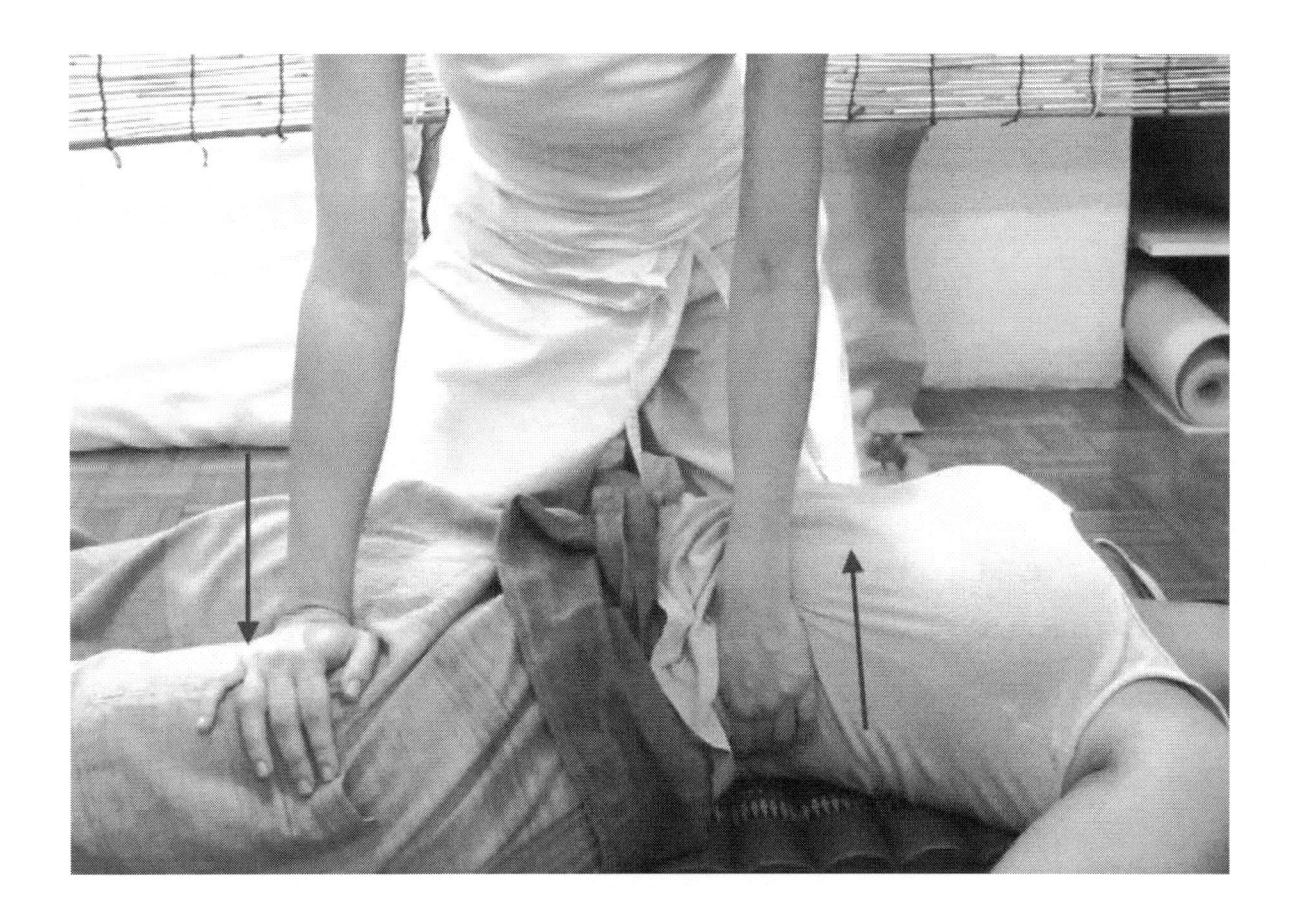

7. Place one hand above the pelvis, and the other on the quadriceps muscle. When the receiver exhales, lift the waist with one hand, and press the quadriceps muscle with the other.

This technique targets the sacrum and the pelvis. It is especially good for anterior pelvic tilt.
.

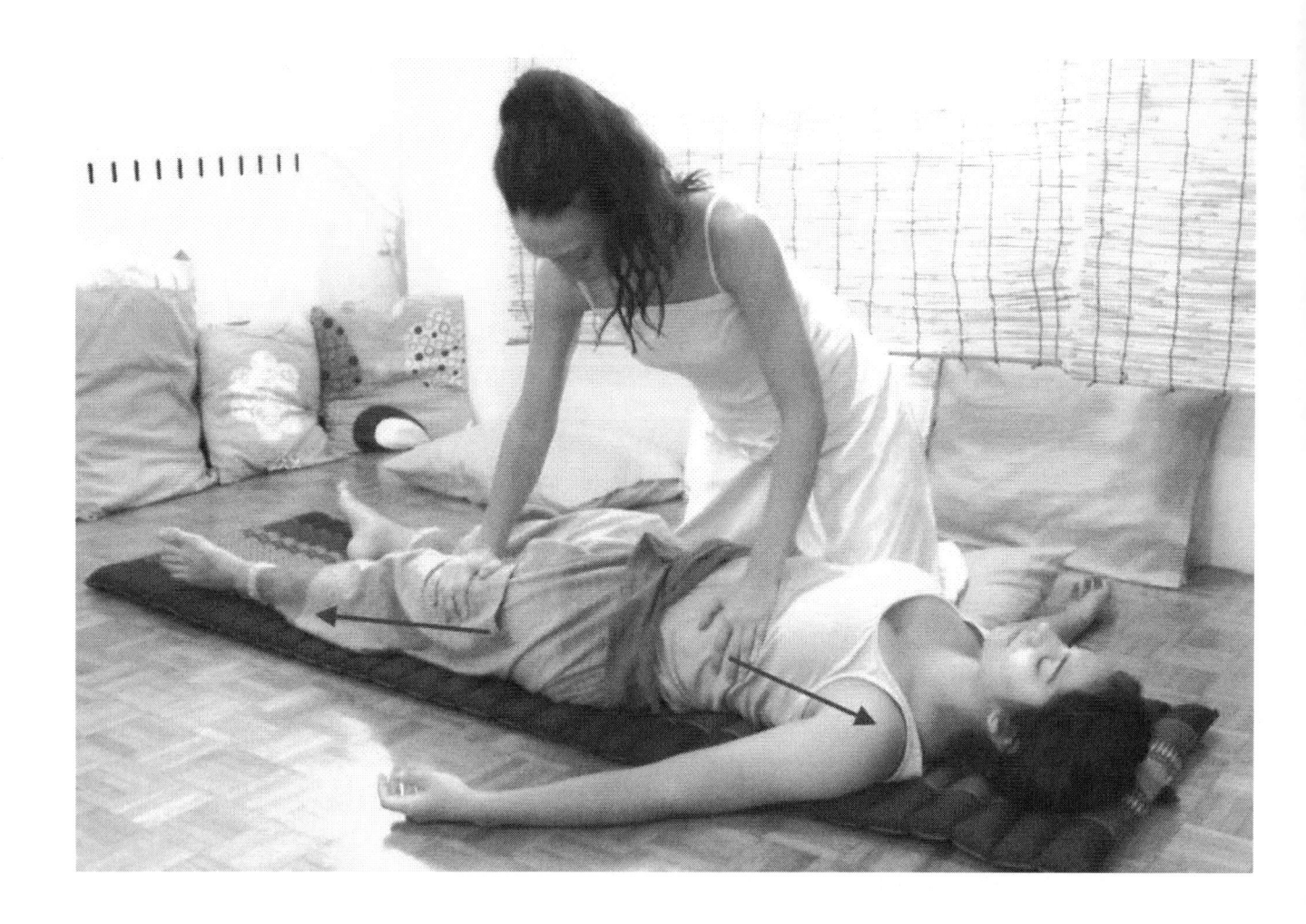

8. Then place one hand on the lower ribs, and one hand on the quadriceps muscle. When the receiver exhales, perform a stretch. This technique is also indicated for lower back pain.

techniques for the thorax

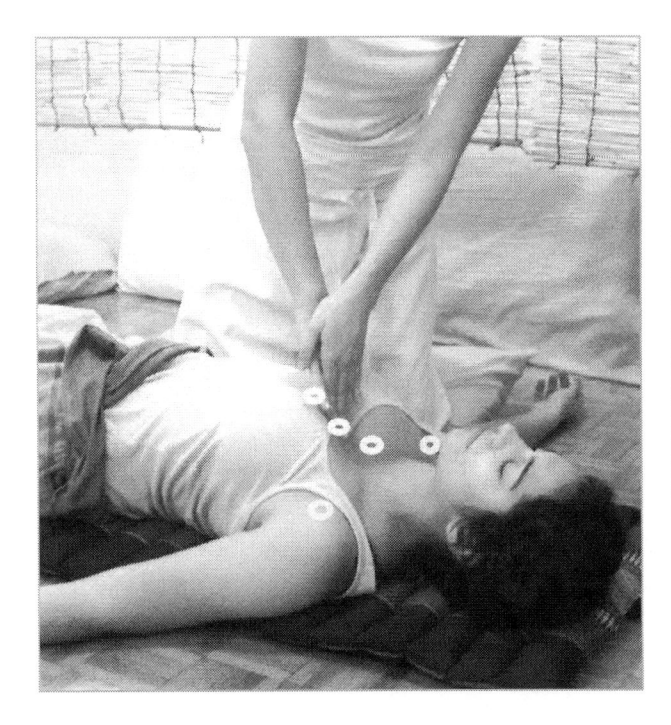

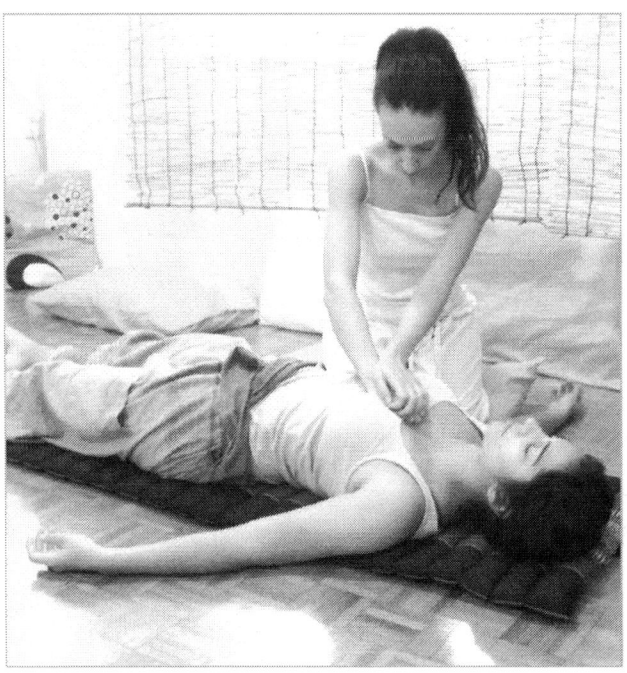

1. Press the Kalatharee Sen and Sumana Sen points on the sternum and under the clavicle bone. This points are indicated for stress and breathing problems.

It is best if you combine these techniques with hot herbal packs. Be sure to add eucalyptus, peppermint and camphor, as these herbs are expectorant and calming for the mind.

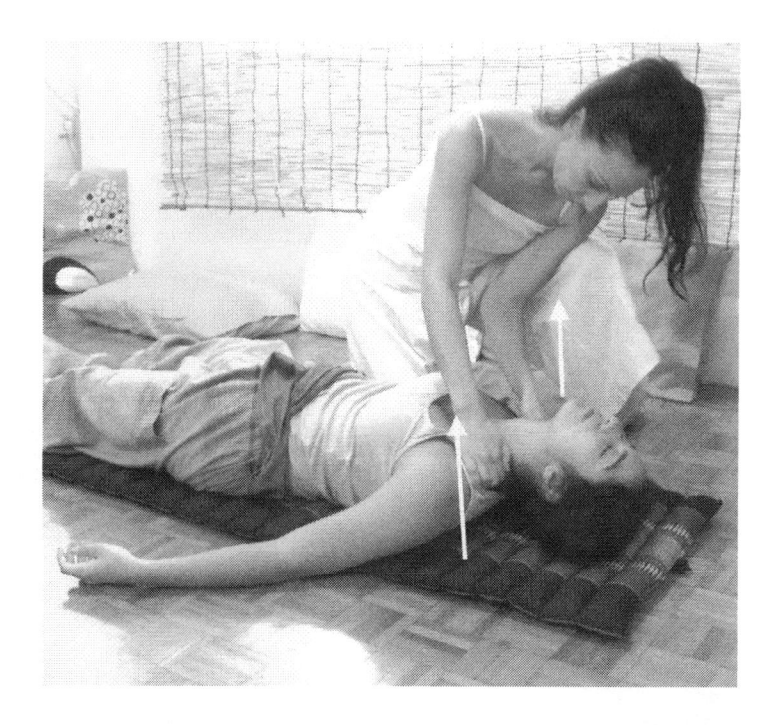

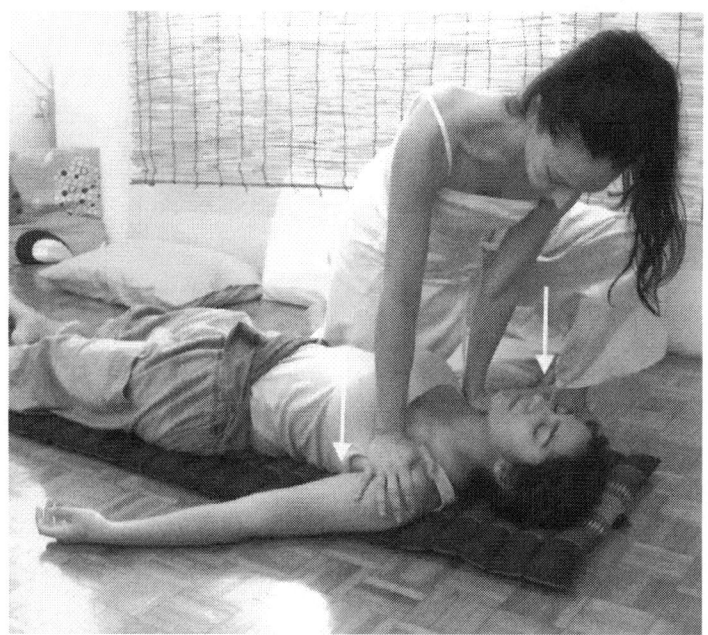

2. Then lift the receiver's torso by grasping her from the trapezoid muscle. Lay her gently on the mat, and press her shoulders with your palms, as she exhales.

Good technique for neck and shoulder pain.

Thus end the techniques for the torso.

what lies underneath

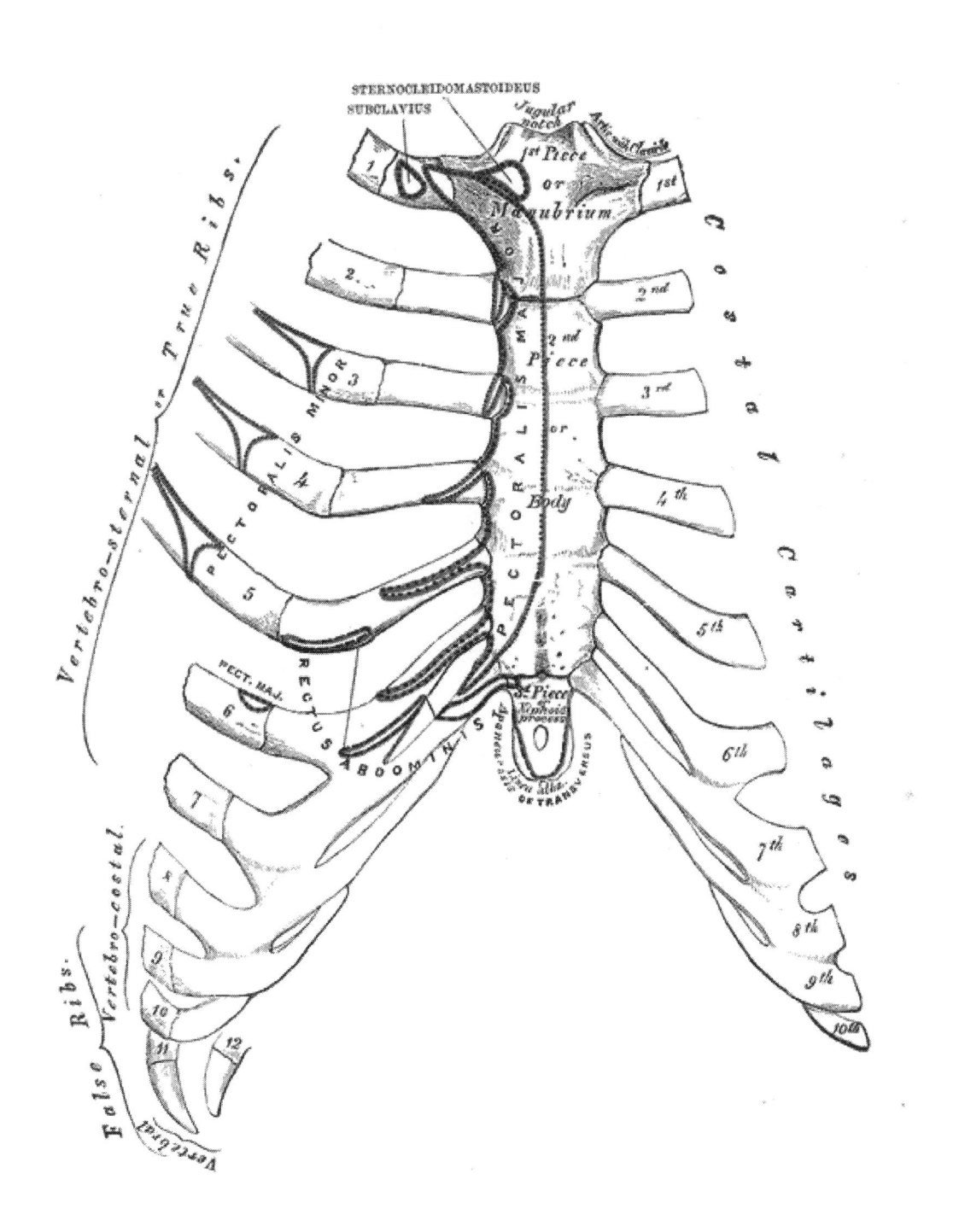

Sternum and ribs

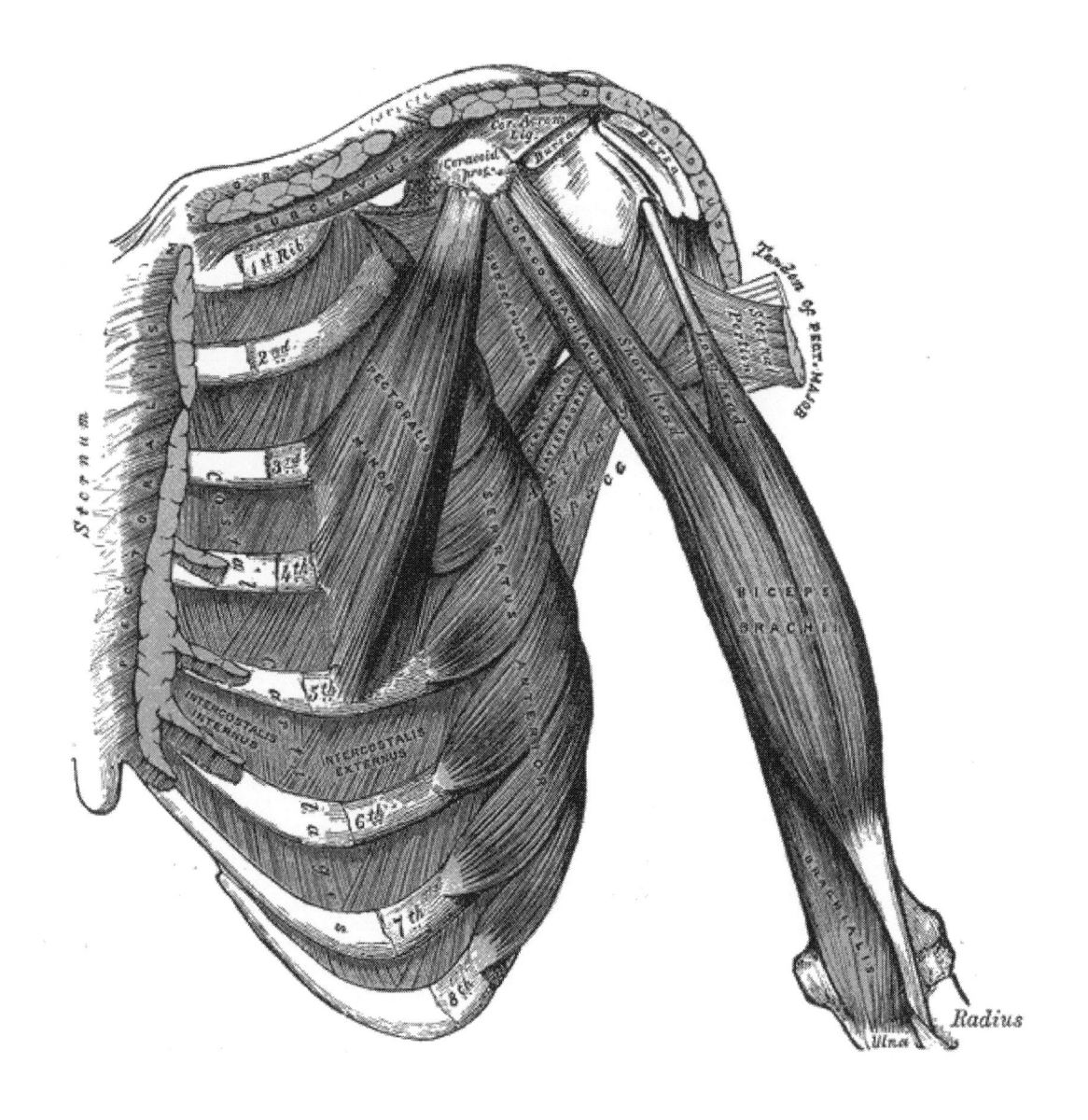

The muscles connecting the arm to the anterior and lateral thoracic walls.

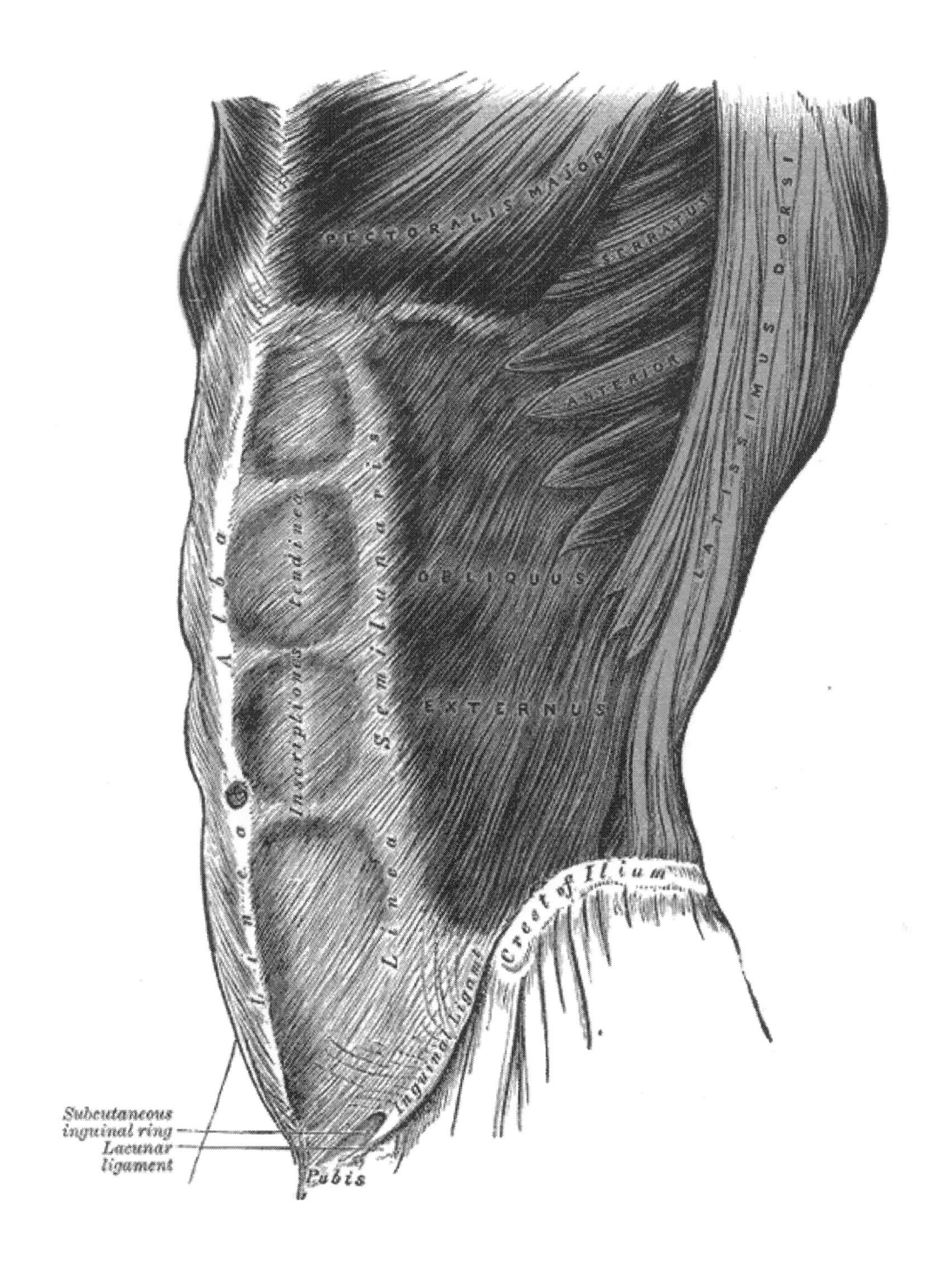

Abdominal muscles

arms & hands

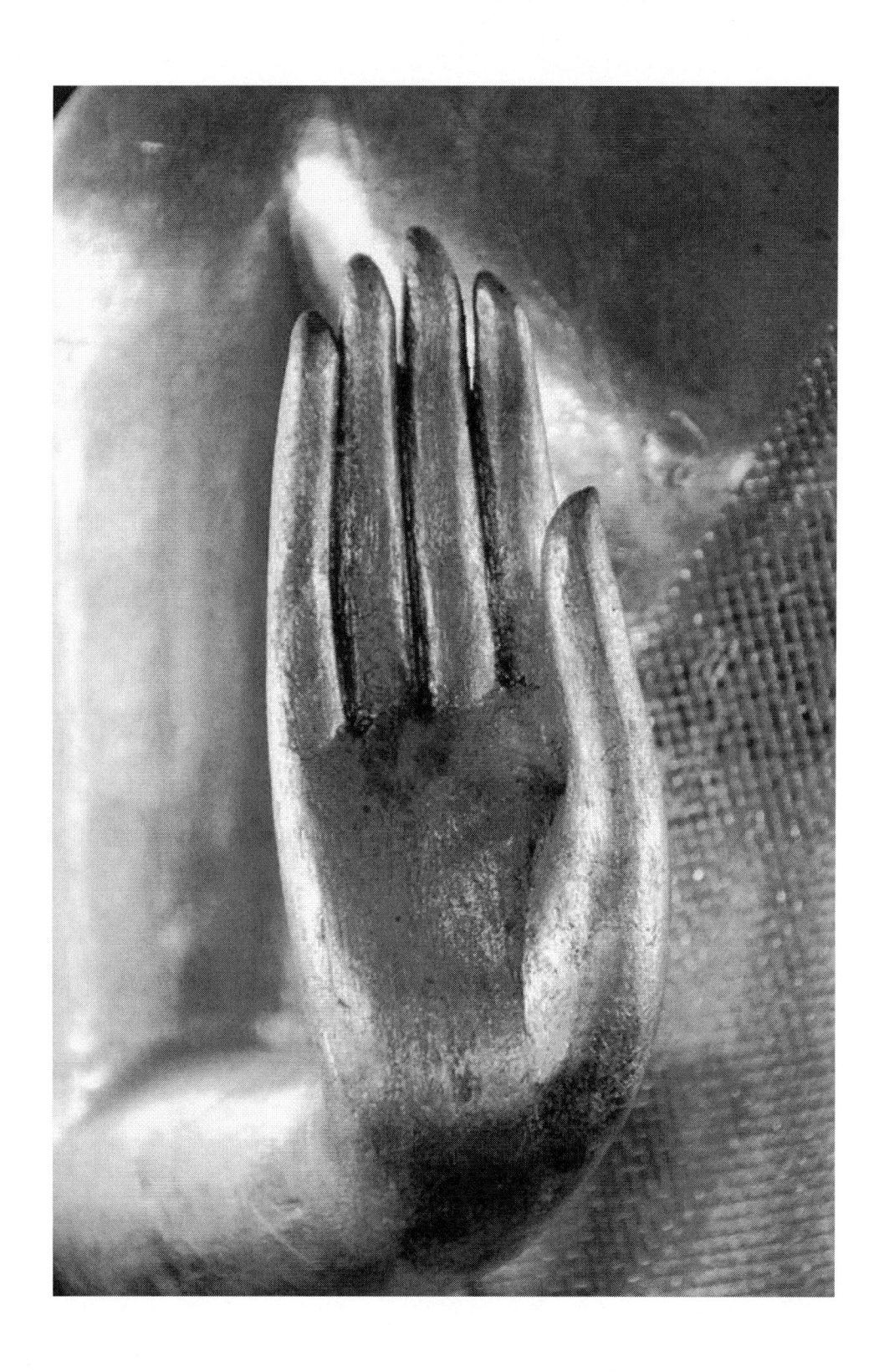

Arm and hand techniques are generally gentle, and can be applied almost to all age groups. They are indicated especially for neck pain (numbness in the arms originates from the neck, as these areas are connected neurologically), stress, shoulder pain, and of course pain localized on the arm and the hand. They work especially well when combined with warm herbal packs and heat rubs.

The *Kalatharee Sen* arm branch has a definite connection to the heart, at an energetic level. Thus, work on this sen can be beneficial for arrythmias – especially if they are due to stress.

Work on the Itha & Pingkala Sen branches of the arms and hands is indicated for tendonitis and overuse disorders.

The therapist should be careful not to apply dynamic arm stretches to clients who have had shoulder dislocation and / or have loose shoulder ligaments or general instability of this area.

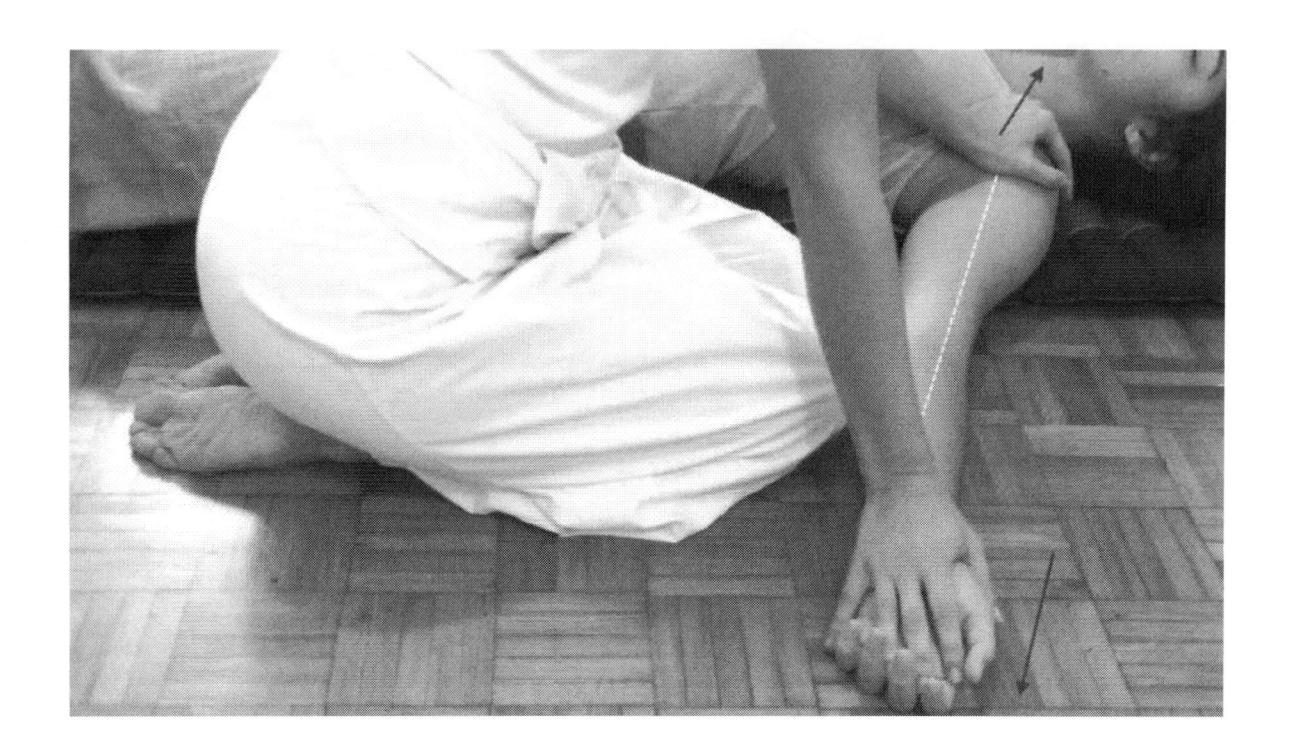

1. Work on the Kalatharee Sen, applying the 5 steps of Jap Sen: stretching, warming, pressing, and again warming and stretching.

In order to apply the stretch properly, place one palm above the receiver's wrist, and one on the receiver's shoulder. Apply the stretch as the receiver exhales.

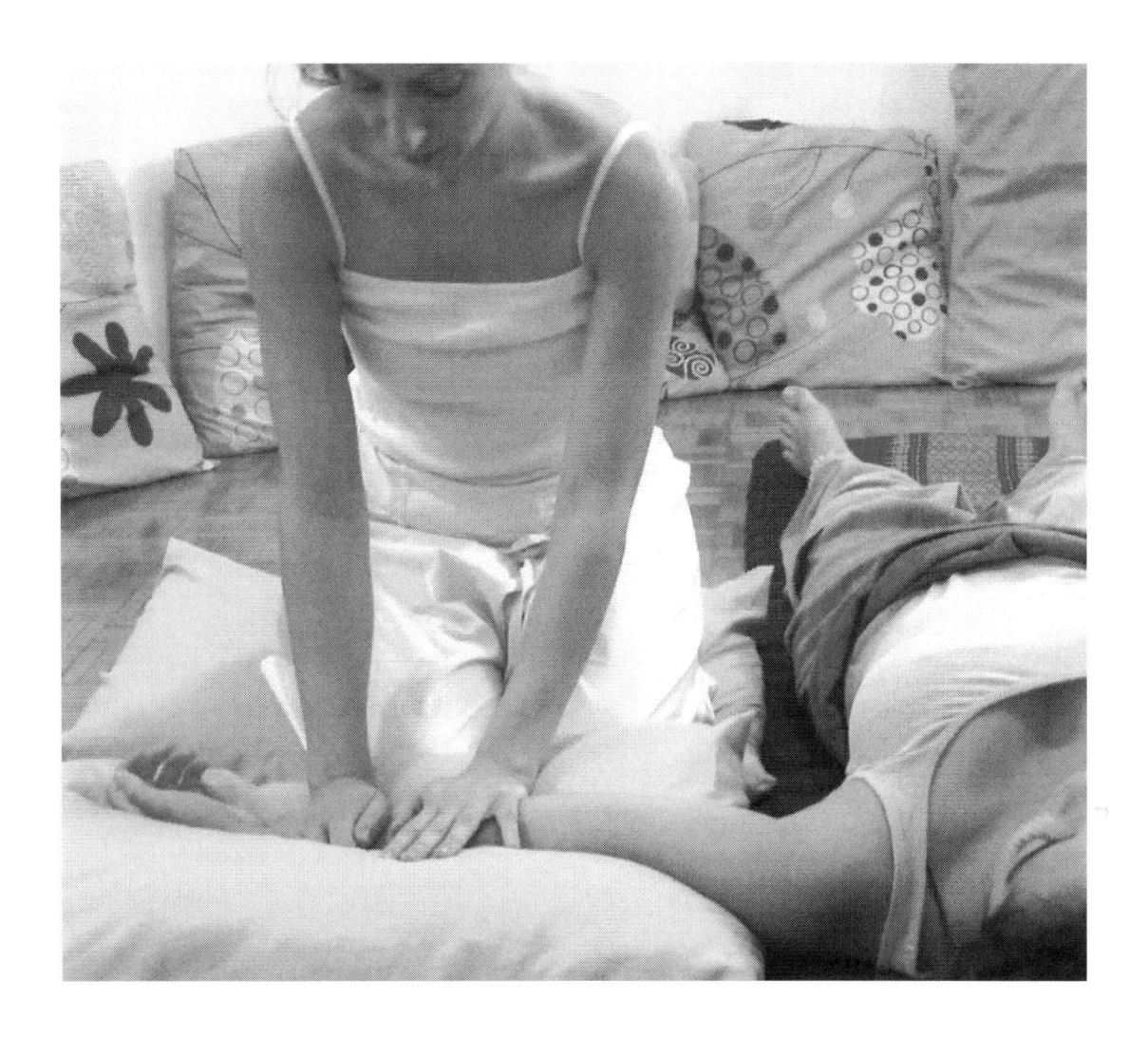

You can also place the receiver's arm on a pillow, for greater comfort.

Photo shows Step 2 & 4 of Jap Sen – that is, warming the meridians.

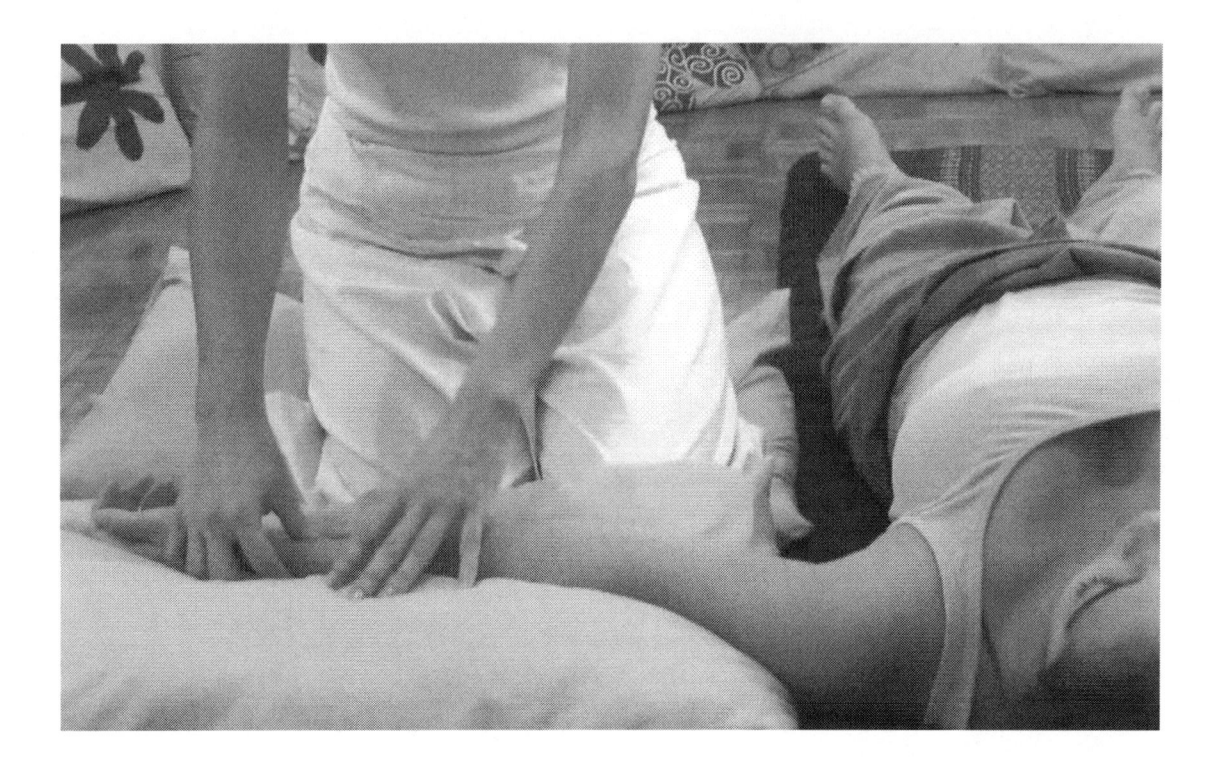

And here you have Step 3 – thumb walking on the meridians.

The therapist should always keep the arms straight, and not break the wrists, in order to prevent tendonitis.

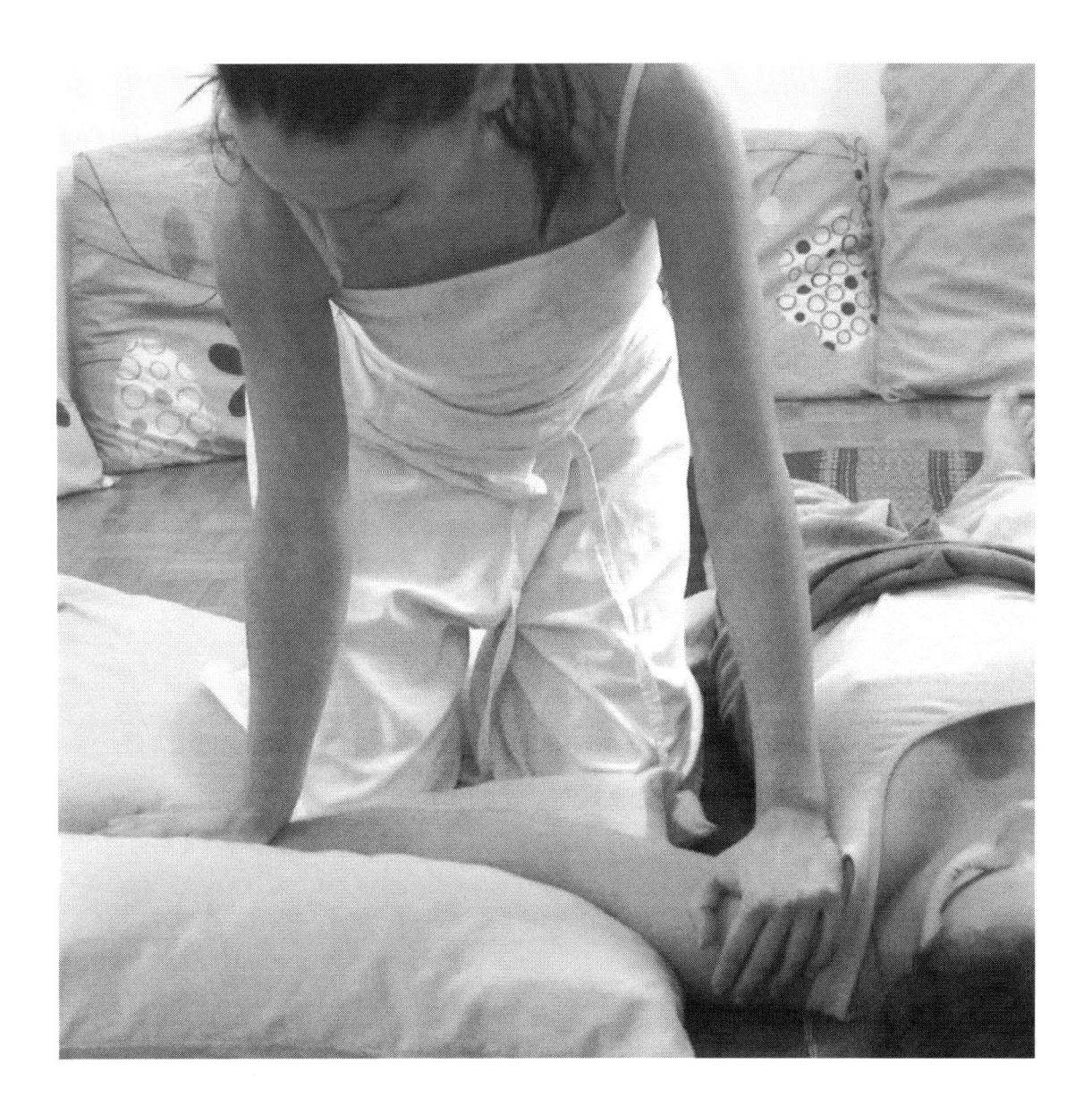

And this is a photo that shows Step 1 and 5 of Jap Sen (that is, stretching and opening the meridian), on the Itha & Pingkala Sen, and with the receiver's arm on a pillow.

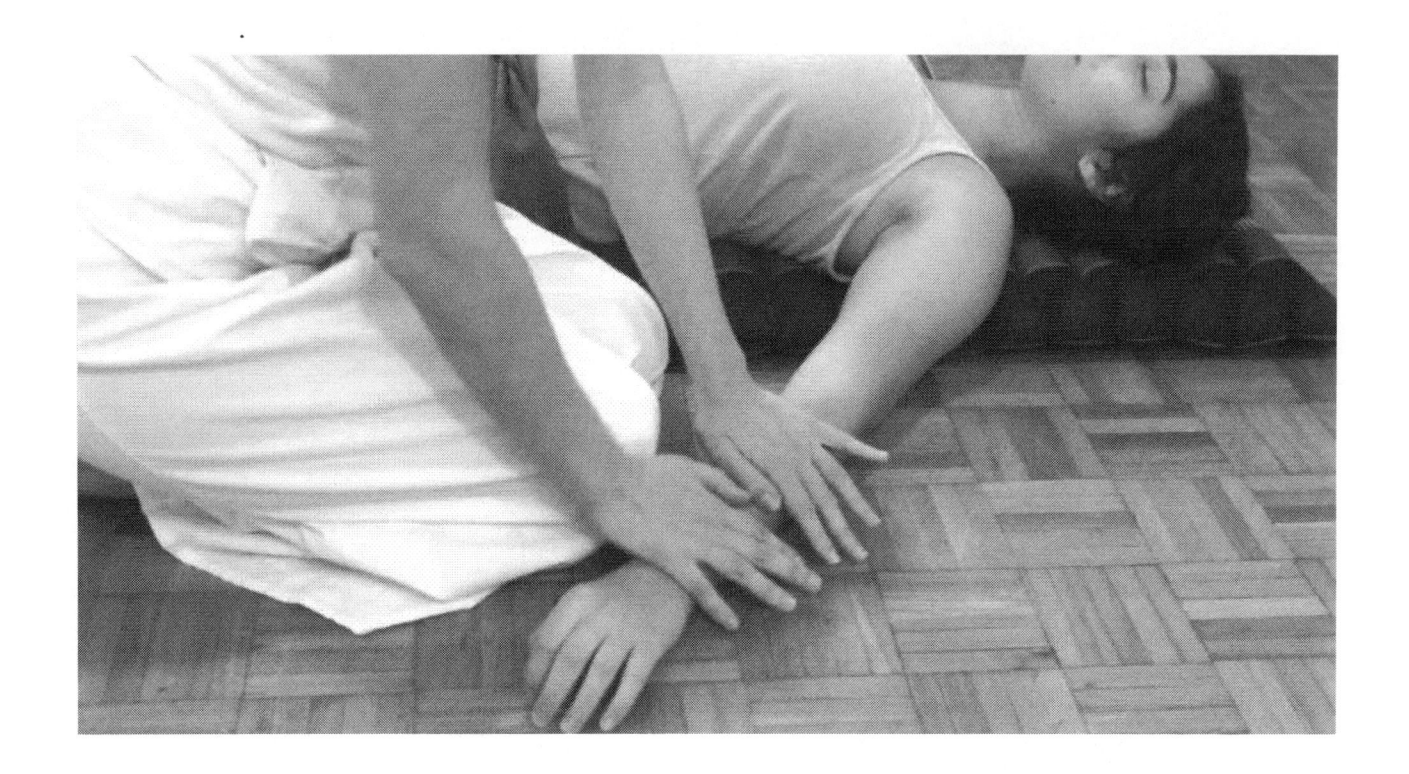

2. This is Step 2 (and / or 4) of 5 of Jap Sen: Palm walking on the meridians.

You can also roll and shake the arm – this will relax tensions in the arm and shoulder area.

Always skip the elbow.

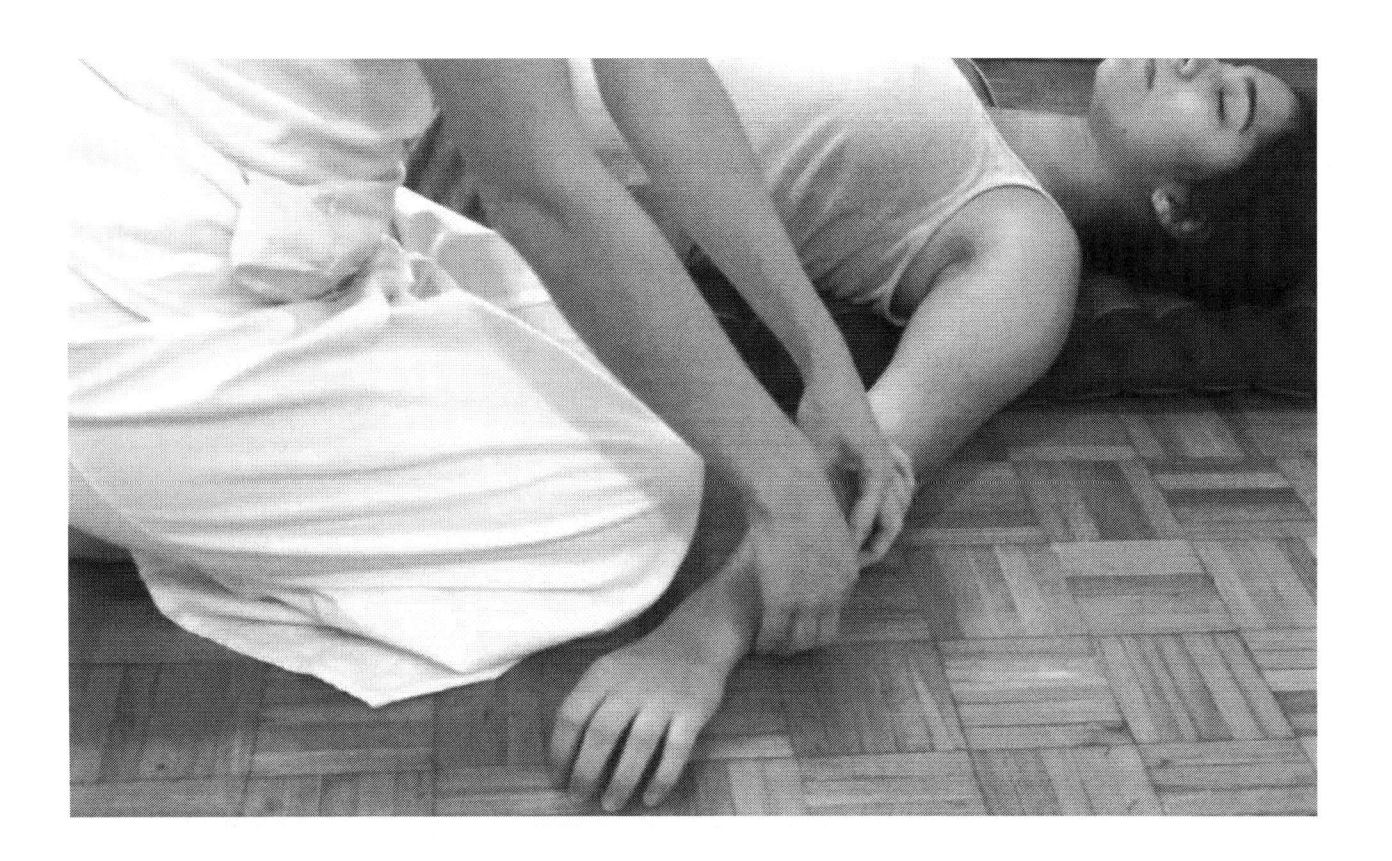

3. This is Step 3 of 5 – thumb walking. Work your way up to the shoulder, on the Itha – Pingkala Sen, and then return to the hand.

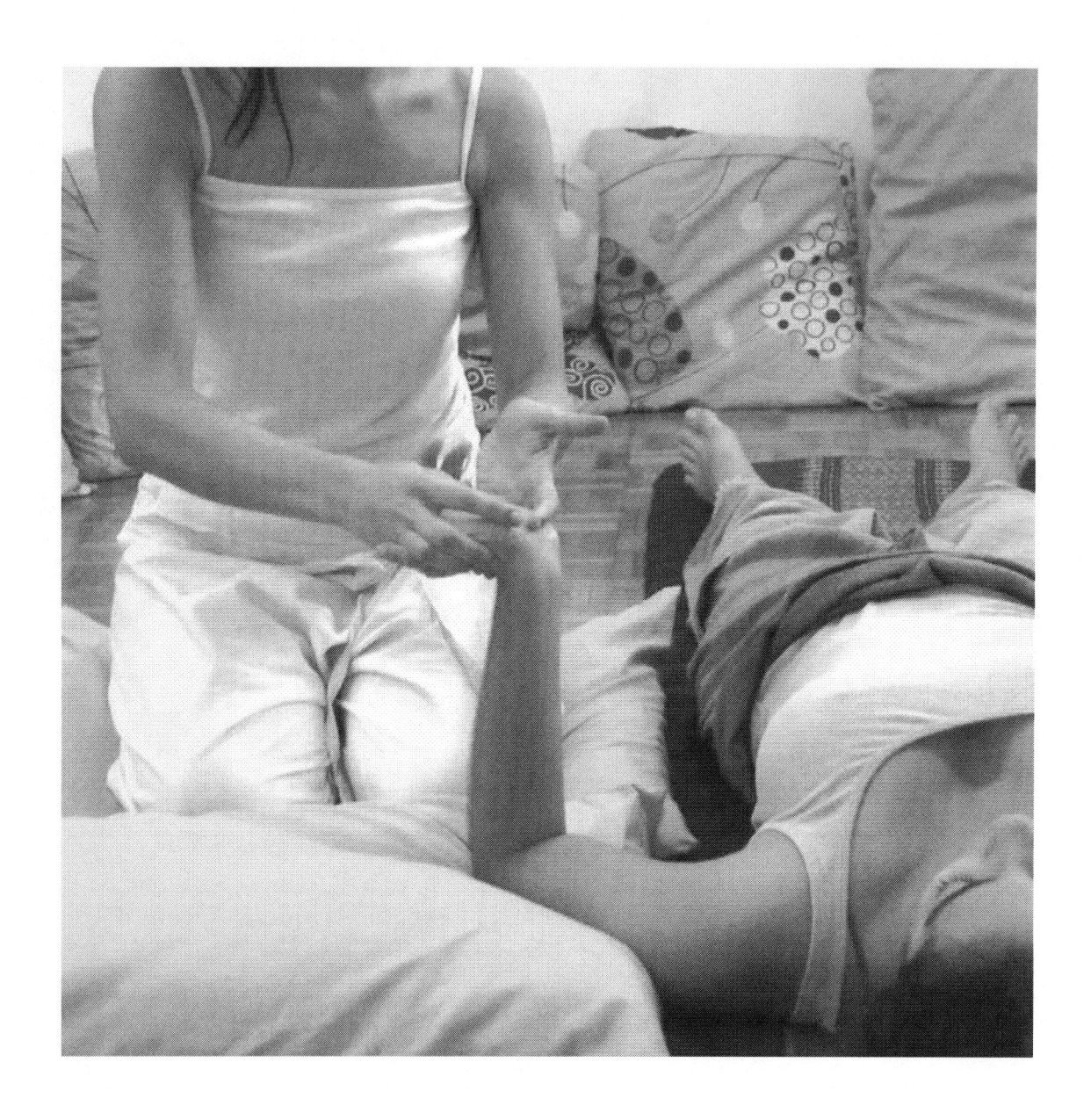

4. Lift the hand and place your small fingers next to the receiver's thumb and small finger, and stretch her palm. From this lock, you can also massage the palm.

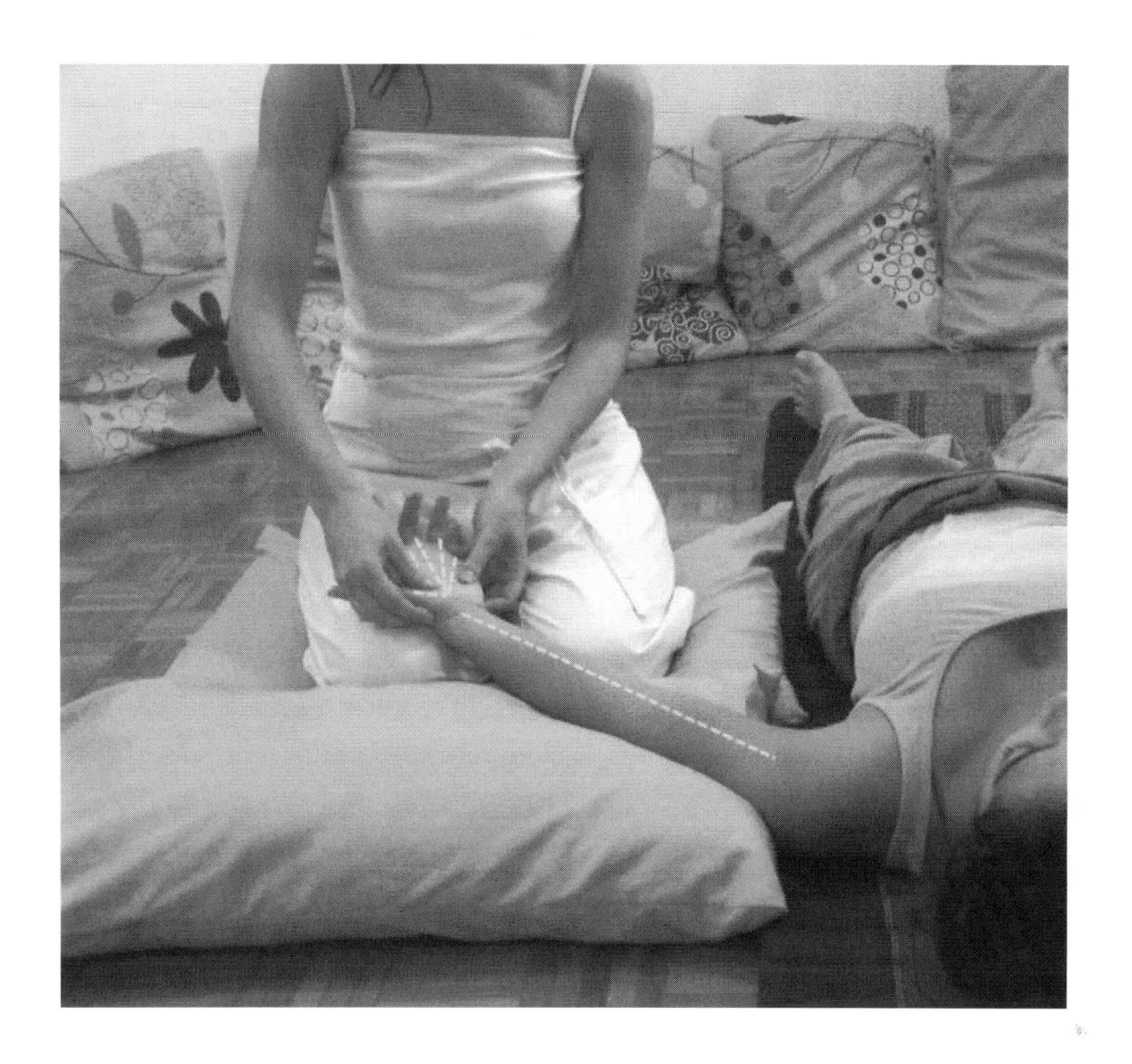

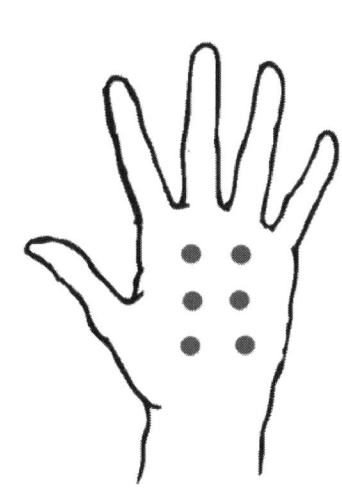

5. Then place the receiver's palm on your thigh, and press the Kalatharee line . You can also press 6 points on the palm (similar to the 6 points of the foot).

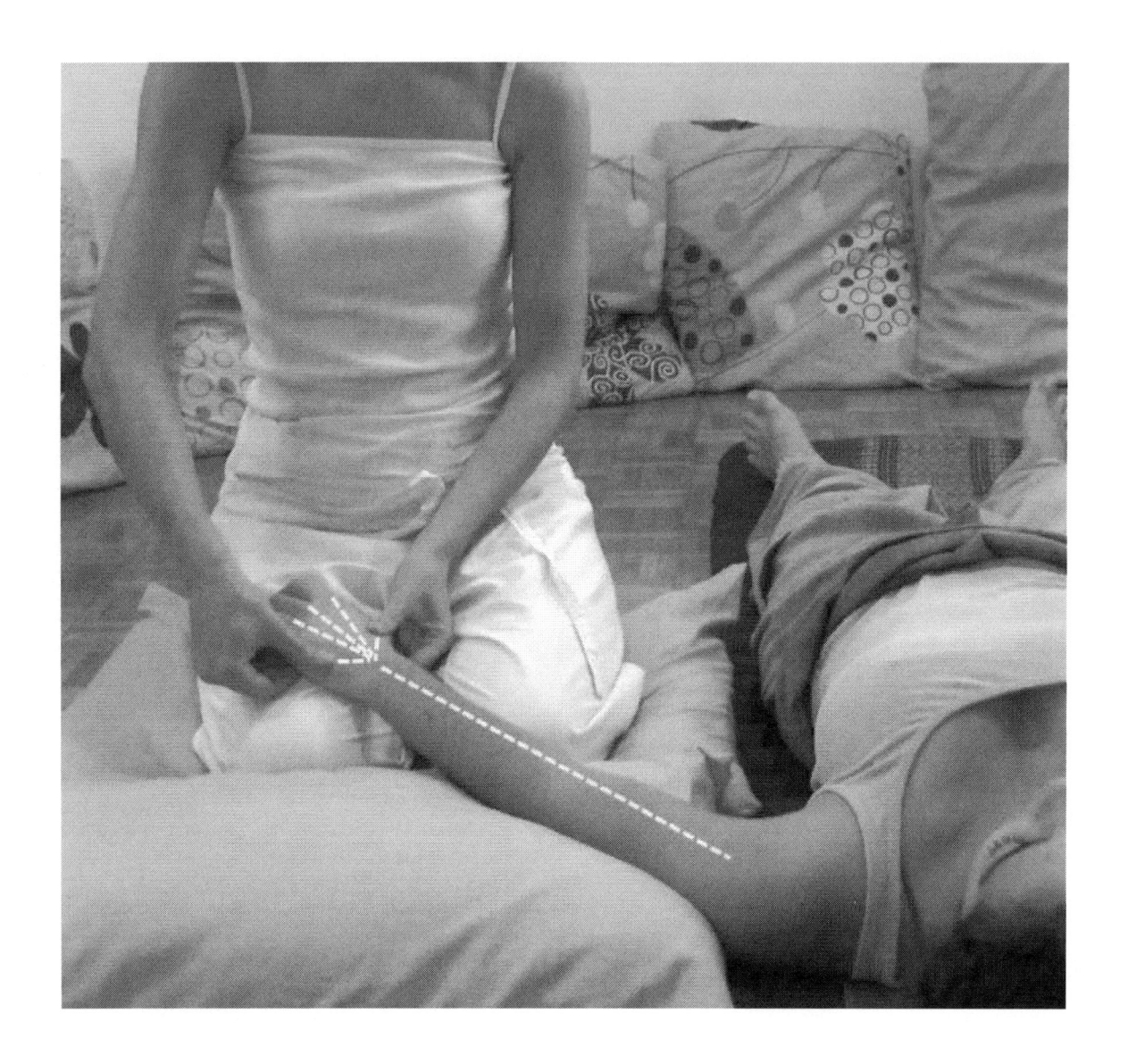

6. Turn the hand, in order to work on the Itha & Pingkala Sen lines on the dorsal aspect of the hand. Do not press – just rub gently the lines.

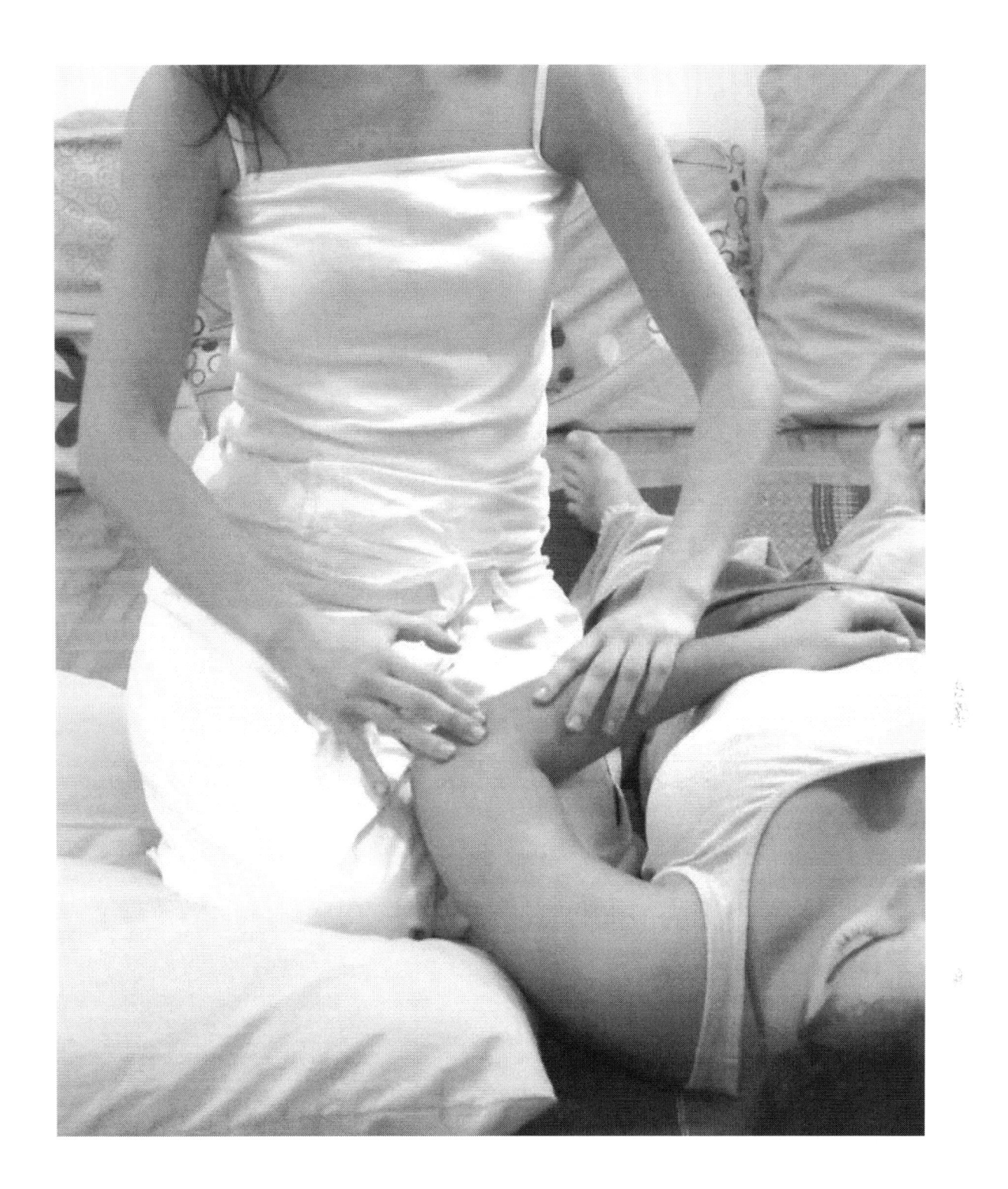

7. Place the receiver's elbow on your thigh, and massage the joint gently.

If the receiver suffers from tennis elbow, you can apply heat rubs and / or herbal compresses.

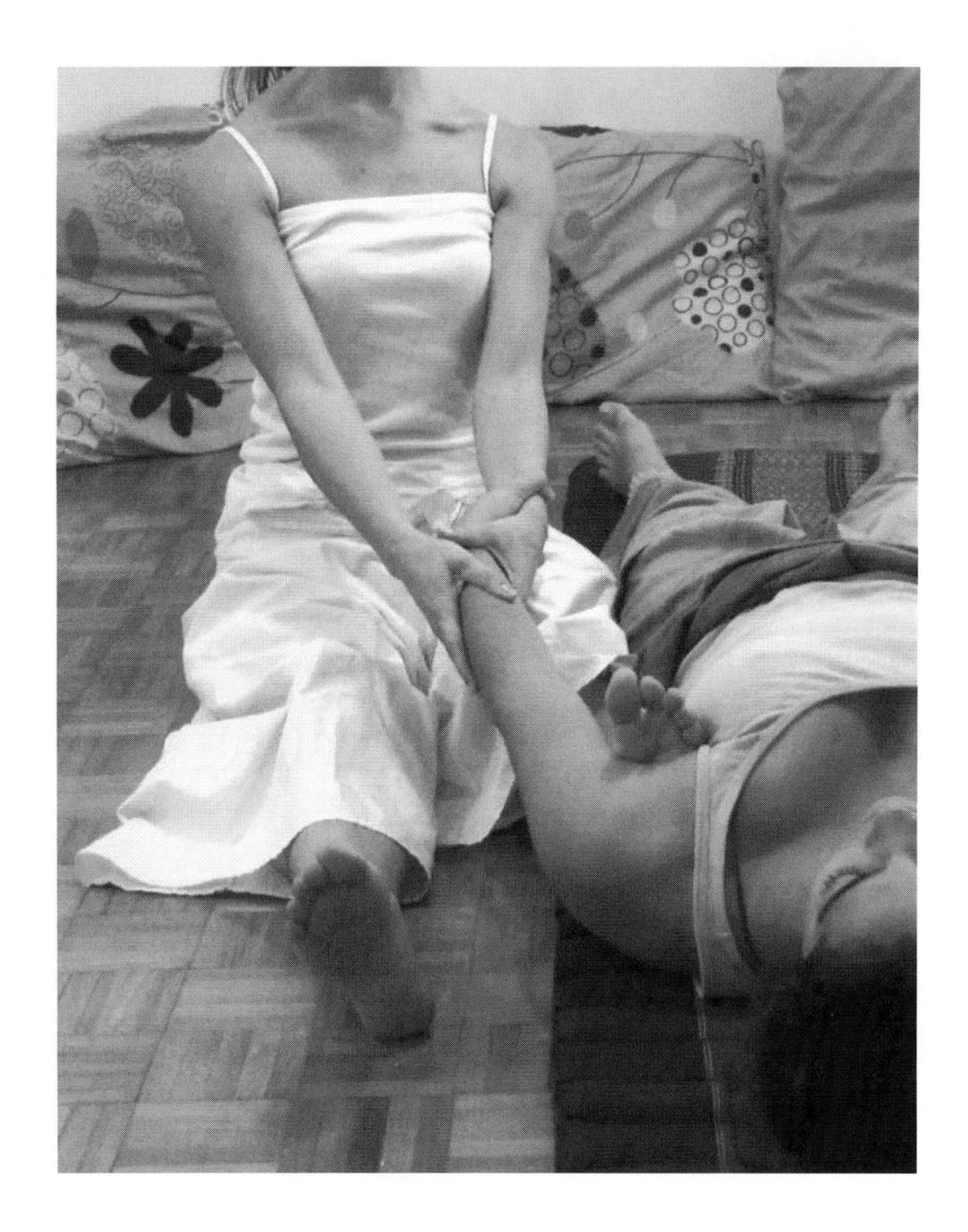

8. Place your foot on the receiver's armpit. Grasp her arm, and stretch it as she exhales.

Do not apply pressure on the armpit.

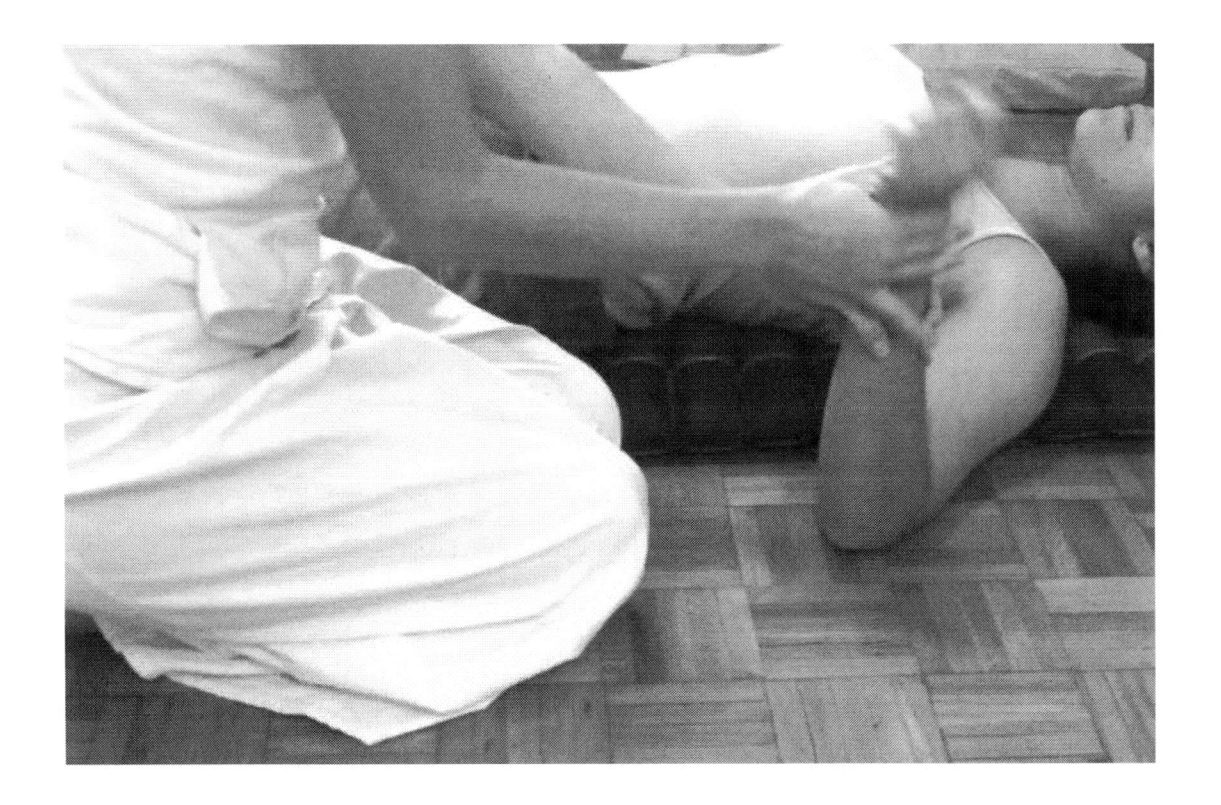

9. Grasp the receiver's wrist and shake it.

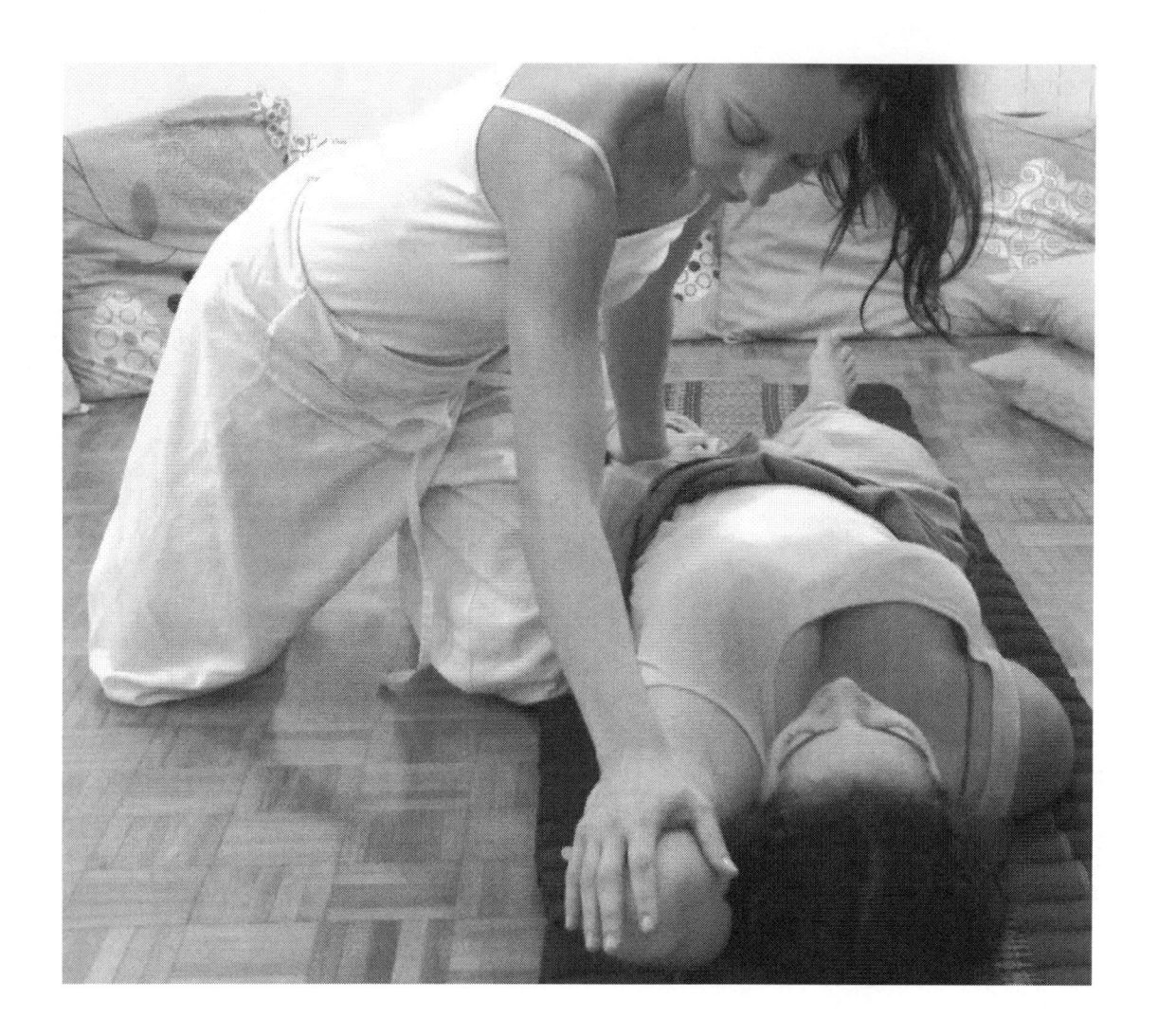

10. Bend the receiver's arm, with her fingers facing her shoulder. Place one hand on the quadriceps muscle, and one hand on the receiver's elbow, and stretch the triceps muscle and the torso, as she exhales.

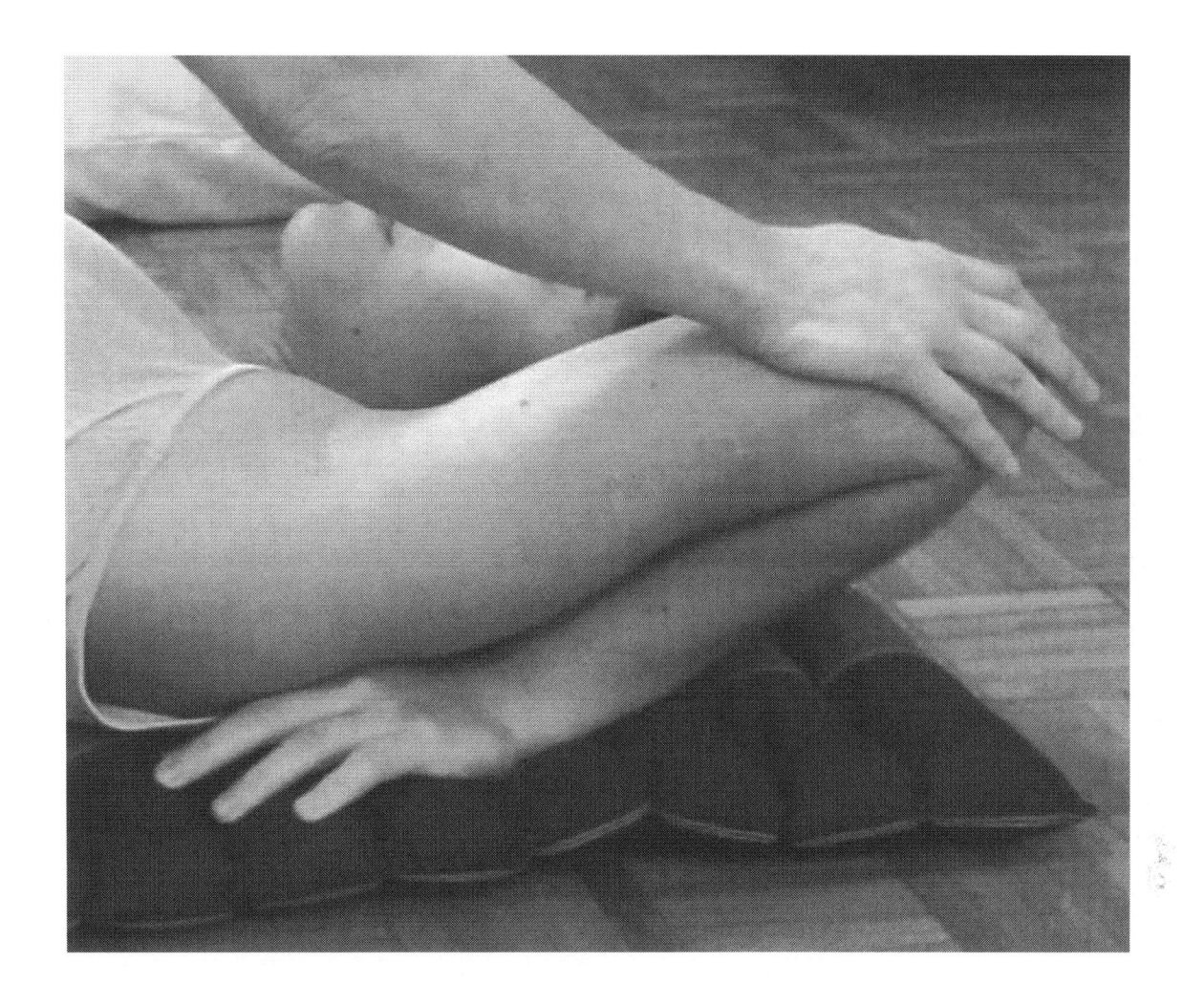

This is how you should grasp the elbow joint. Place the center of your palm on the joint, and push the elbow in a direction parallel to the floor. Never push the elbow downwards.

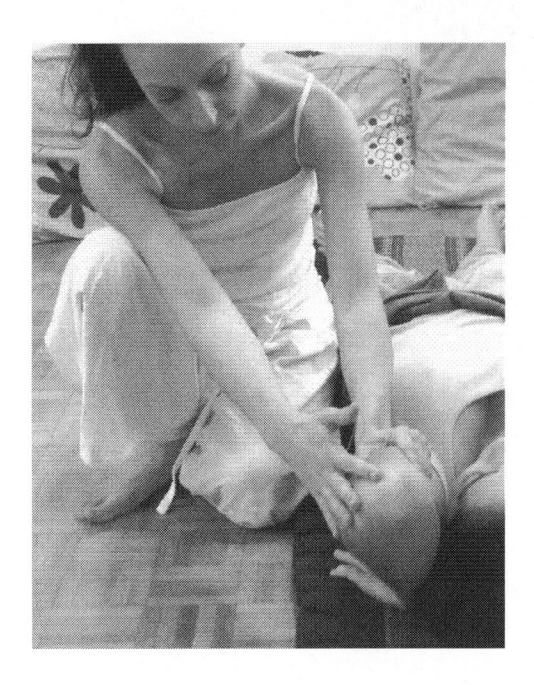

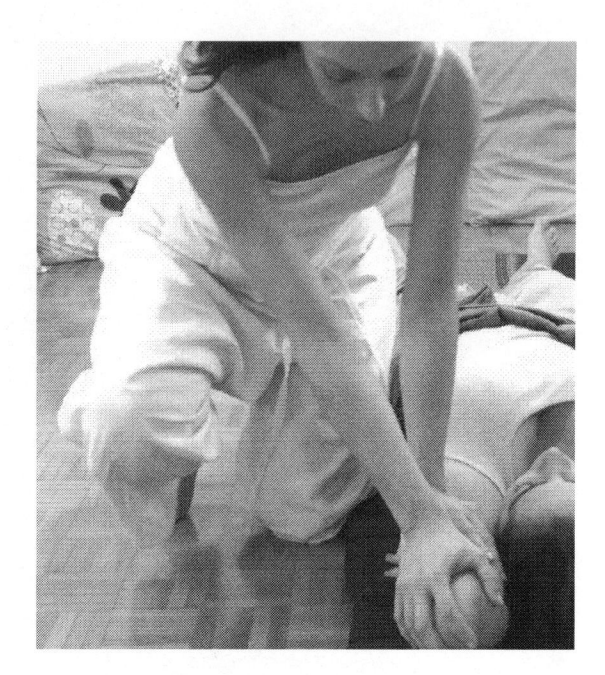

11. In this position, you can also work on the triceps muscle. You can massage the muscle, and even apply myofascial release techniques.

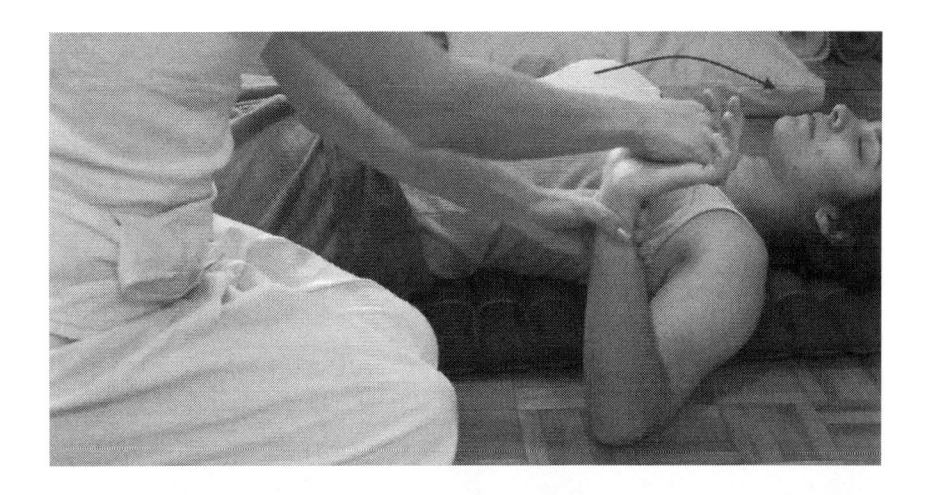

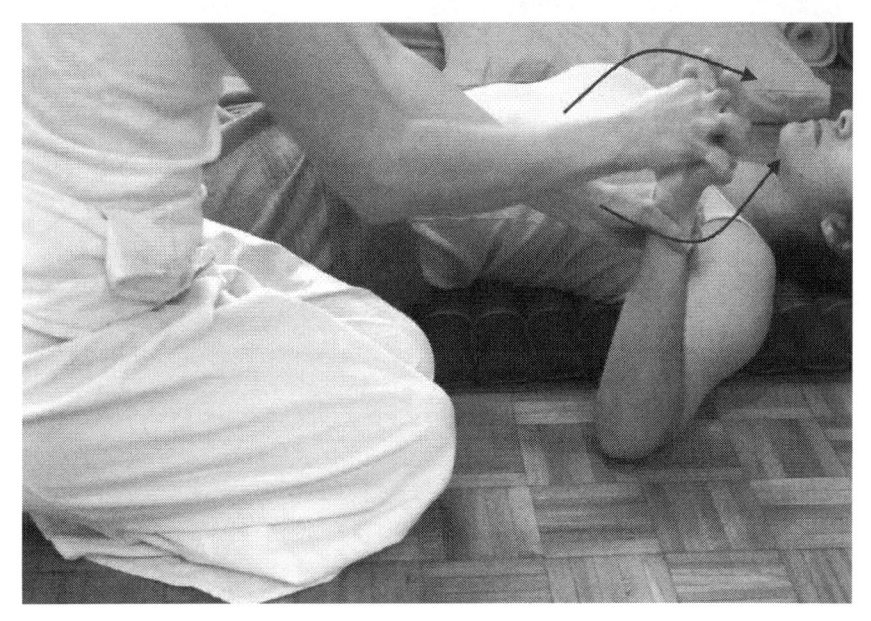

12. Grasp the receiver's hand by interlocking your fingers in theirs. Stretch the hand and rotate the wrist joint.

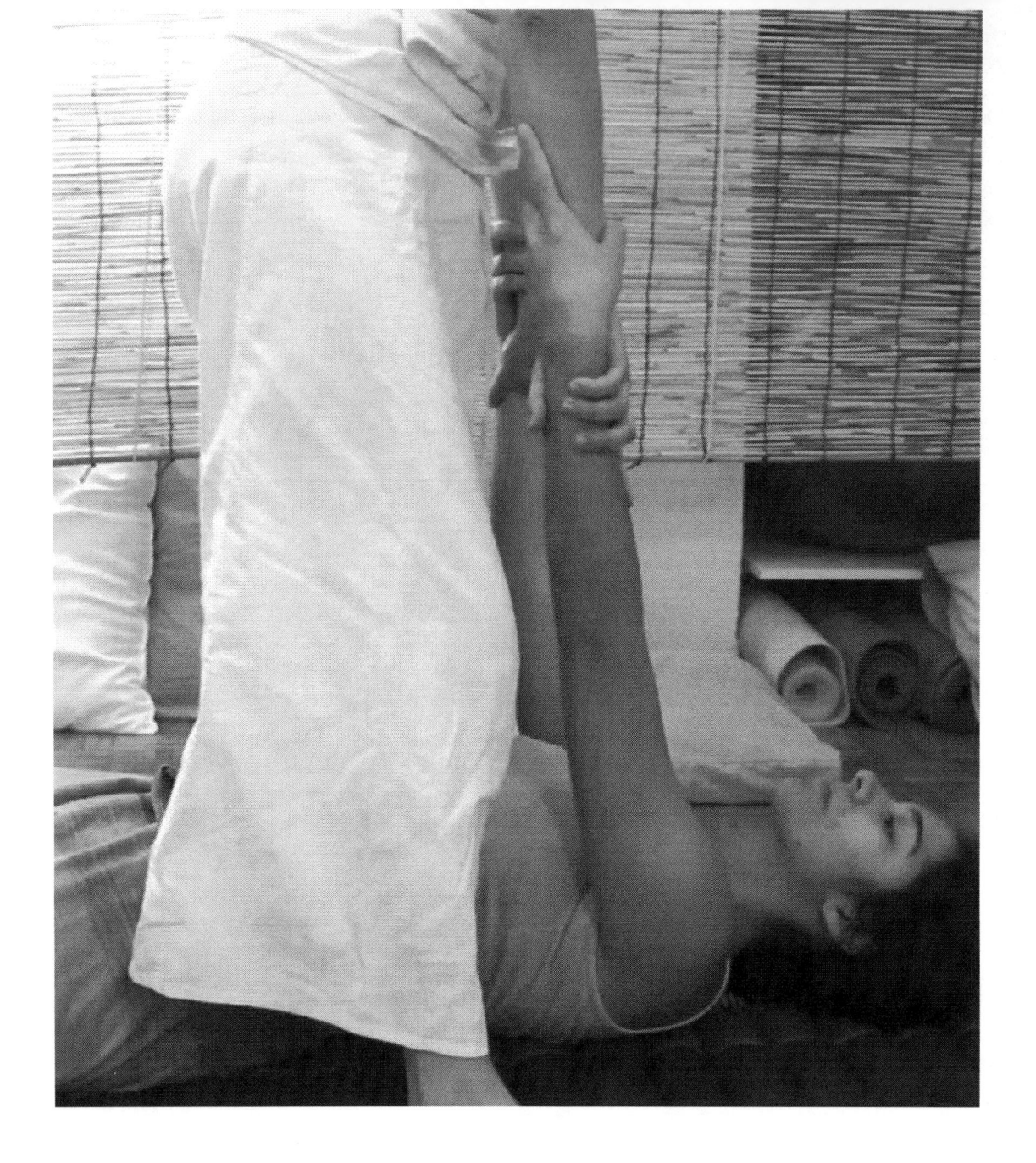

13. Then stand above the receiver, and grasp her arms. Lift her arms alternatively. When you place one arm on the ground, let the receiver rest for 2-3 seconds, before lifting her other arm.

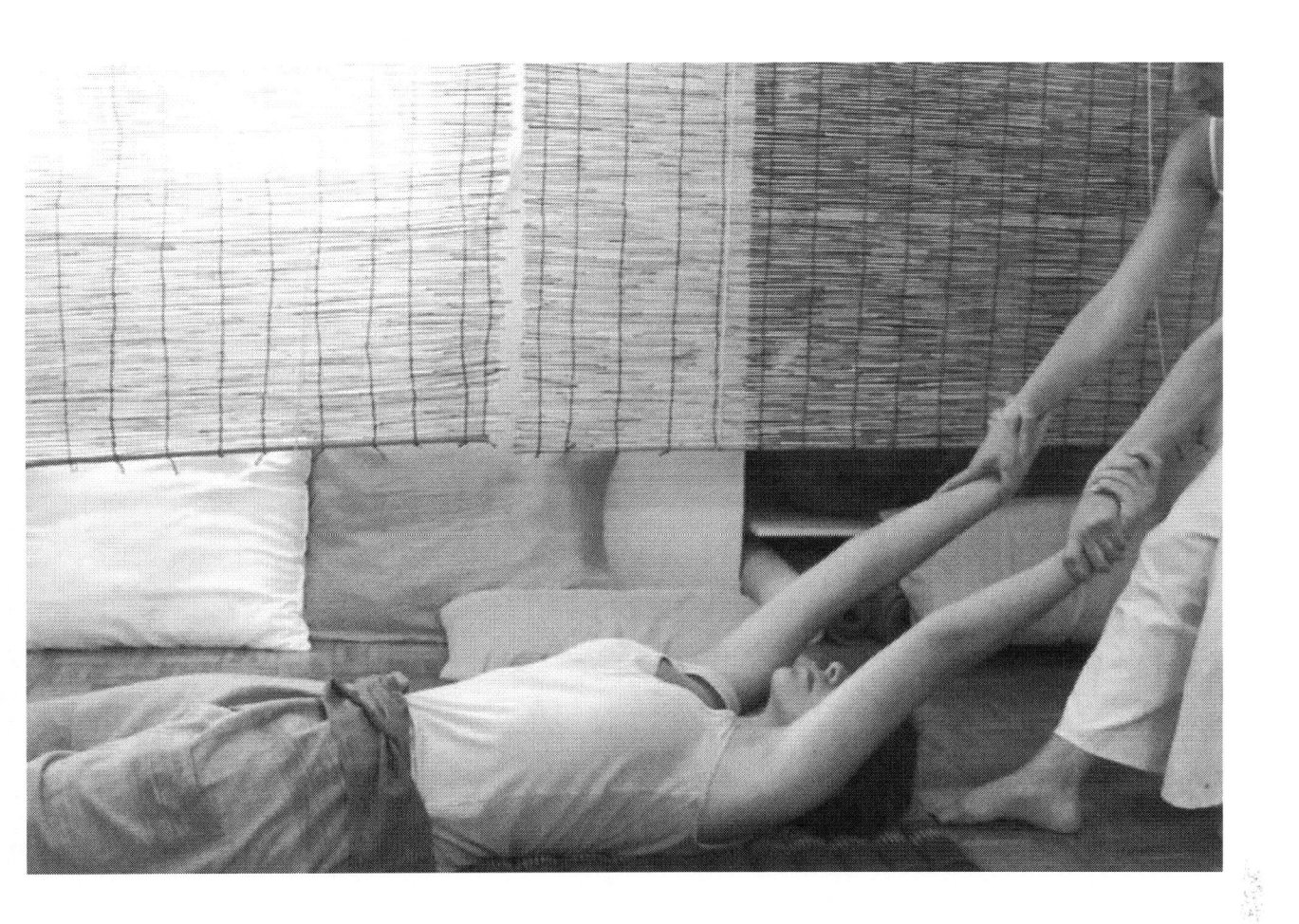

14. Then grasp the receiver's arms behind her head, and pull them in order to stretch the torso, as she exhales.

This is an excellent technique for kyphosis, breathing problems and neck / shoulder pain due to shortened muscles.

what lies underneath

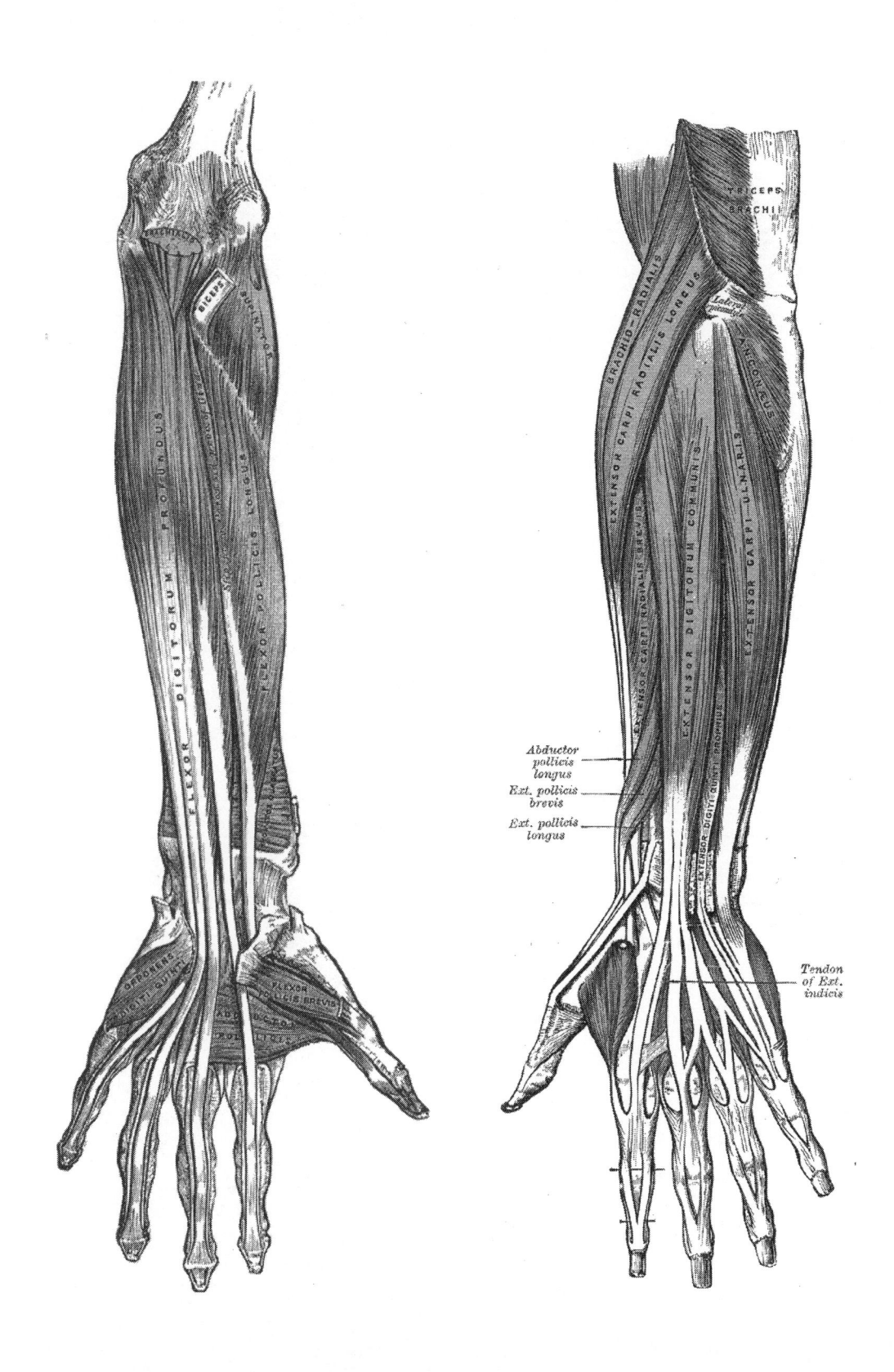

Forearm muscles

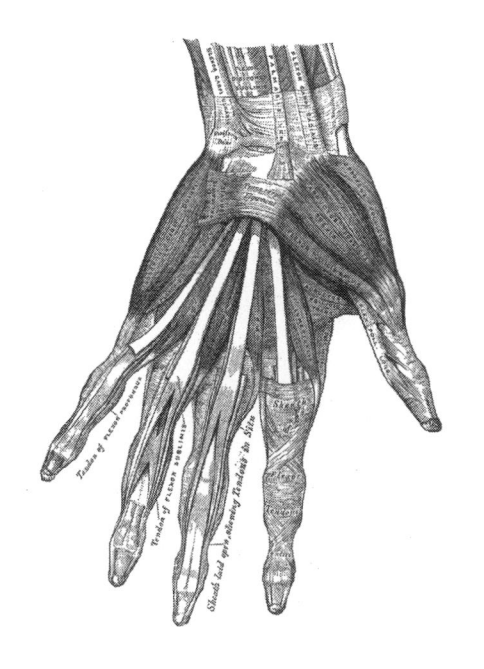

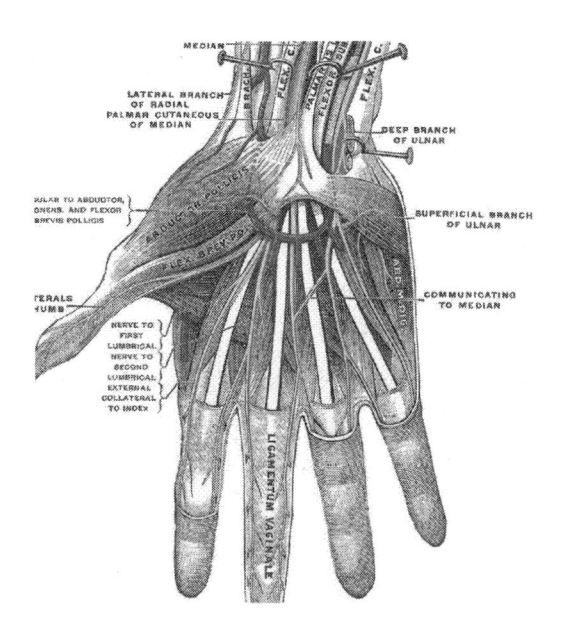

Hand muscles

Hand nerves

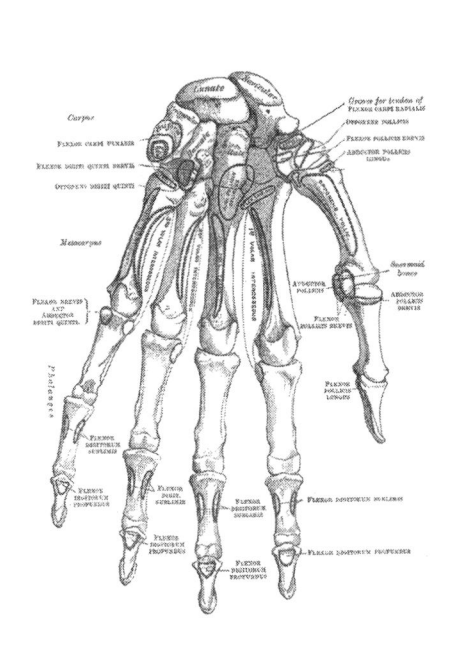

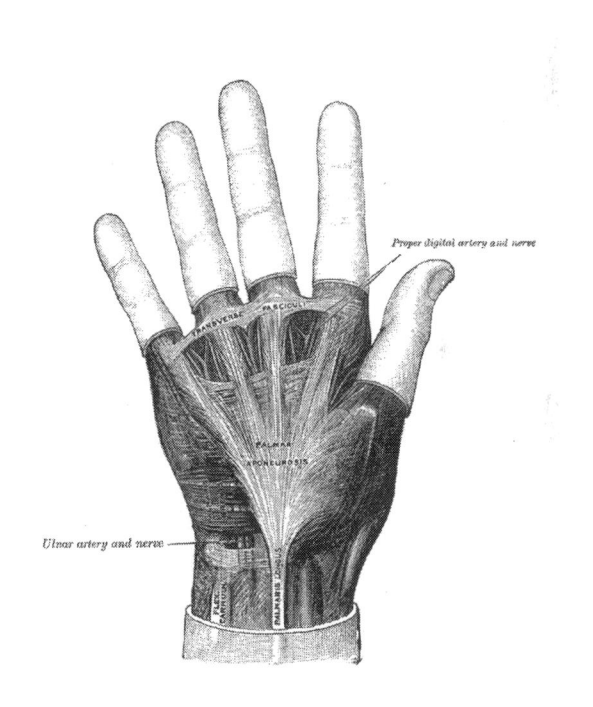

Bones of the hand

The palmar aponeurosis

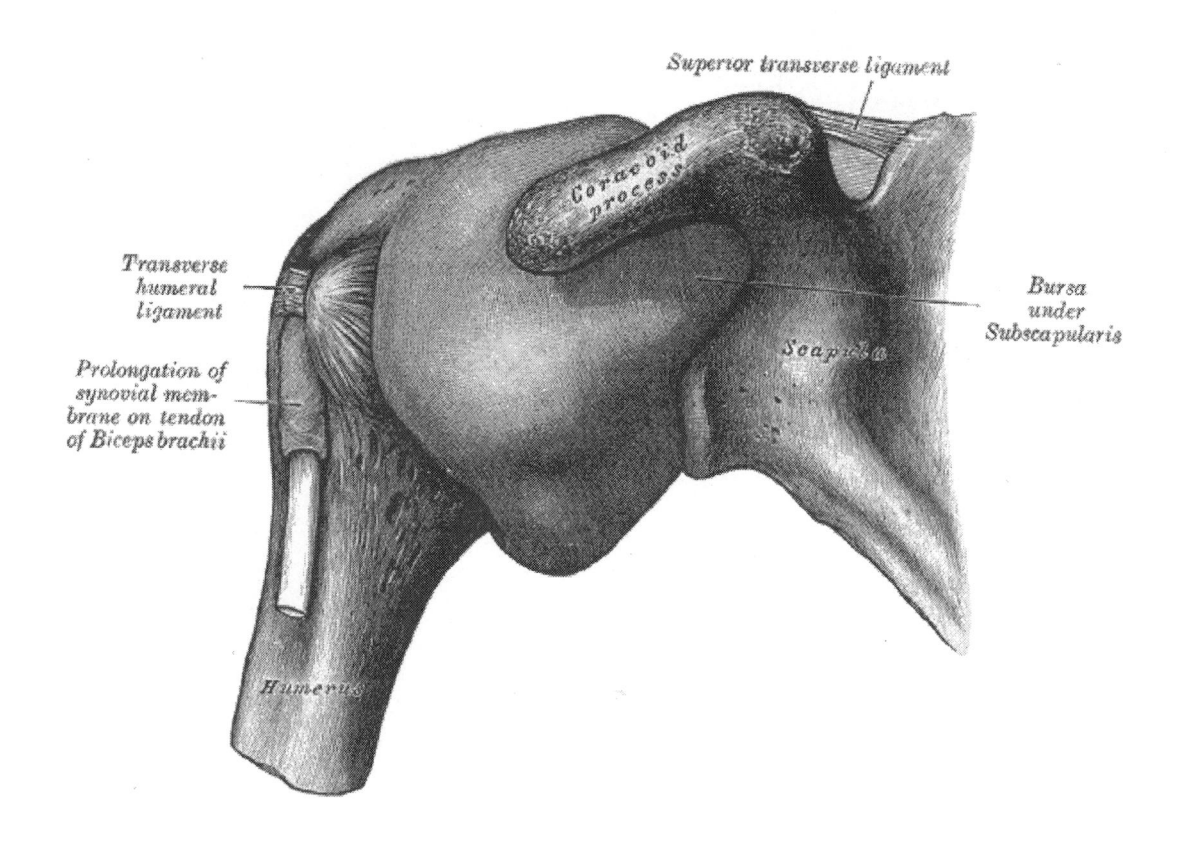

Shoulder joint

side position

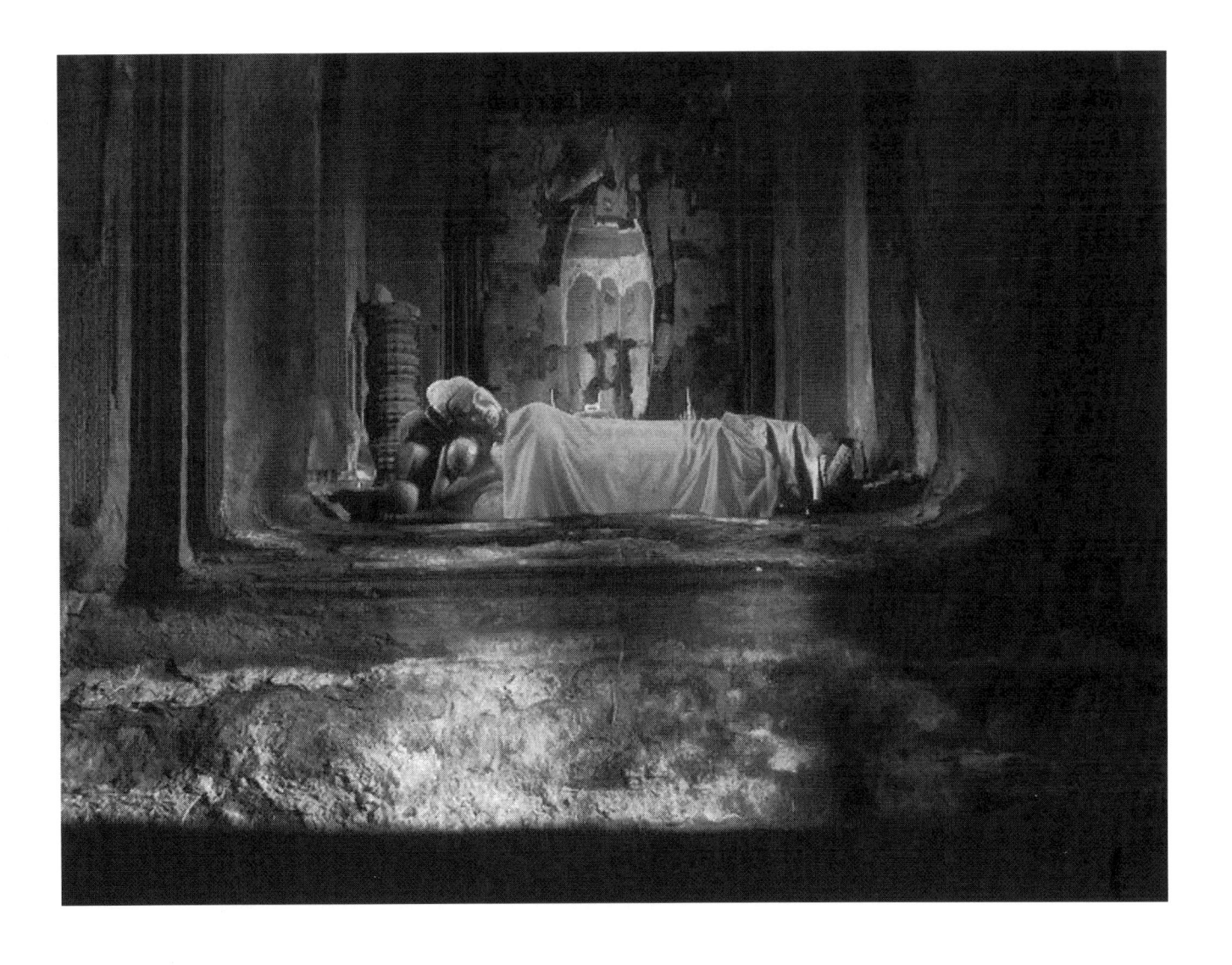

The side position is perhaps the most important position of Thai Massage, as it gives us the opportunity to work on the whole body. Actually, a Thai Massage session can be comprised solely by the side position. Moreover, it is a very comfortable position for the receiver, especially for people with lower back problems, as it respects all the spinal curves.

You will need 4 pillows – one for your own knees, and 3 for the receiver. Specifically, one should be placed under her knee, one under her arm, and one under her head, for proper support (see next page).

The side position is also ideal for pregnant women.

Any technique applied to the one side of the body, should be applied on the other side too. The therapist should also be very cautious when performing back bends to clients with degenerated discs and / or spinal stenosis.

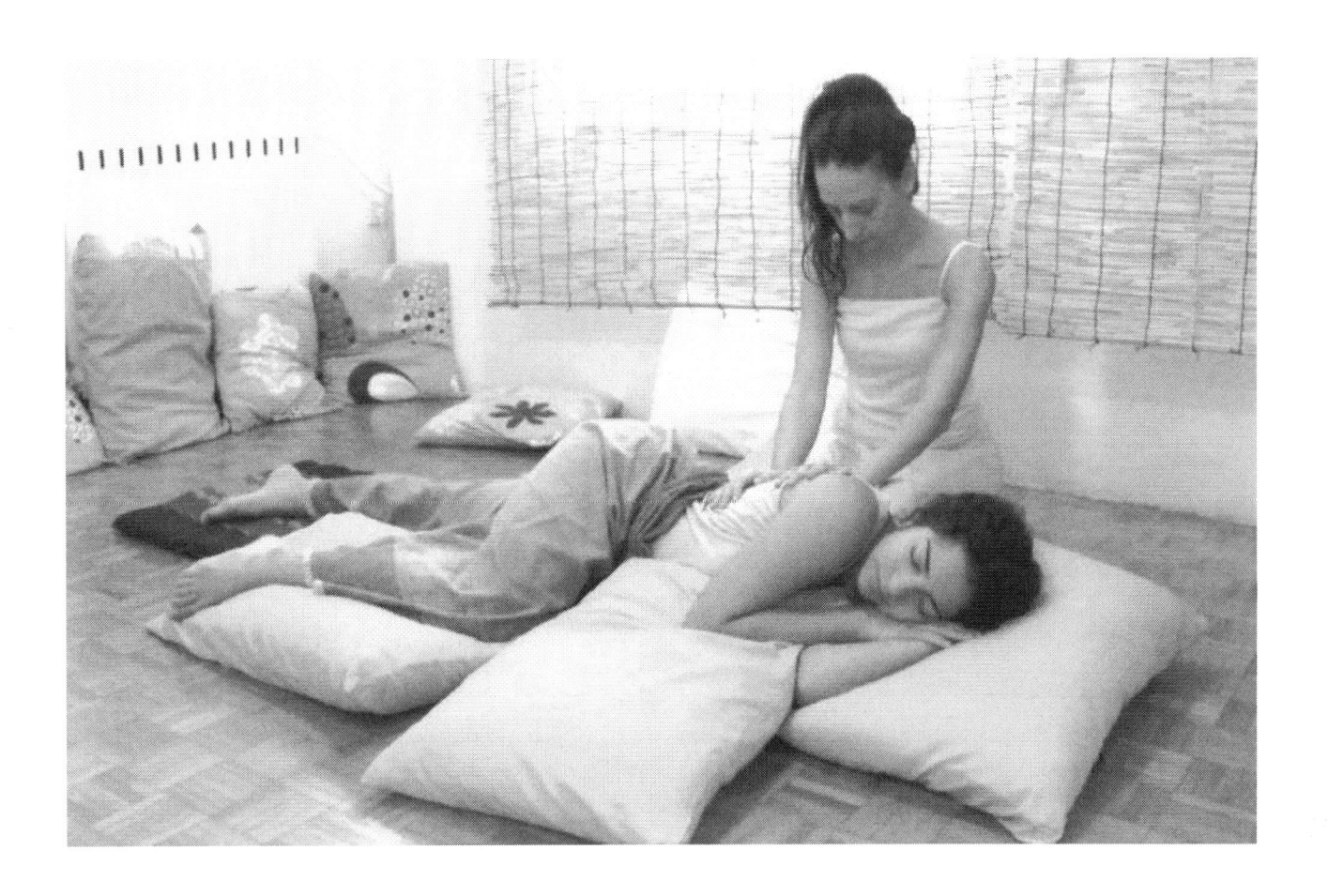

This is the proper setting for the side position, and the placement of pillows.

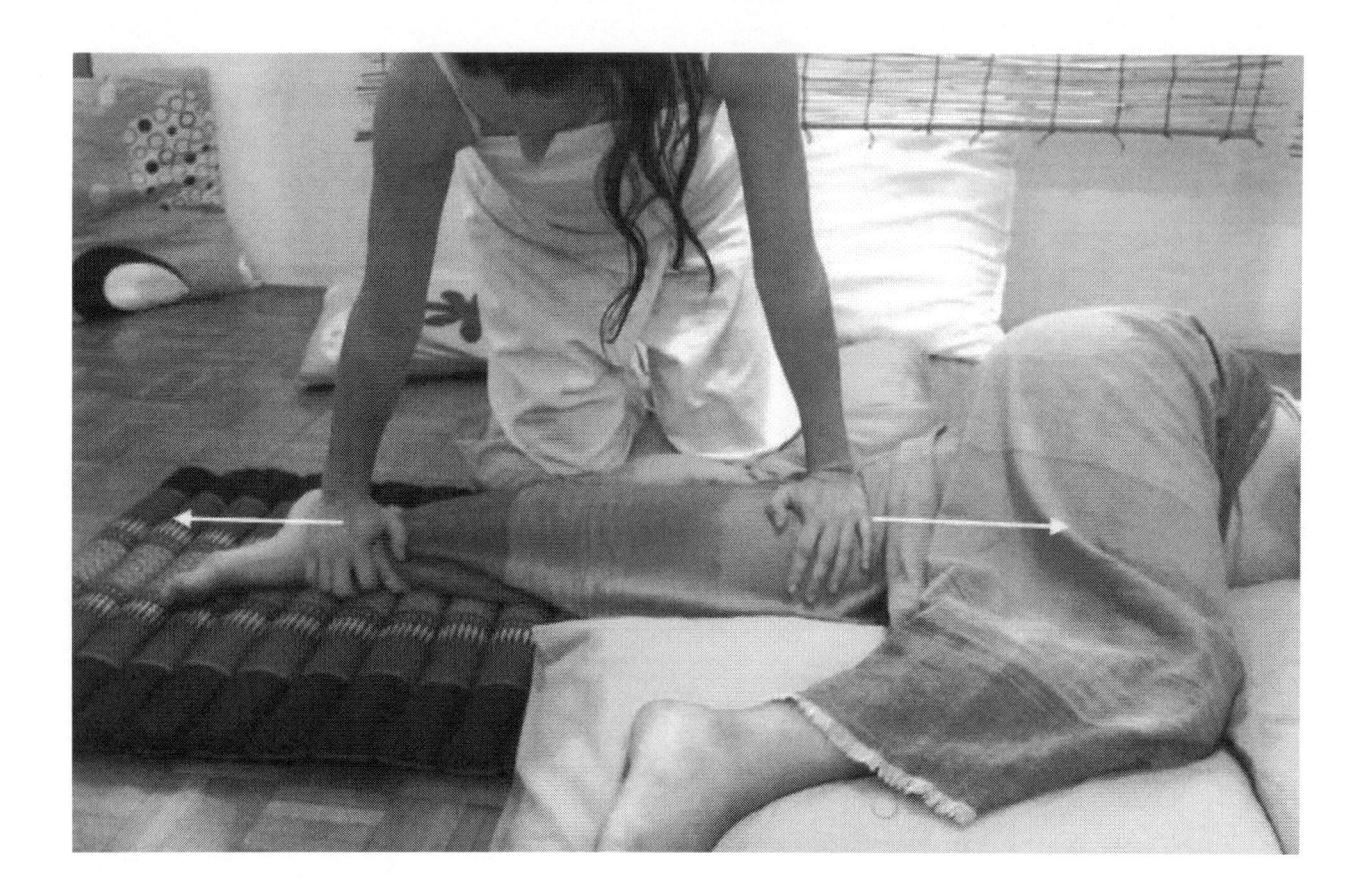

1. Begin by working on the *Kalatharee Sen* on the inner side of the leg. You can also work on the Sahatsarangsi and Tawaree lines.

The photo shows Step 1, that is stretching (opening) the meridian.

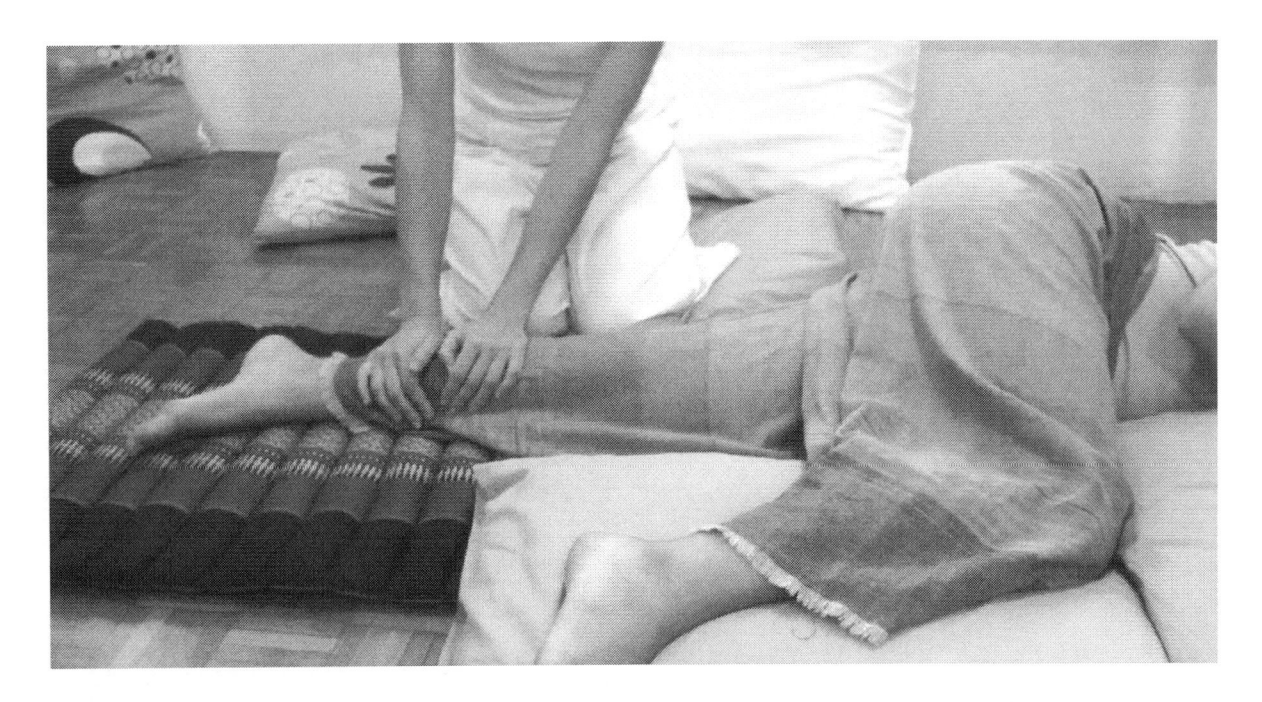

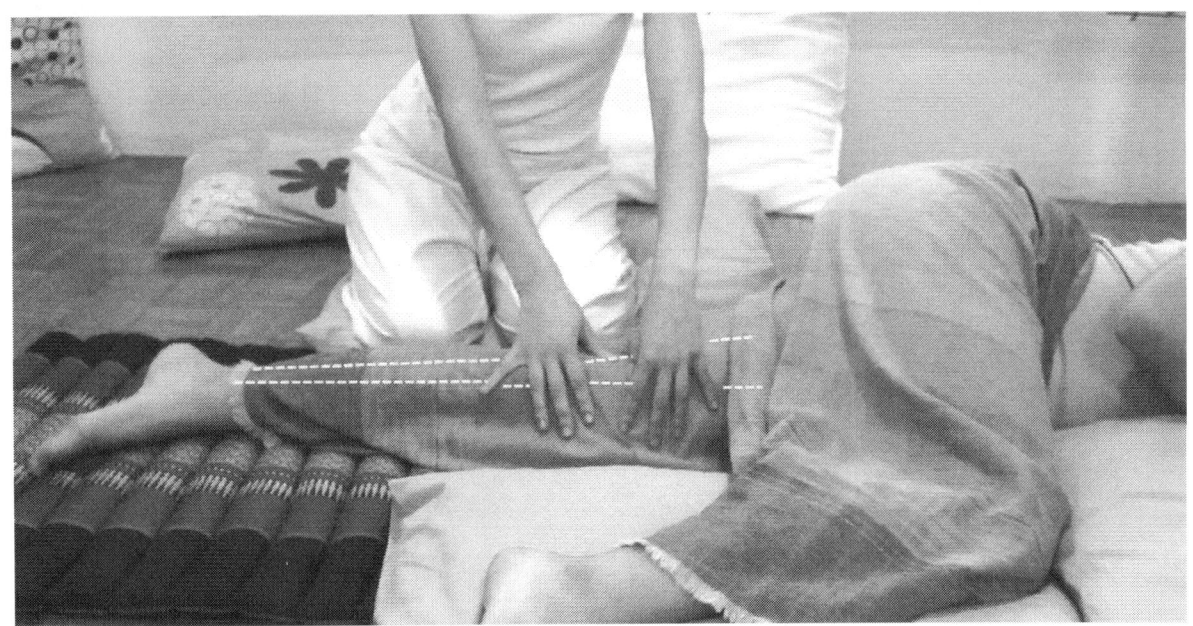

These photos show the palm walking (Steps 2 and 4) and thumb walking techniques of Jap Sen.

It is always a good idea to do Jap Sen before applying any other technique, as this warms the muscles and ensures the safe performance of the following techniques.

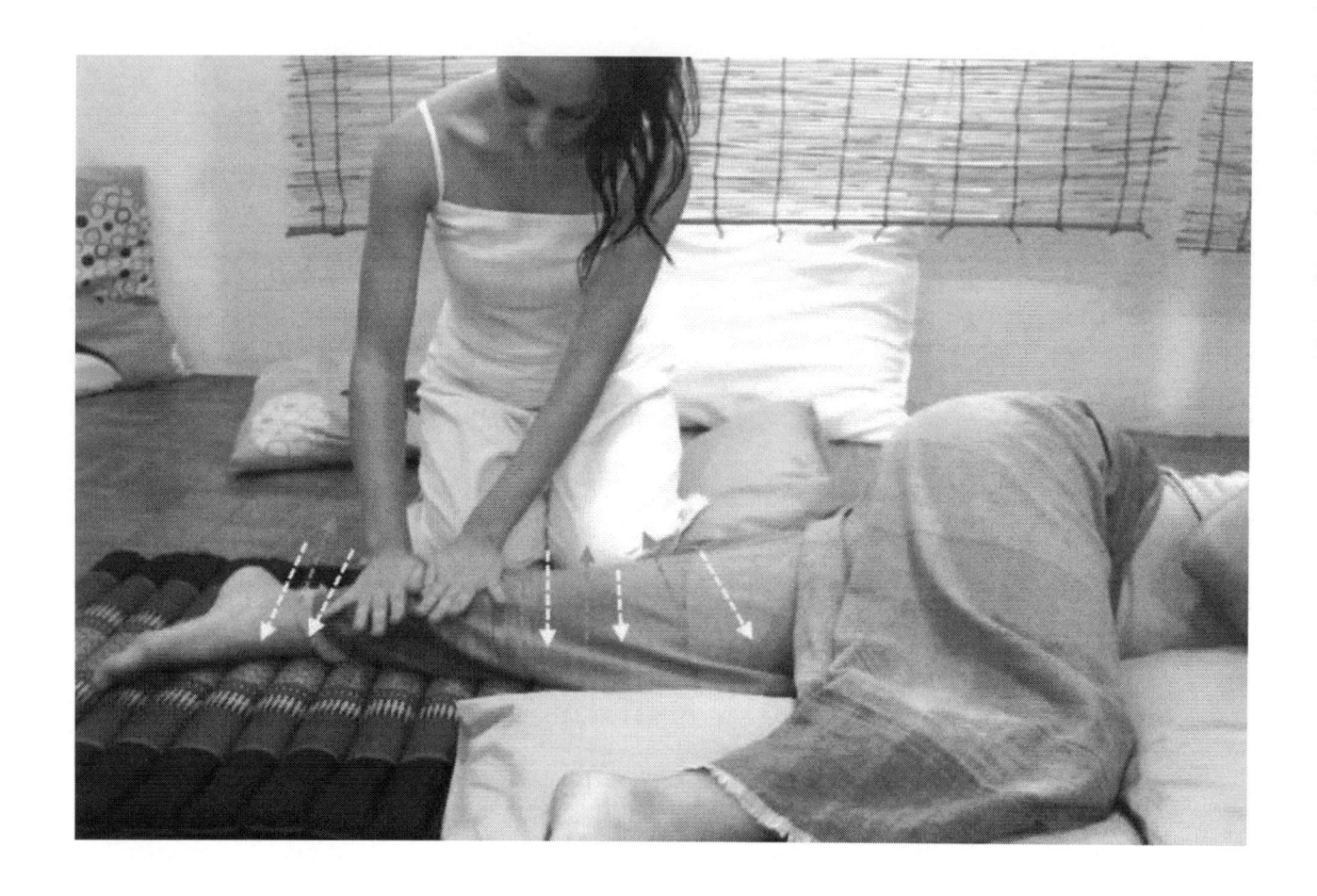

2. Then rock the receiver's leg with your hands.

Start from the lower leg, and continue to the thigh. As always, skip the knee.

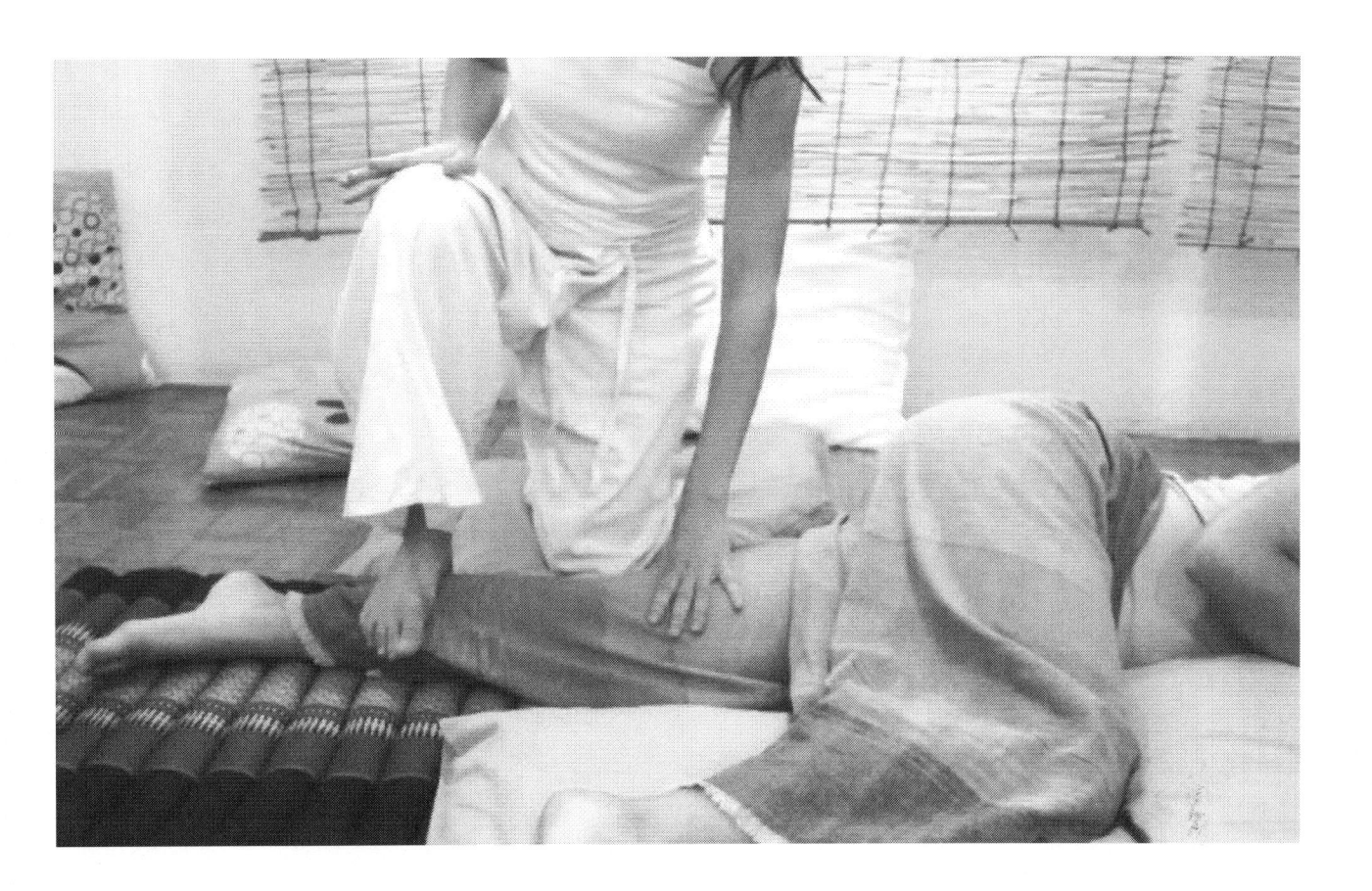

3. ... and press the leg with the transverse arch of your foot. You can also roll the leg with your foot, instead of your hand, if you so wish.

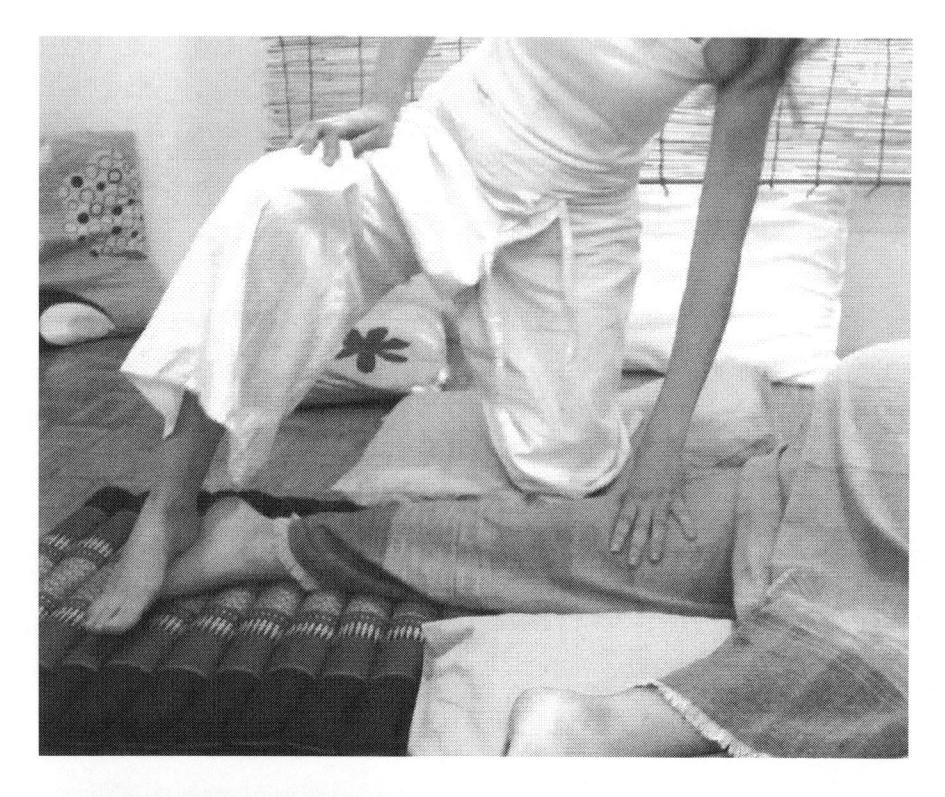

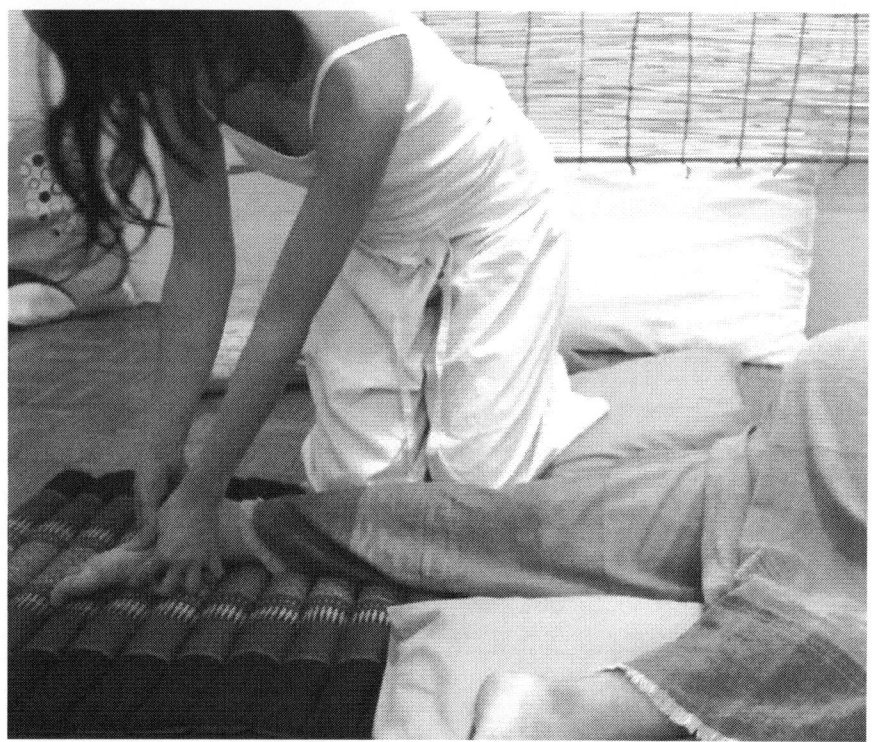

4. Then press the receiver's foot with your foot, and then with your thumbs.

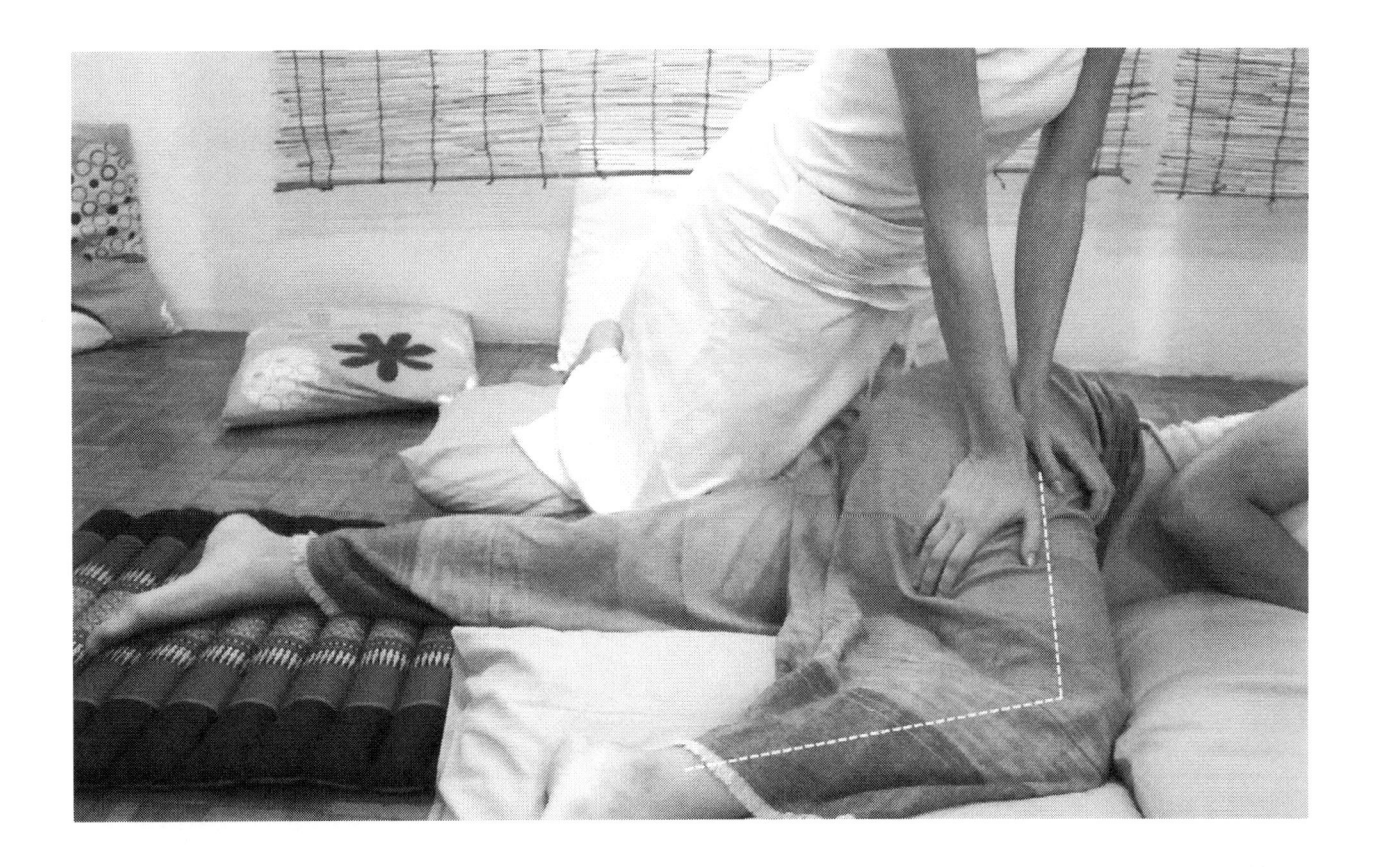

5. Now work on the 3rd outer line of the leg – that's *Itha & Pingkala Sen*. Do "butterfly presses" with your palms.

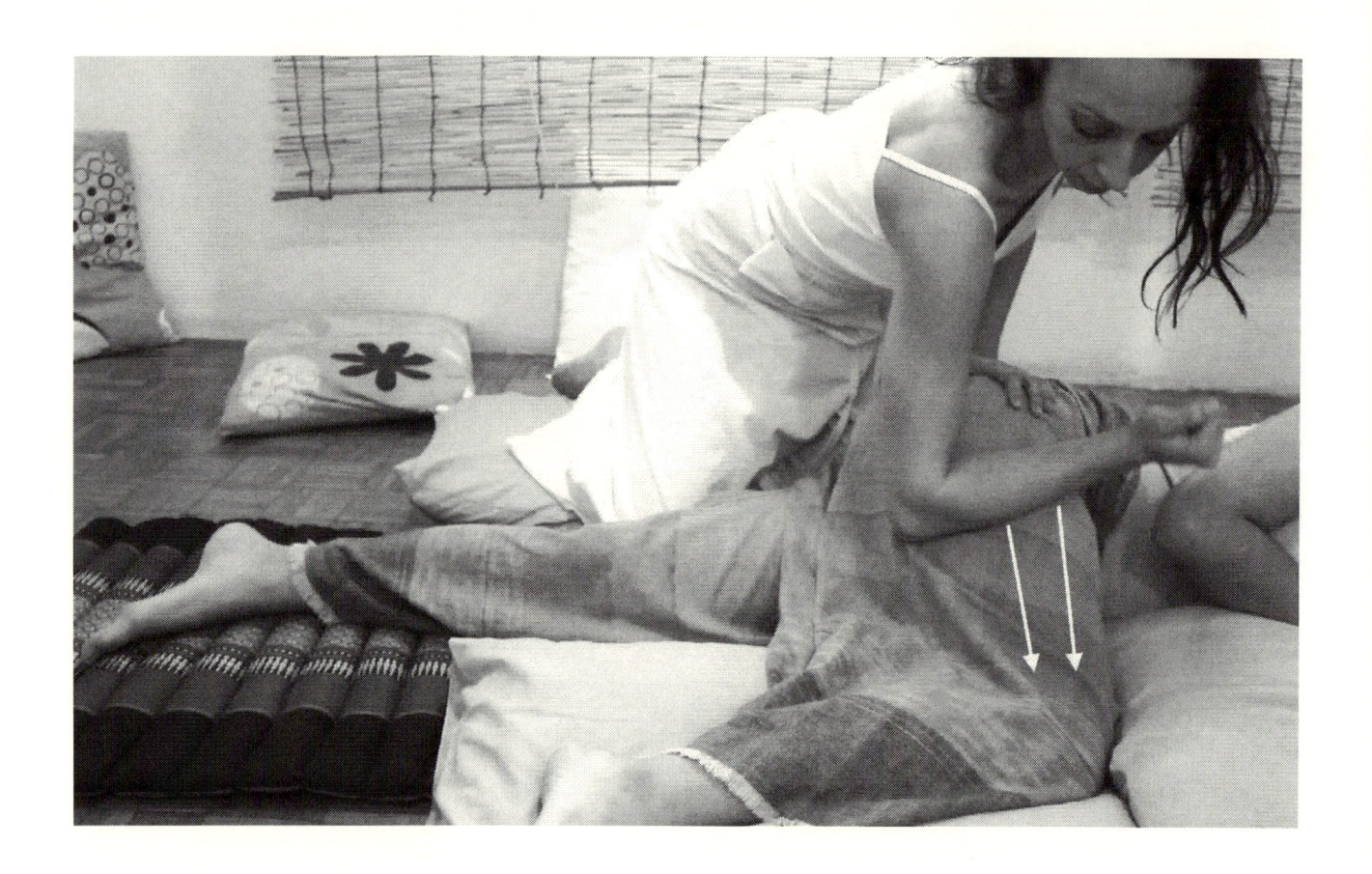

6. You can also work on the iliotibial band, by rolling firmly your forearm. Great technique for iliotibial band syndrome (ITBS).

> The iliotibial band is a thick band of fascia, extending from the outside of the pelvis, over the hip and knee, and inserting just below the knee.
>
> ITBS can result from training habits (especially excessive running), anatomical abnormalities, or muscular imbalances.

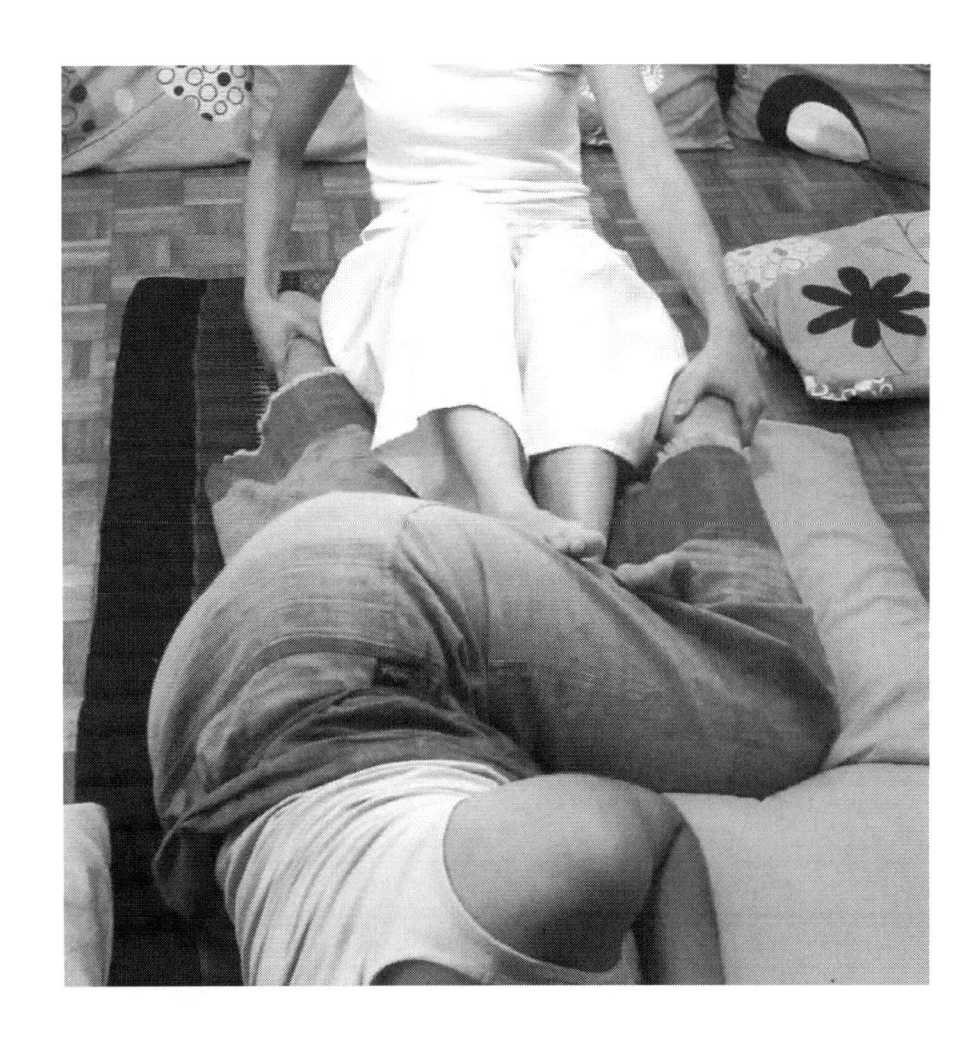

7. Then sit between the receiver's legs, and walk with your feet on the posterior thigh muscles. The presses should be done with the transverse arch of the feet.

Your grip (of the receiver's legs) should be firm, but not too tight.

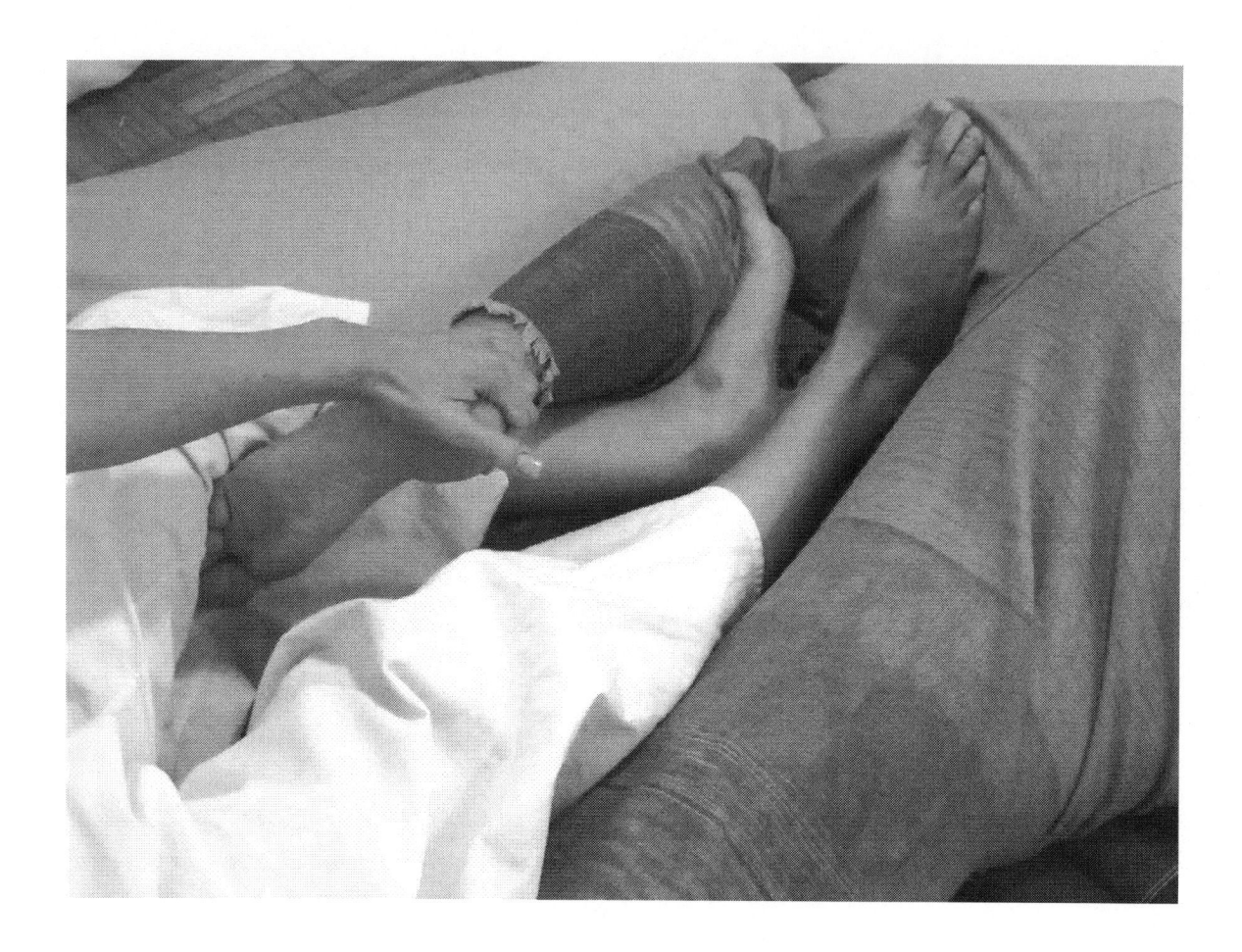

8. Actually from this position you can apply all the similar techniques of the supine position, that involve leg locks.

Lock the receiver's foot in your knee joint. Grasp her heel and other leg, and repeat the previous foot presses, with one foot. Simultaneously, pull the other leg of the receiver.

This is similar to technique 10 of the single leg techniques.

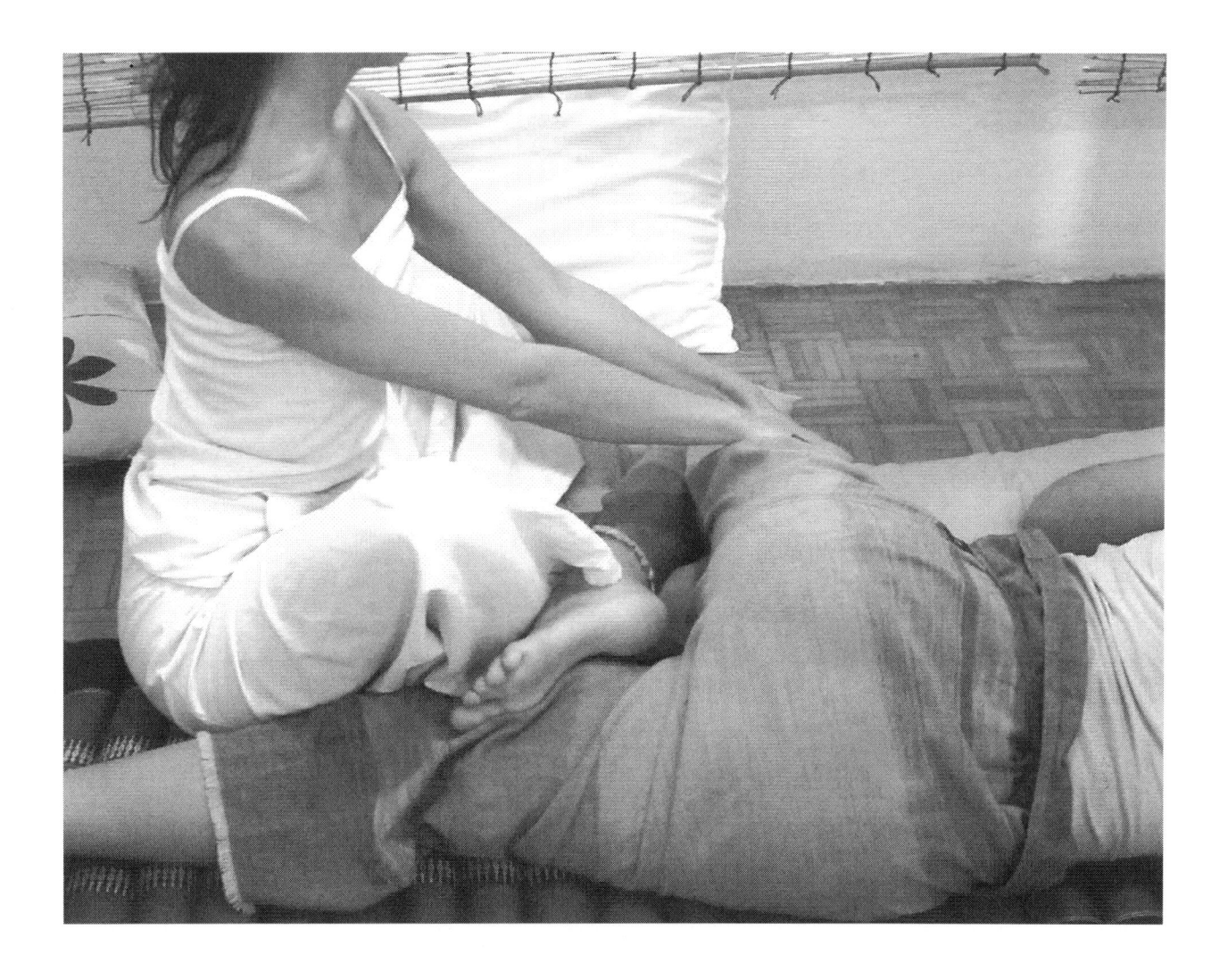

9. You can also work on the quadriceps muscle, by stabilizing the leg with a lock. This is similar to technique 11 of the single leg techniques.

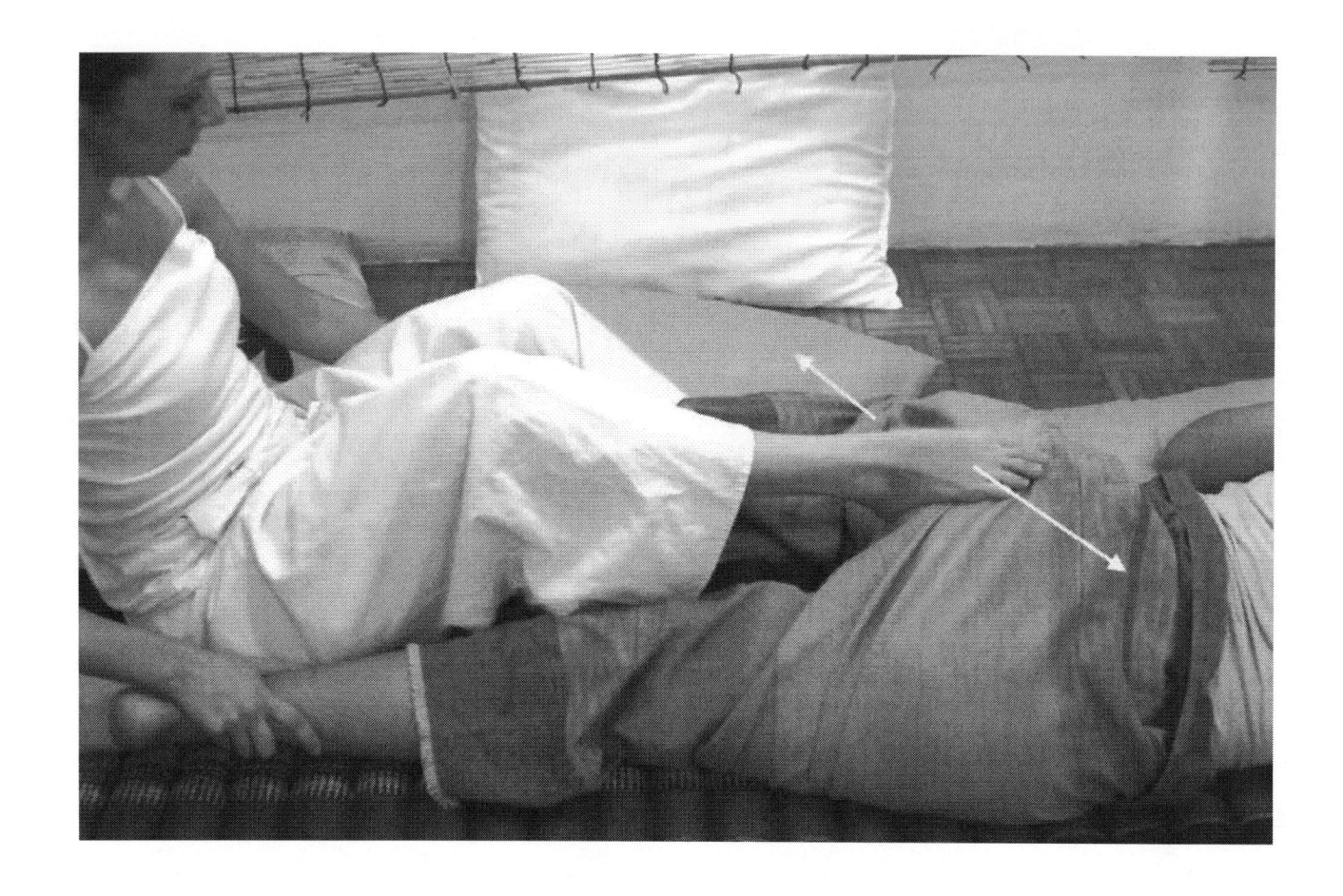

10. Place one foot on the gluteus muscle, and one foot on the knee joint, and apply a light stretch on the posterior thigh muscles.

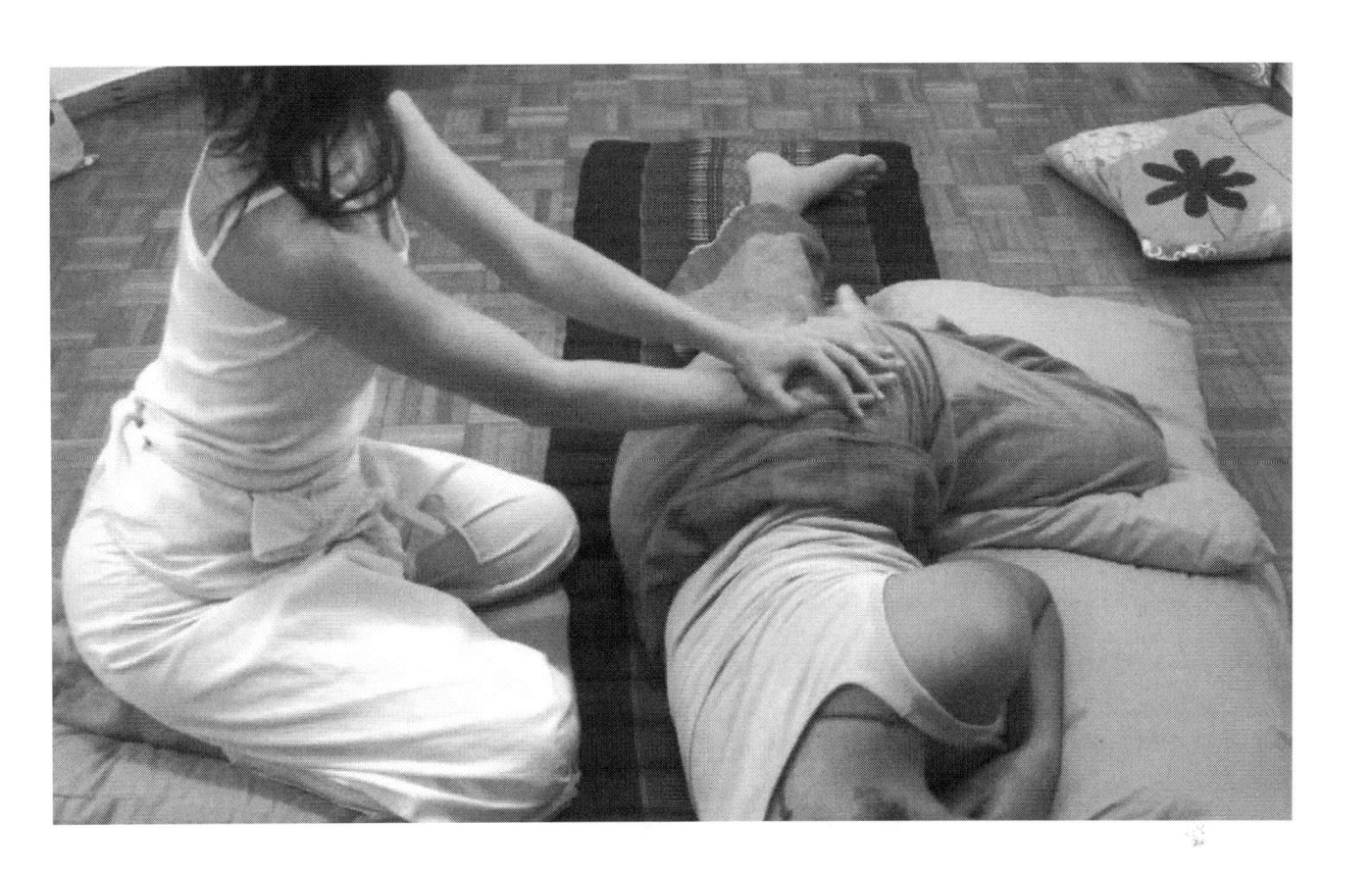

11. Work on the gluteus muscle, trying to "detach" it from the surrounding tissues.

This is a very good technique for sciatica and lower back pain.

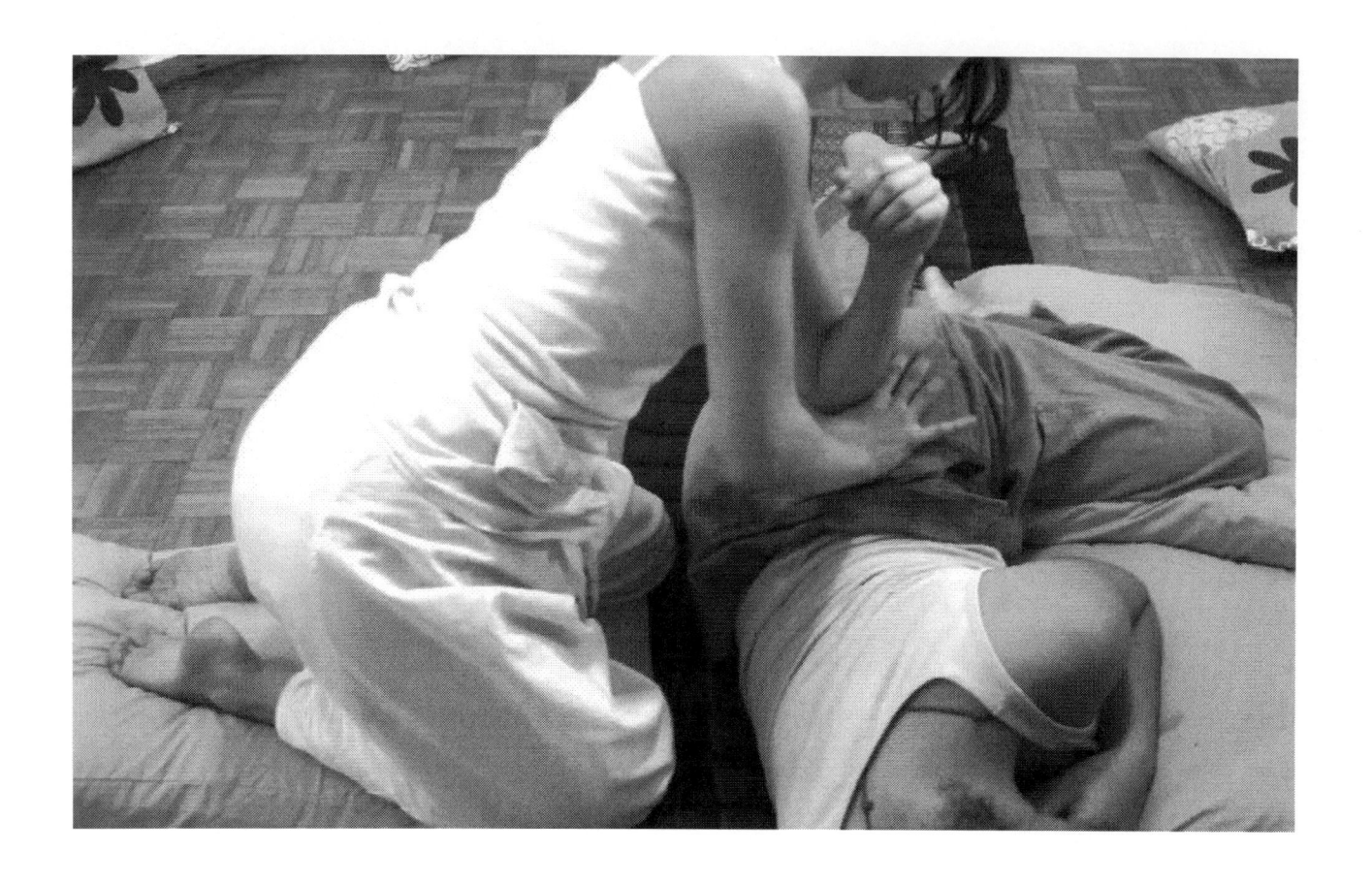

12. You can also work with your elbow on this area.

Be careful not to apply too strong pressure on the area – the sciatic nerve passes from this area. Actually, elbow work is recommended only in larger and heavier clients.

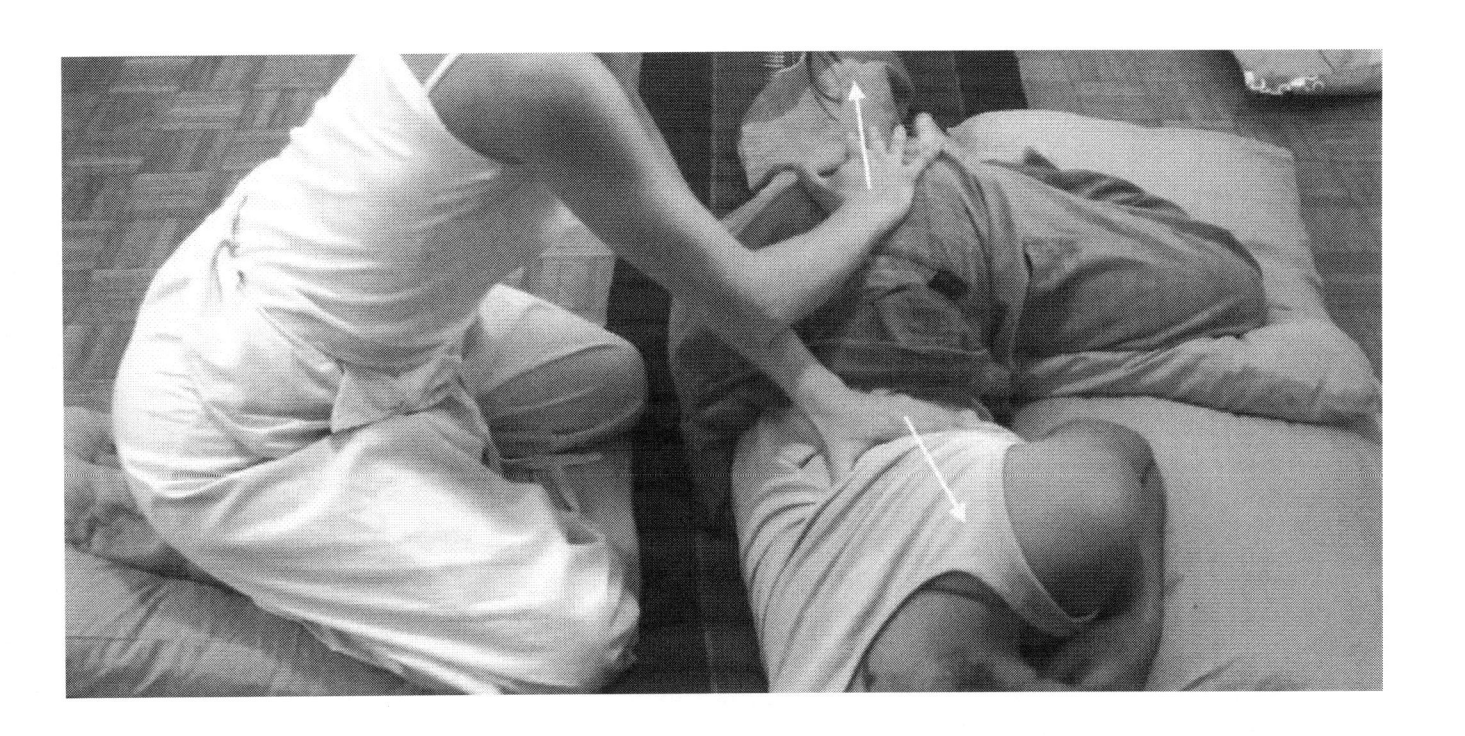

13. Place one palm on the gluteus, and one palm above the pelvis. At exhaling, apply a light stretch.

This technique decompresses the lumbar spine, and is indicated for degenerated discs.

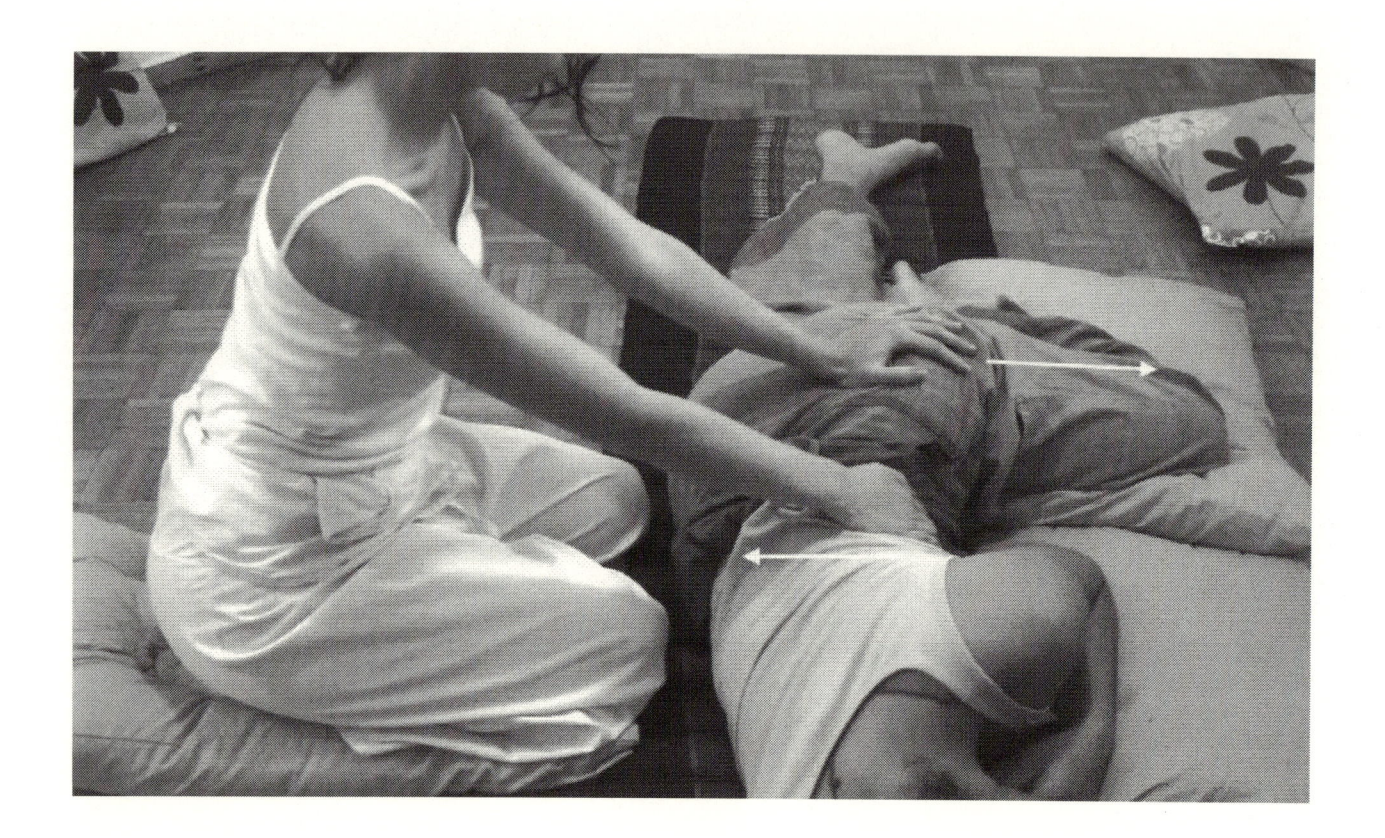

14. Place one hand on the gluteus, and one hand above the pelvis, and move your hands in opposite directions. Apply greater pressure to the hand on the gluteus.

Actually, this technique targets the sacrum and the sacroiliac joint.

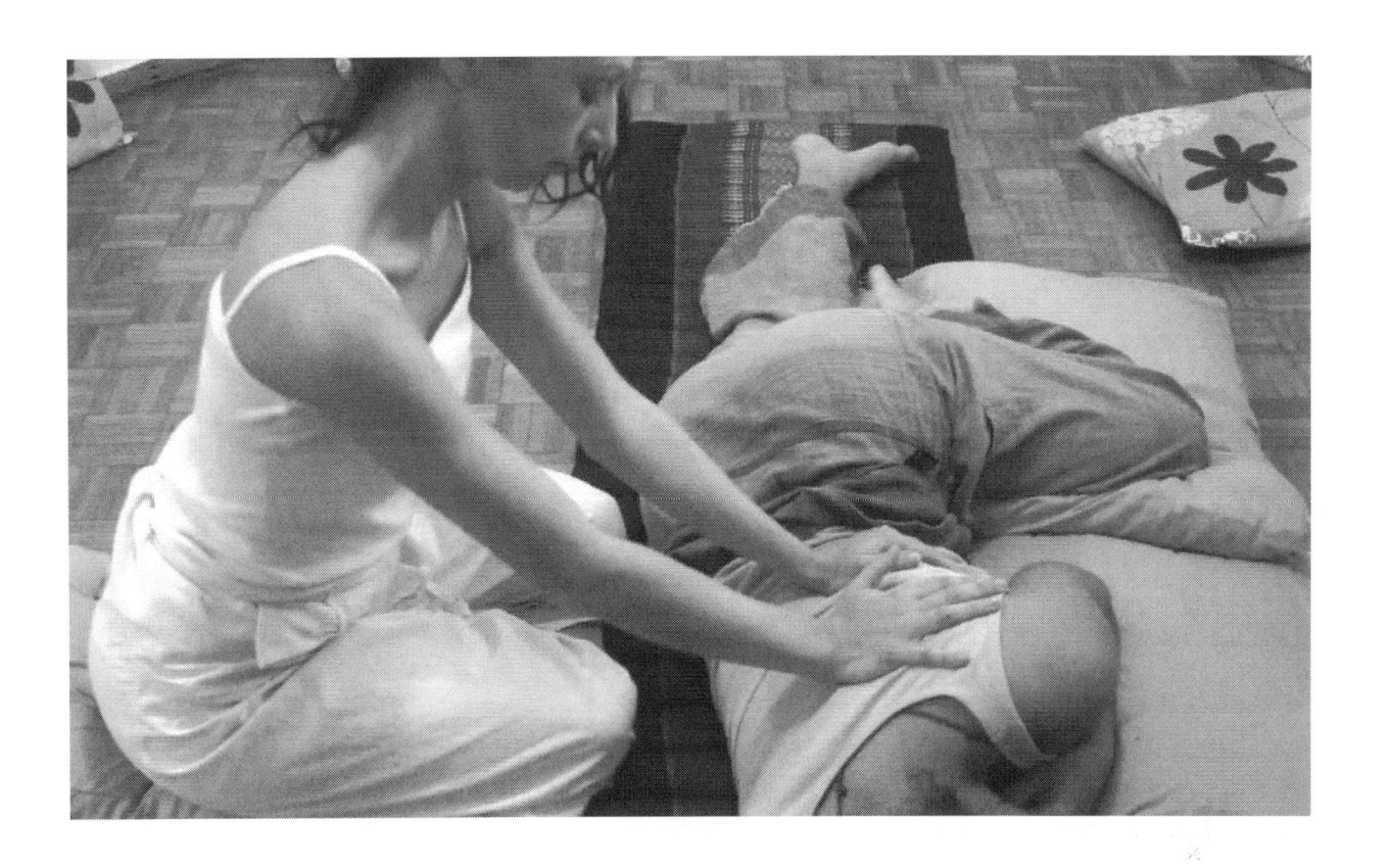

15. Then walk with your palms on the receiver's back, following the *Itha & Pingkala Sen* lines.

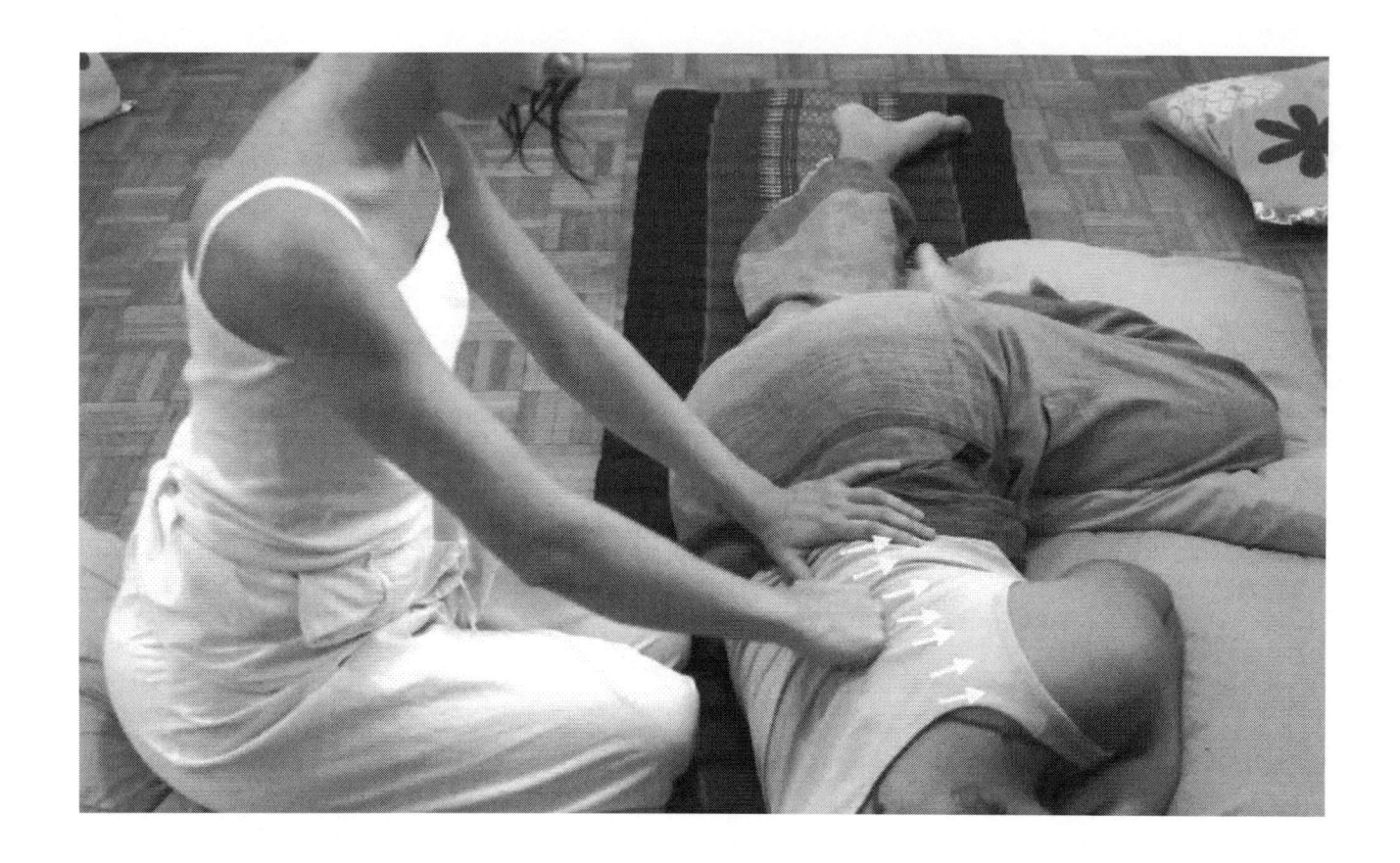

16. Now do deep tissue work next to the spine. Work with your knuckles and do transverse friction massage.

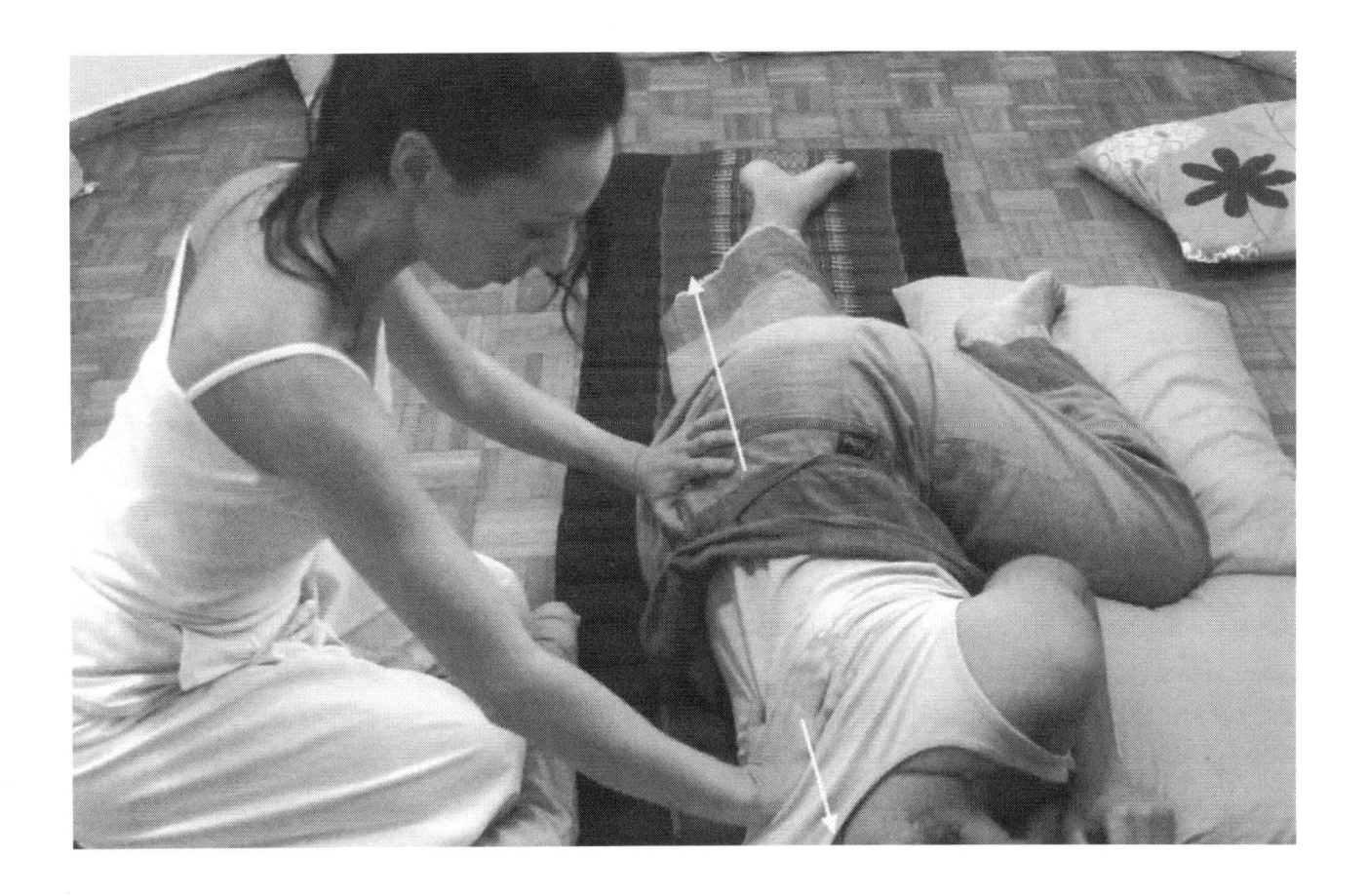

17. Place one hand on the sacrum, and one hand at the end of the thoracic spine, and perform a light stretch of the lumbar spine.

Actually, the stretch is performed with the hypothenar eminence. Hold the stretch for 5-6 seconds, and apply hot herbal compresses.

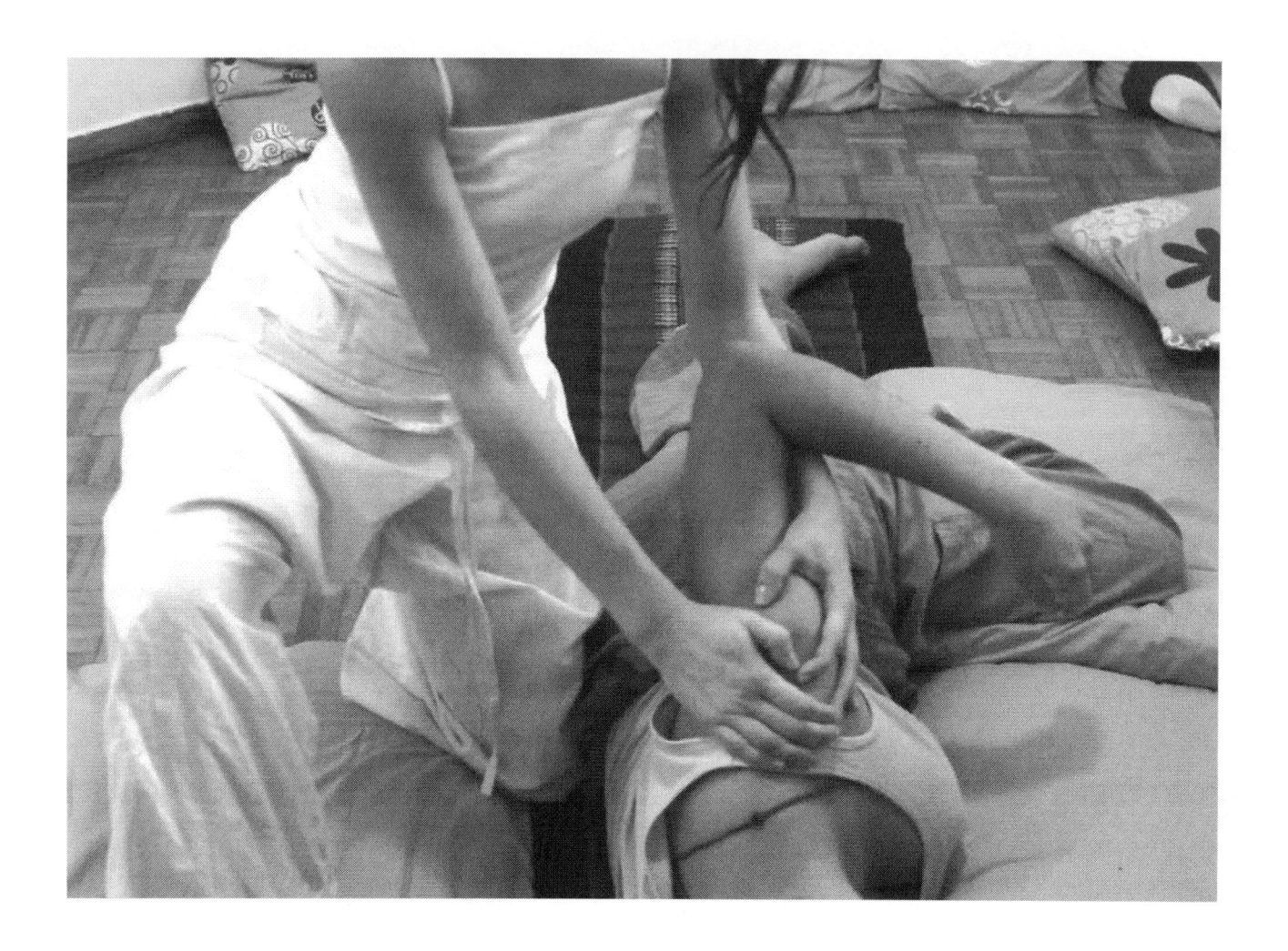

18. Grasp the receiver's shoulder and rotate it. Then fall back with your body weight, applying a stretch on the neck muscles.

While rotating the shoulder, you may hear cricking sounds. This may mean that the shoulder joint is unstable. In this case, you should not pull the shoulder, especially upwards or laterally.

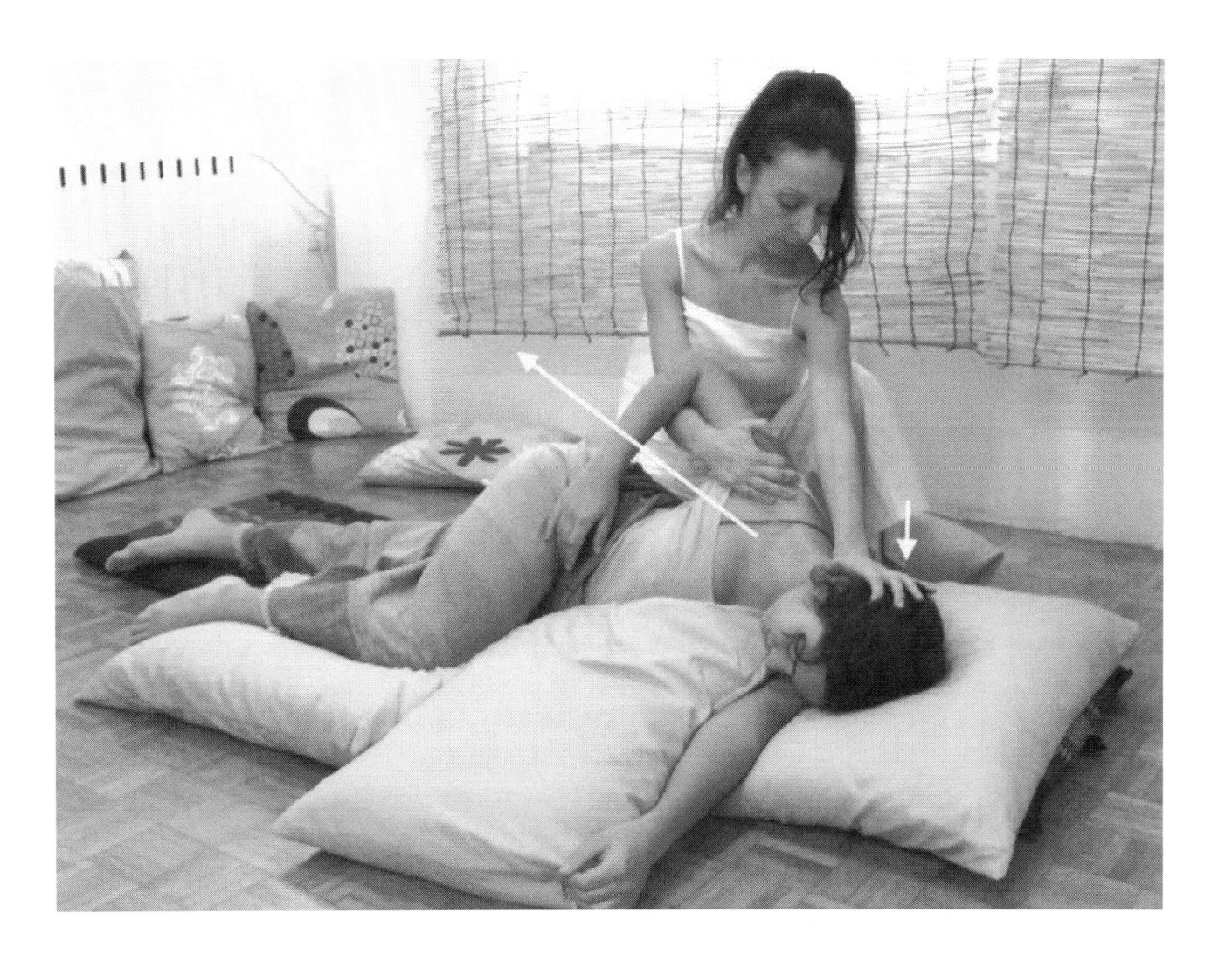

19. Then, place one hand on the mastoid process gently, and pull back the receiver's shoulder, as she exhales.

Good technique for neck pain due to shortened muscles.

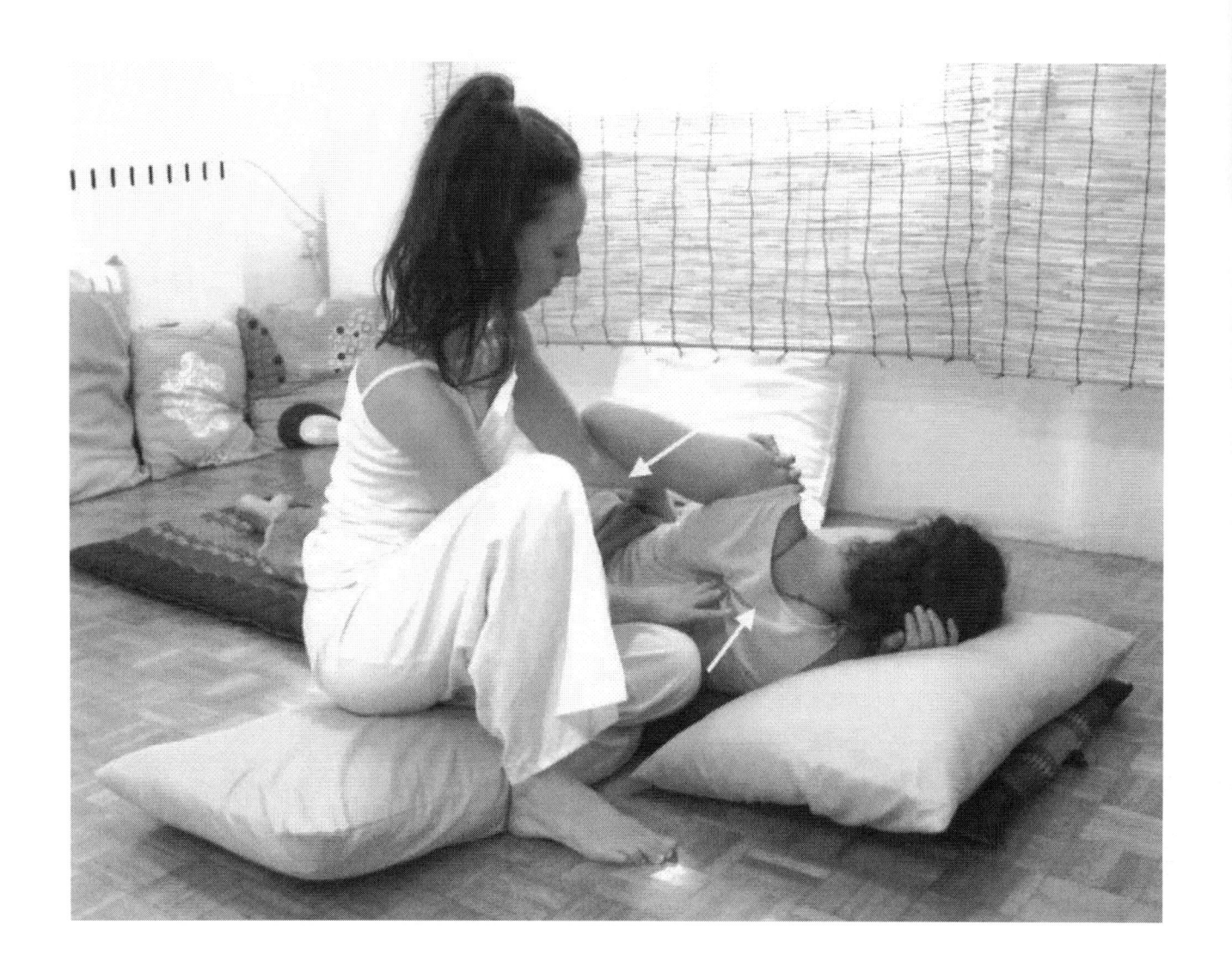

20. Place one palm in front of the receiver's clavicle. Insert your fingertips in the scapula, as you pull it back.

Move your fingers in many spots around the scapula, and stay 3-4 seconds on each "insertion".

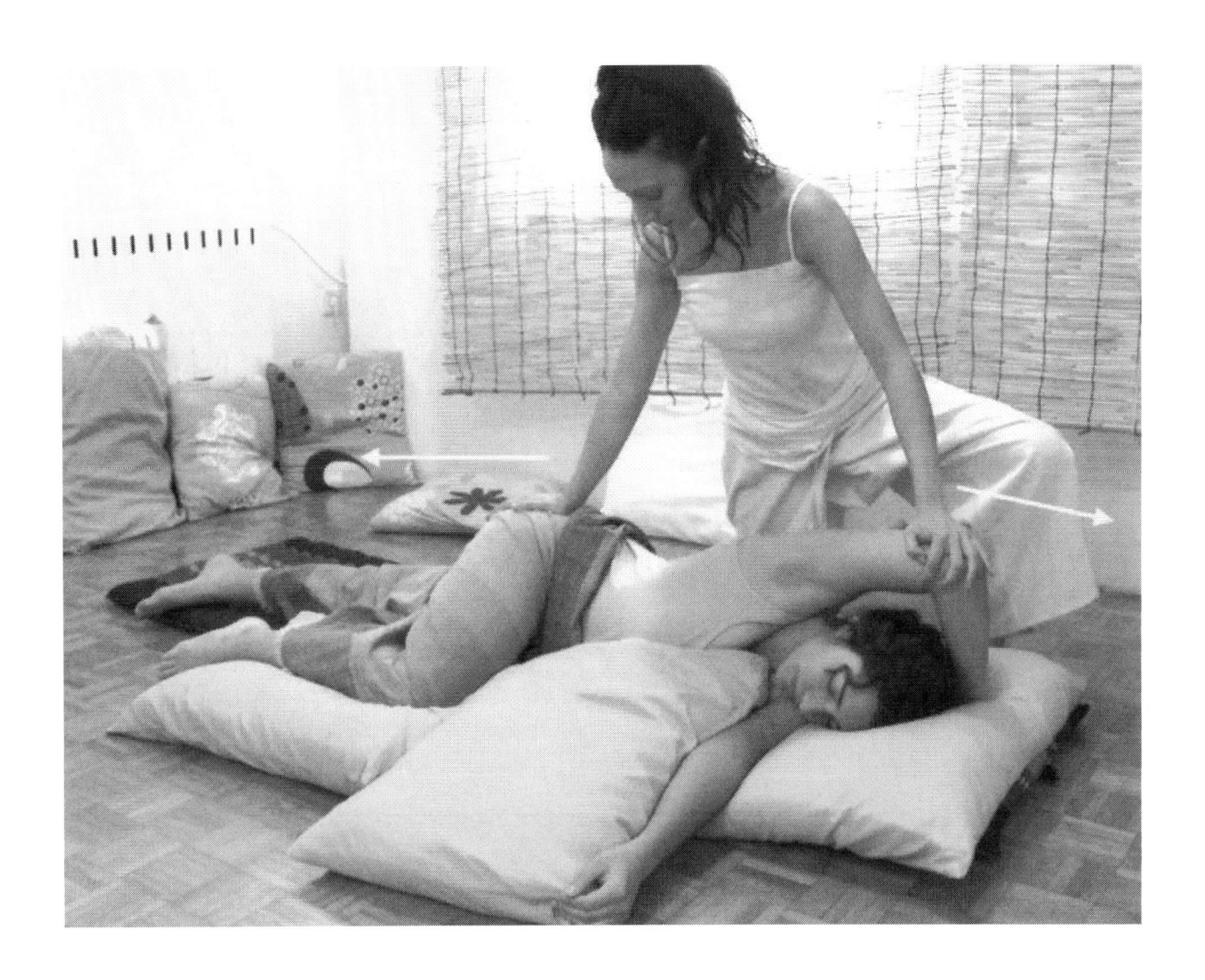

21. Place the receiver's hand above her head, with her fingers towards her shoulder. Then place one hand on her elbow, and one hand below the pelvis, and apply a stretch, as the receiver exhales.

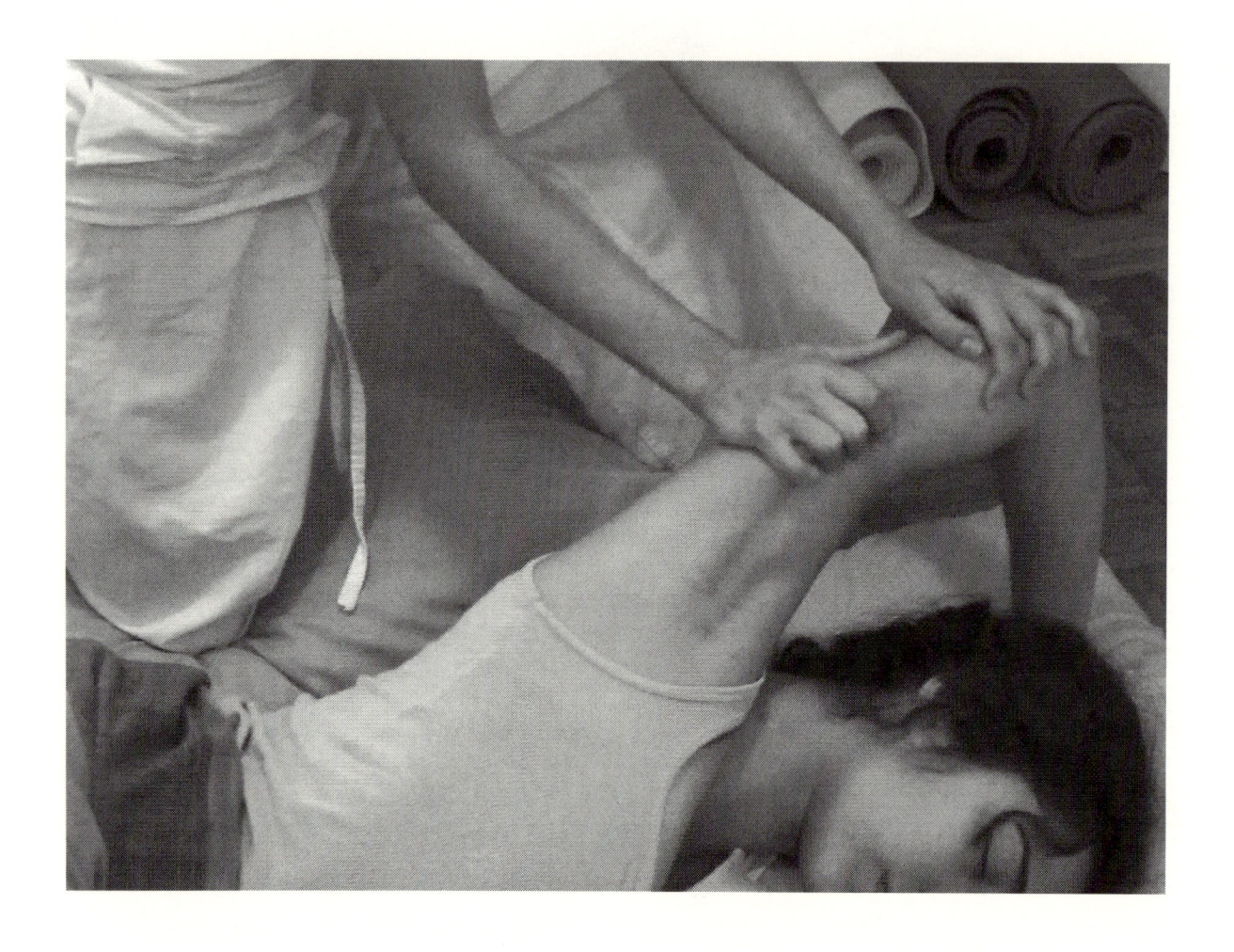

22. You can also work on the triceps muscle from this lock. Try to "separate" the muscle from the surrounding tissue, and do some decent kneading.

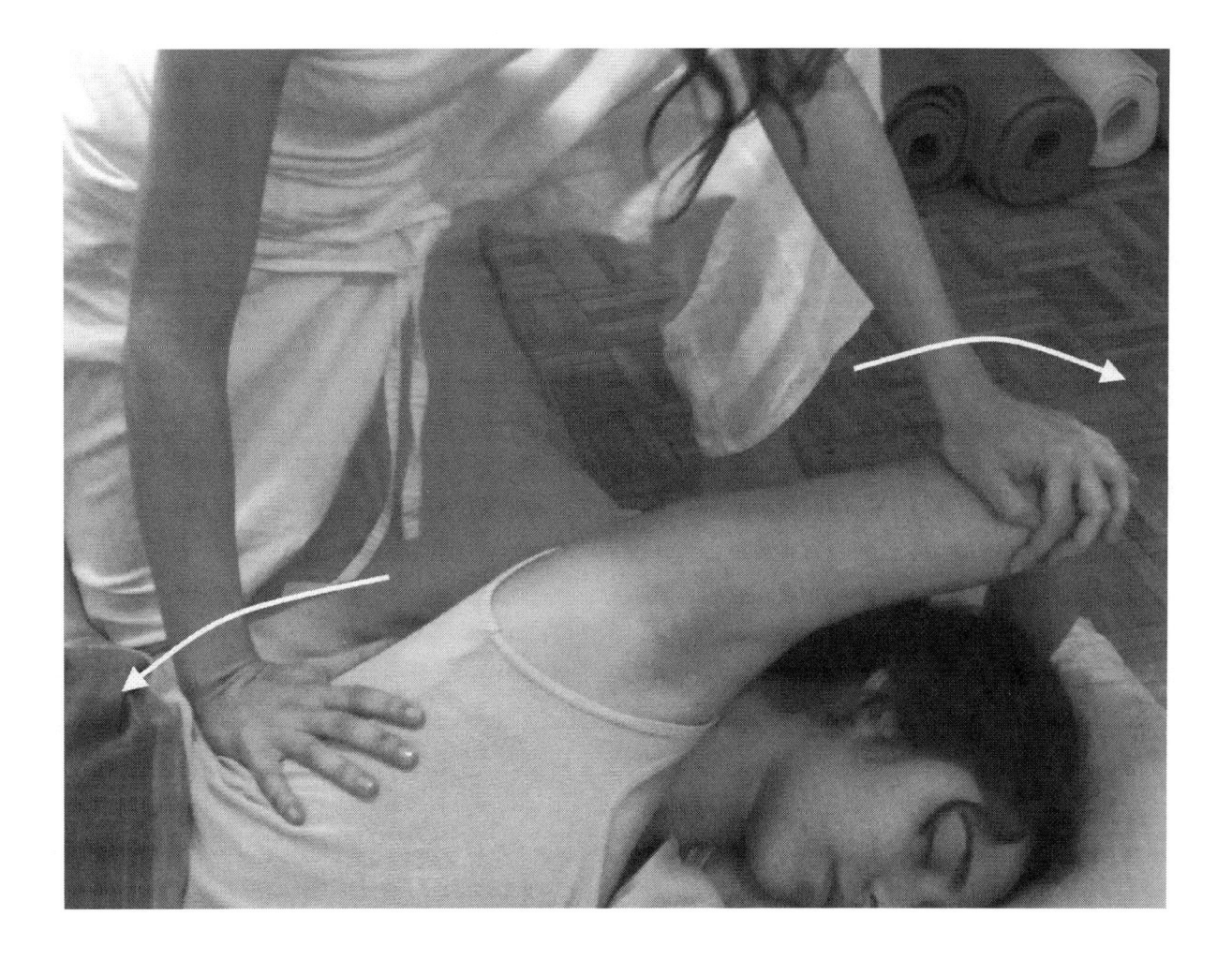

23. In the previous lock, place one hand on the elbow joint, and on the teres major. Open the rotator cuff by pressing down the teres major with the hypothenar eminence.

You can also place your hand lower on the ribs, in order to "open" the rib cage.

This is an excellent technique for kyphosis and chronic breathing problems.

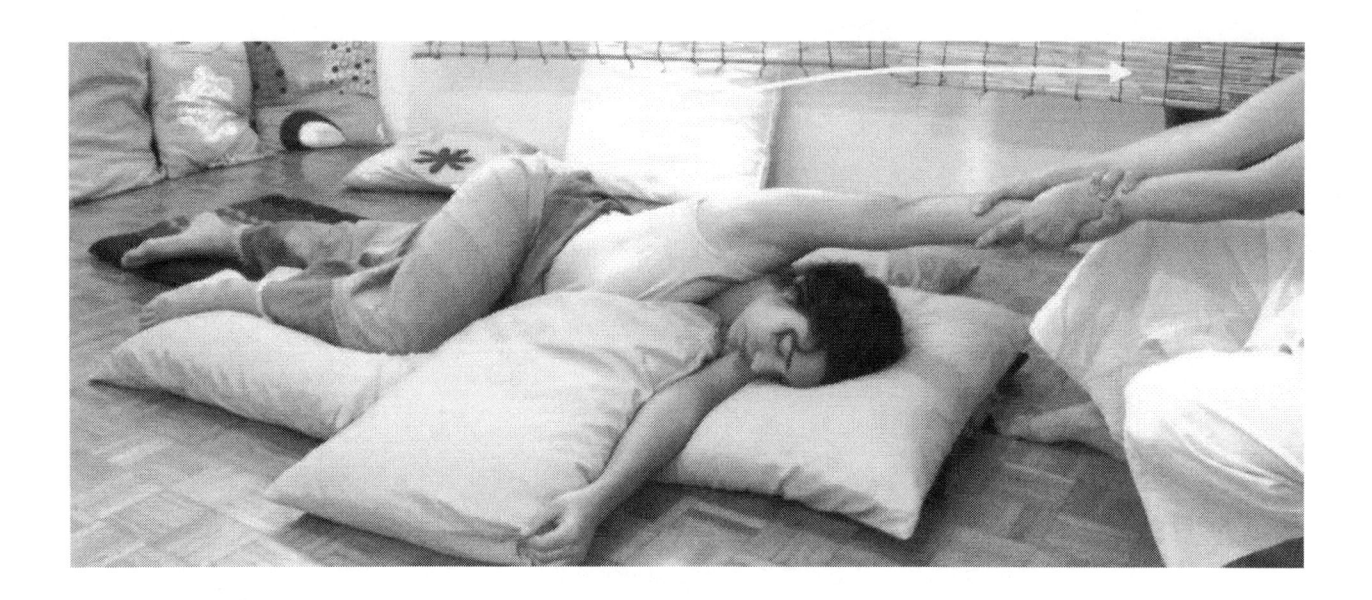

24. Grasp the receiver's arm, and pull it backwards, in order to open the ribs and the thoracic spine.

Do not apply this technique if the client has unstable shoulder joint.

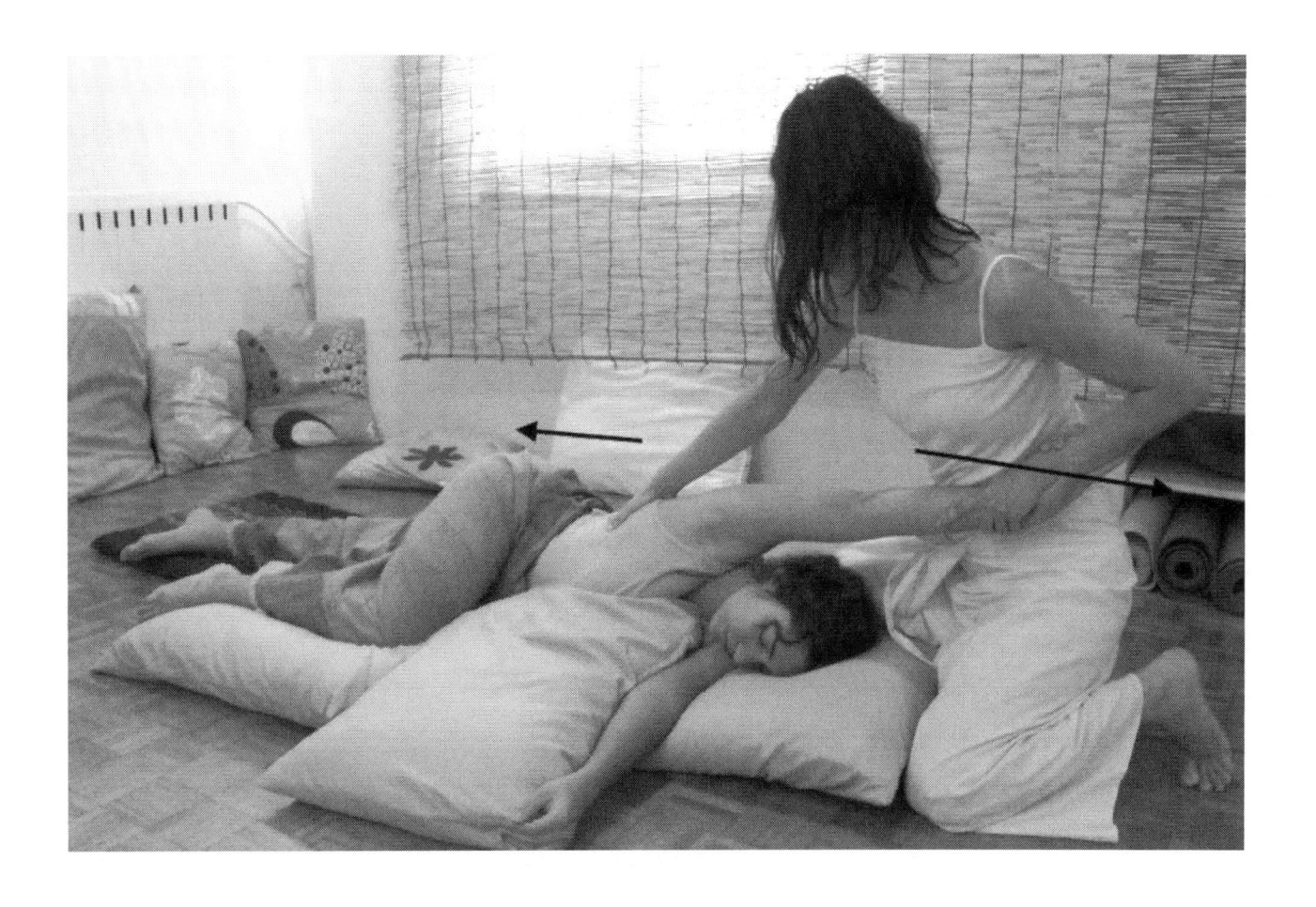

25. Then push downwards the teres major, in order to release the rotator cuff muscles.

This is similar to technique 23. The difference is that technique 23 allows more focused work on the rotator cuff and the rib area. This one is a rather more general stretch.

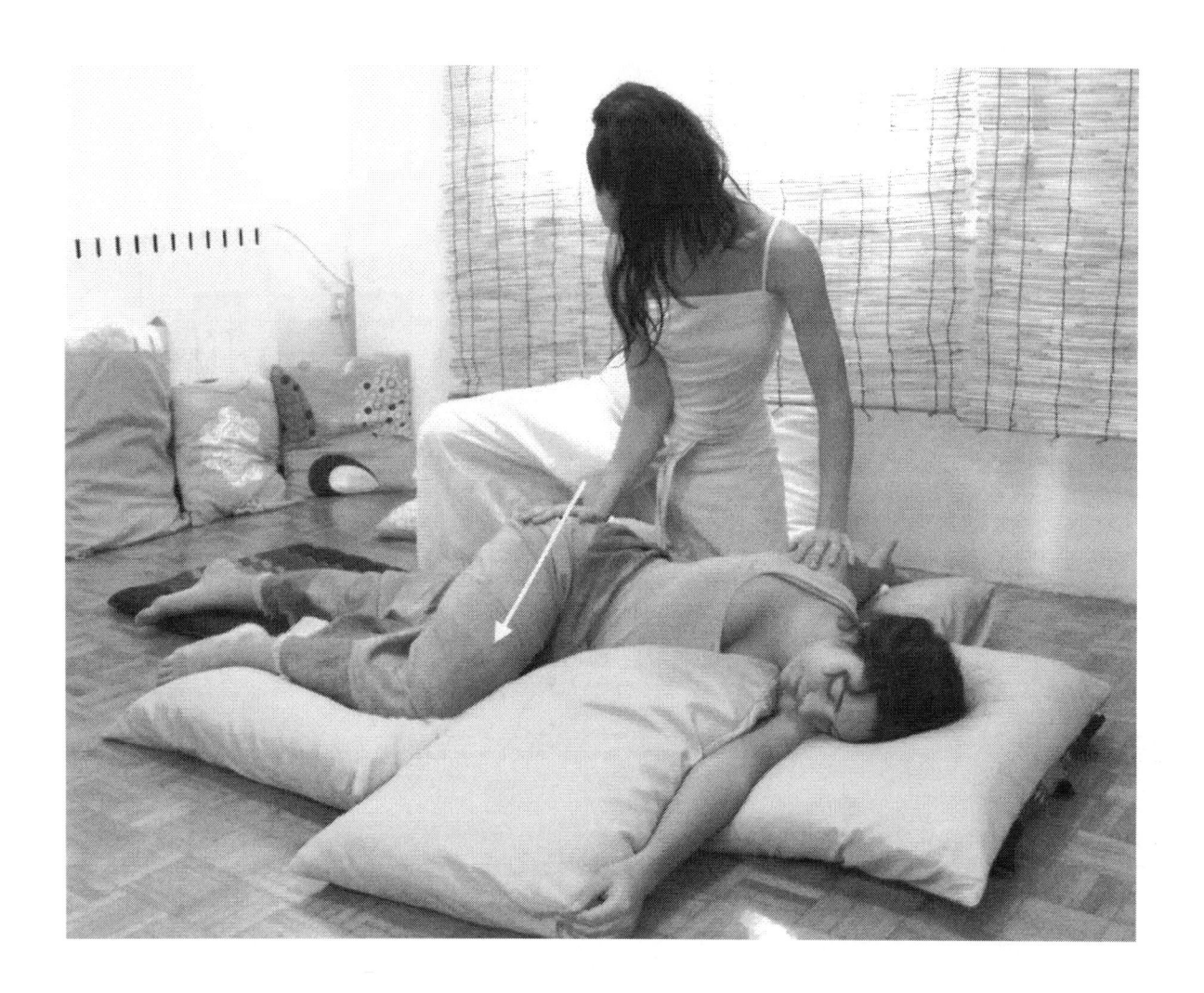

26. Hold down gently the receiver's shoulder. Place your other hand on the gluteus muscle, and push it forward. This is a corrective technique for the sacroiliac joint.

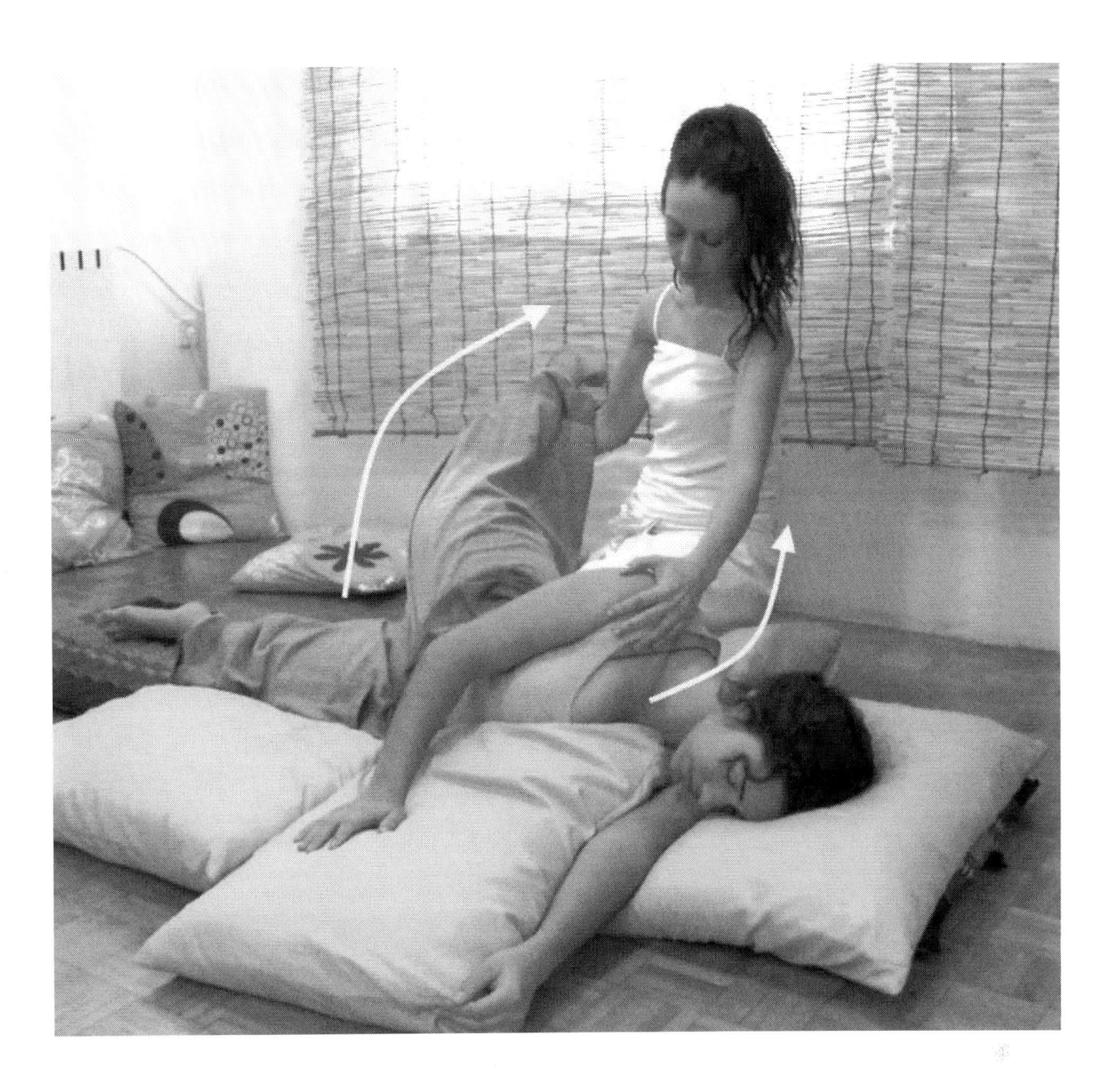

27. Grasp the receiver's leg with one hand, and her shoulder with the other. Place your knee above her pelvis, and apply a "bow" stretch as she exhales.

Do not press your knee on the receiver's body. The knee just stabilizes the technique. Actually, pressing the knee would be painful.

For proper body alignment, the receiver's thigh should be parallel to the ground. Do not lift the thigh higher in order to make the lift easier for you.

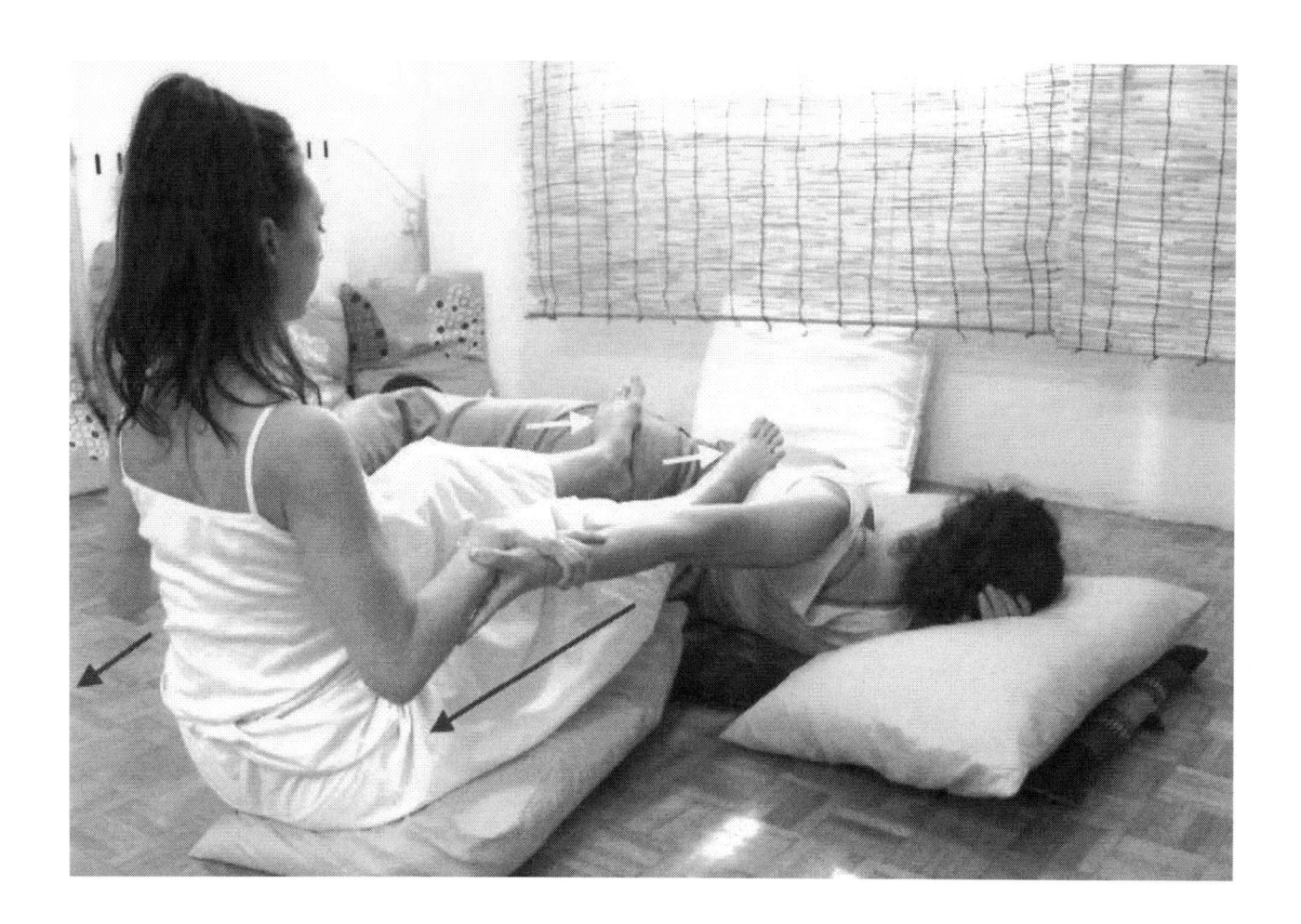

28. Place one foot above the pelvis, and one foot on the gluteus muscle. Grasp the receiver's leg and arm, and perform a stretch as she exhales.

Do not press your foot that is on the kidneys, on the receiver's body. You can press slightly the other foot.

This technique targets the sacrum and misalignments on this area.

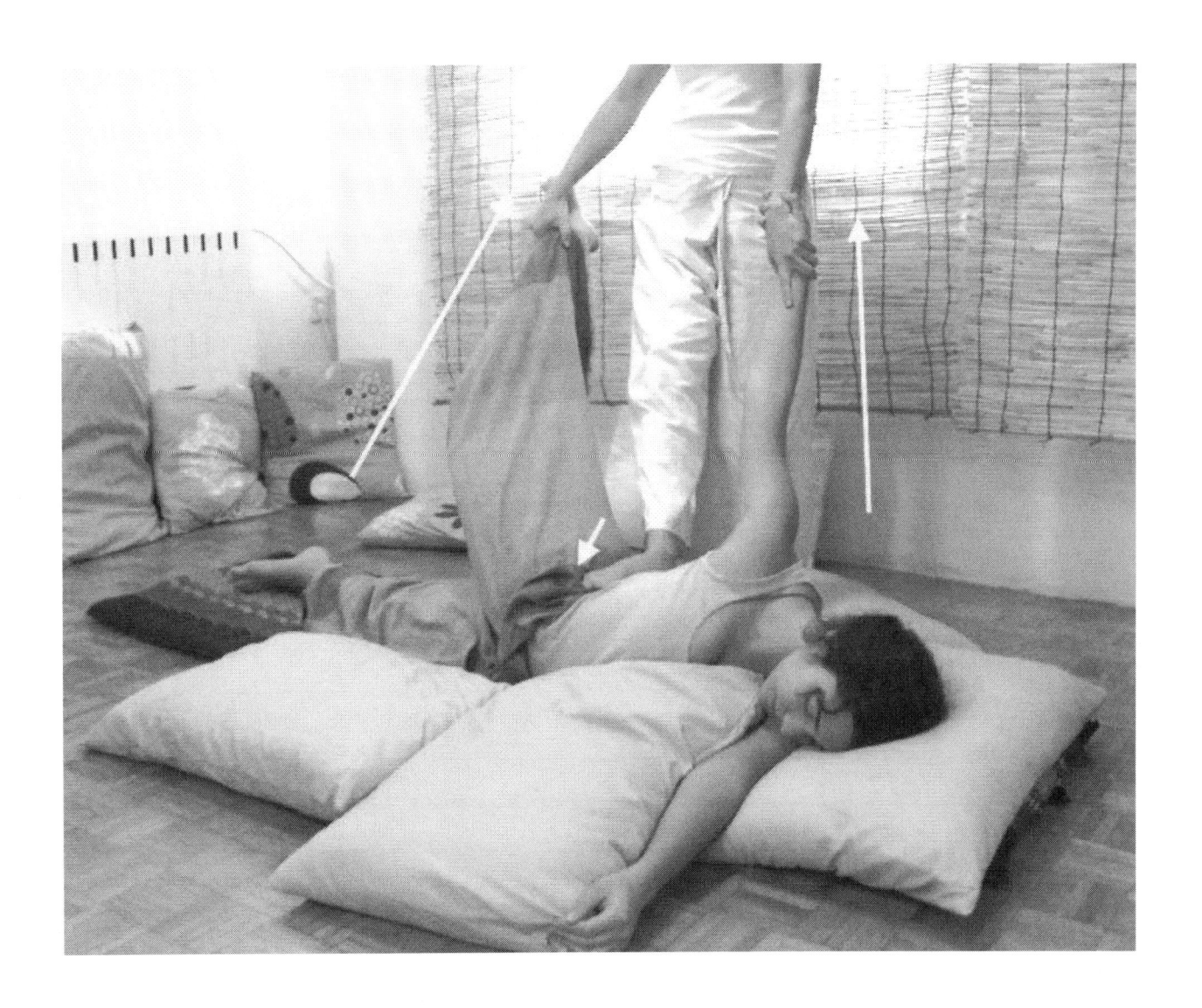

29. Then stand, and place your foot above the receiver's pelvis.

Grasp the receiver's leg and arm, and perform a stretch.

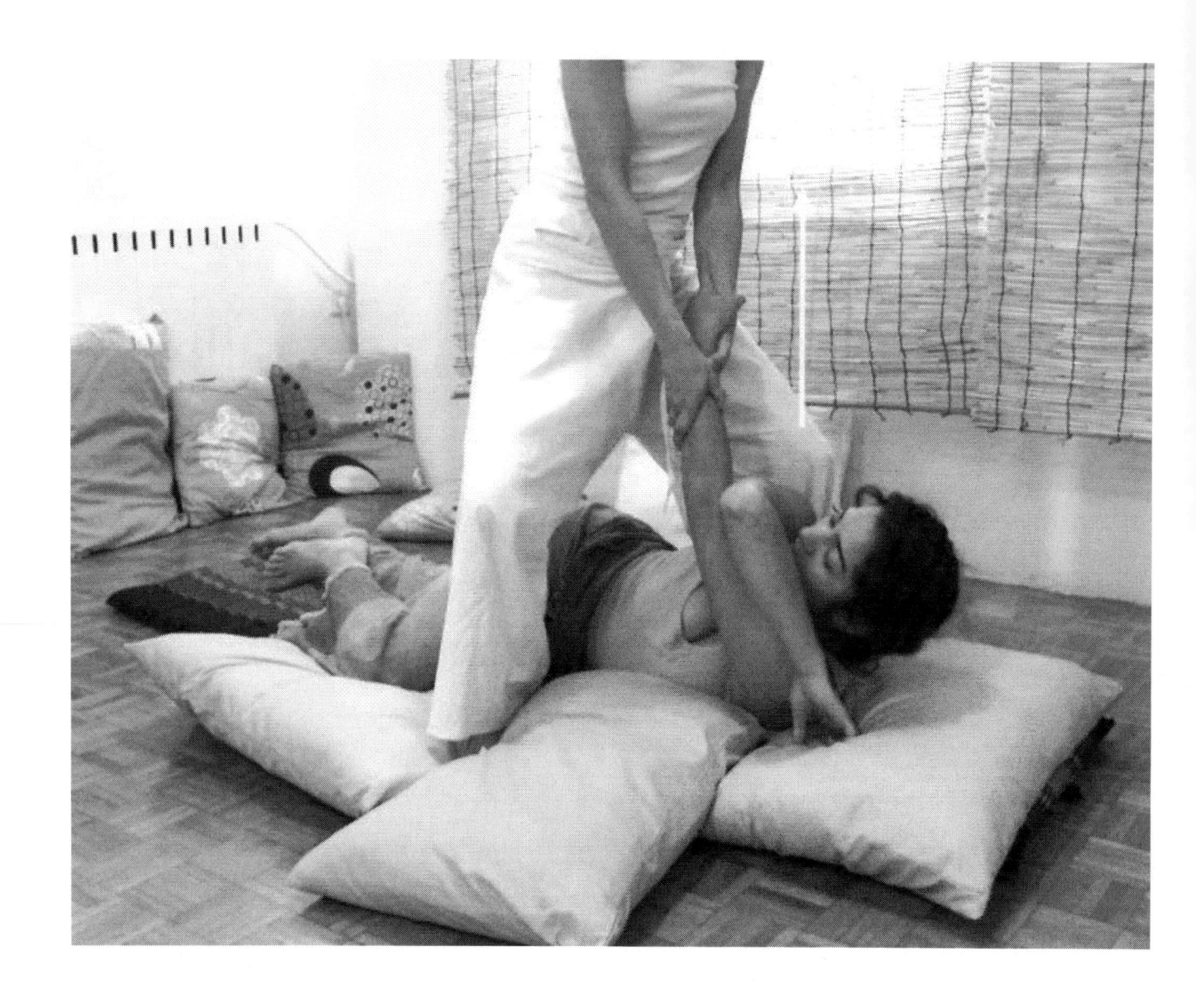

30. Stand above the receiver, grasp her arm, and pull it upwards as she exhales.

Do not perform this technique if the shoulder joint is unstable. It is also contraindicated for osteoporotic patients.

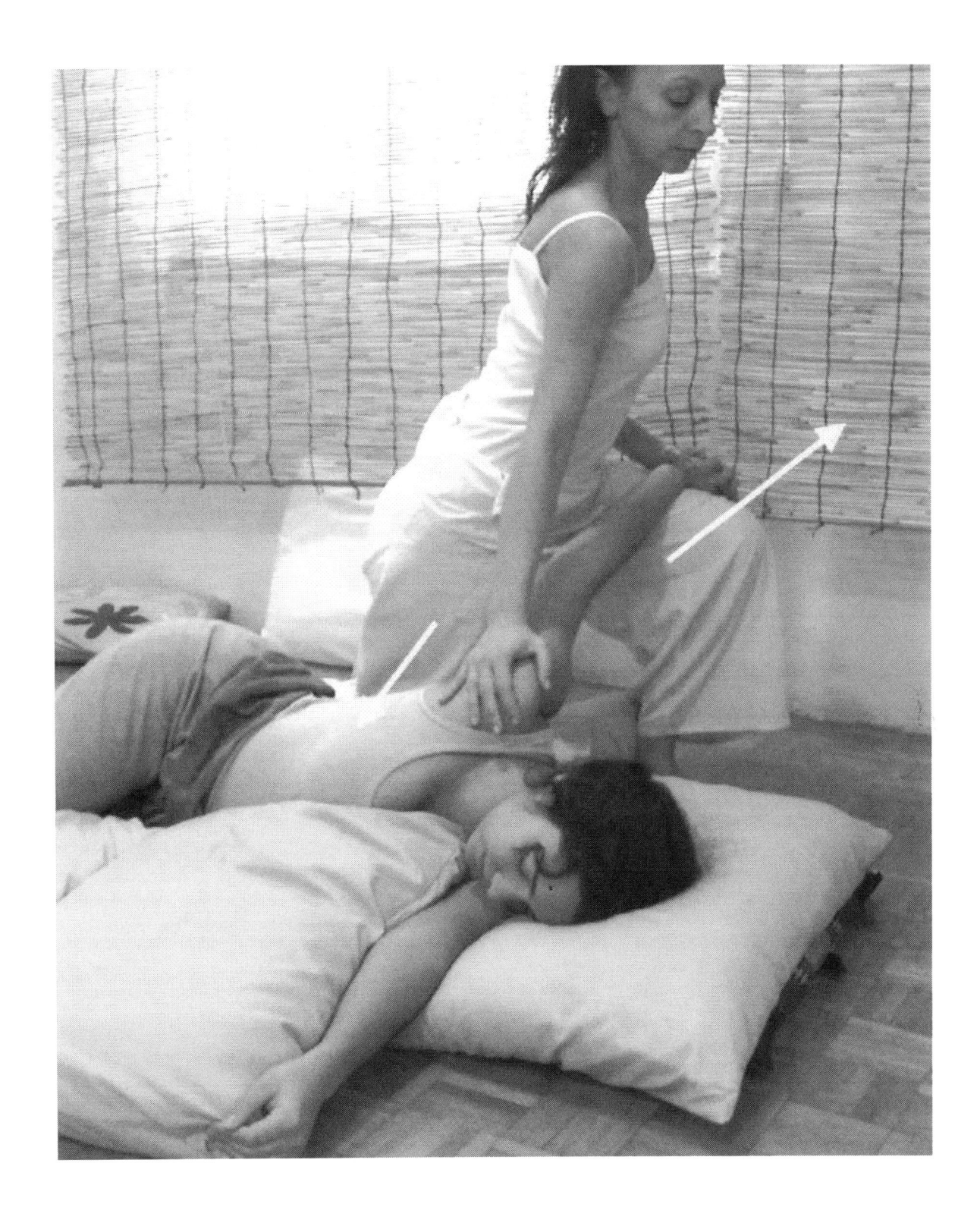

31. You can also work on the arms from the side position. It is possible to work on the Kalatharee Sen, at the interior part of the arm.

In order to work on the *Kalatharee Sen*, place the receiver's hand on your thigh. Now place one hand on her wrist, and one hand next on her shoulder. Perform the stretch as you exhale.

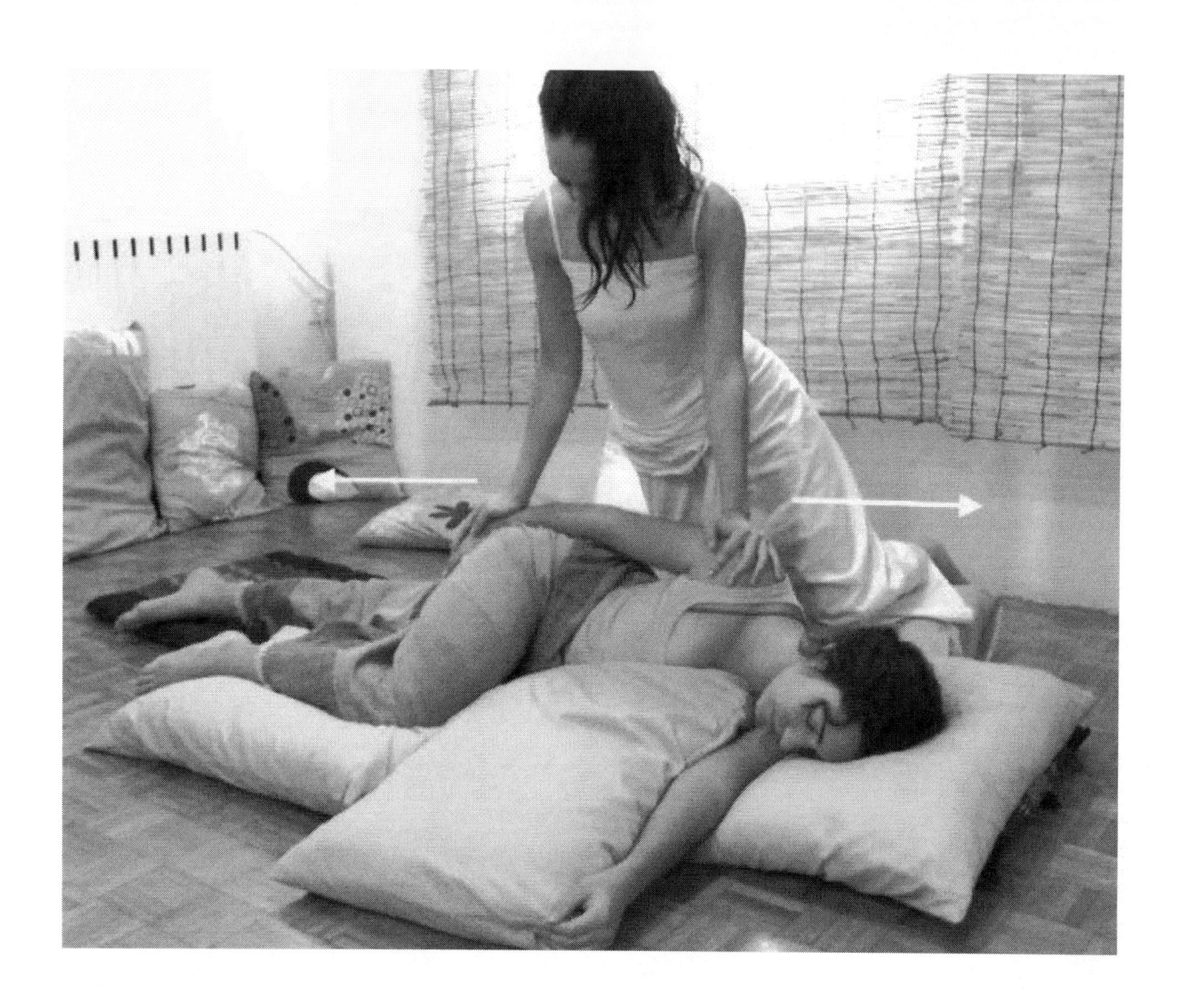

32. You can also work on the *Itha & Pingkala Sen* on the external part of the arm.

Apply all 5 Steps of Jap Sen. The photo shows Step 1 (and 5) – stretching and "opening" the meridian.

prone position

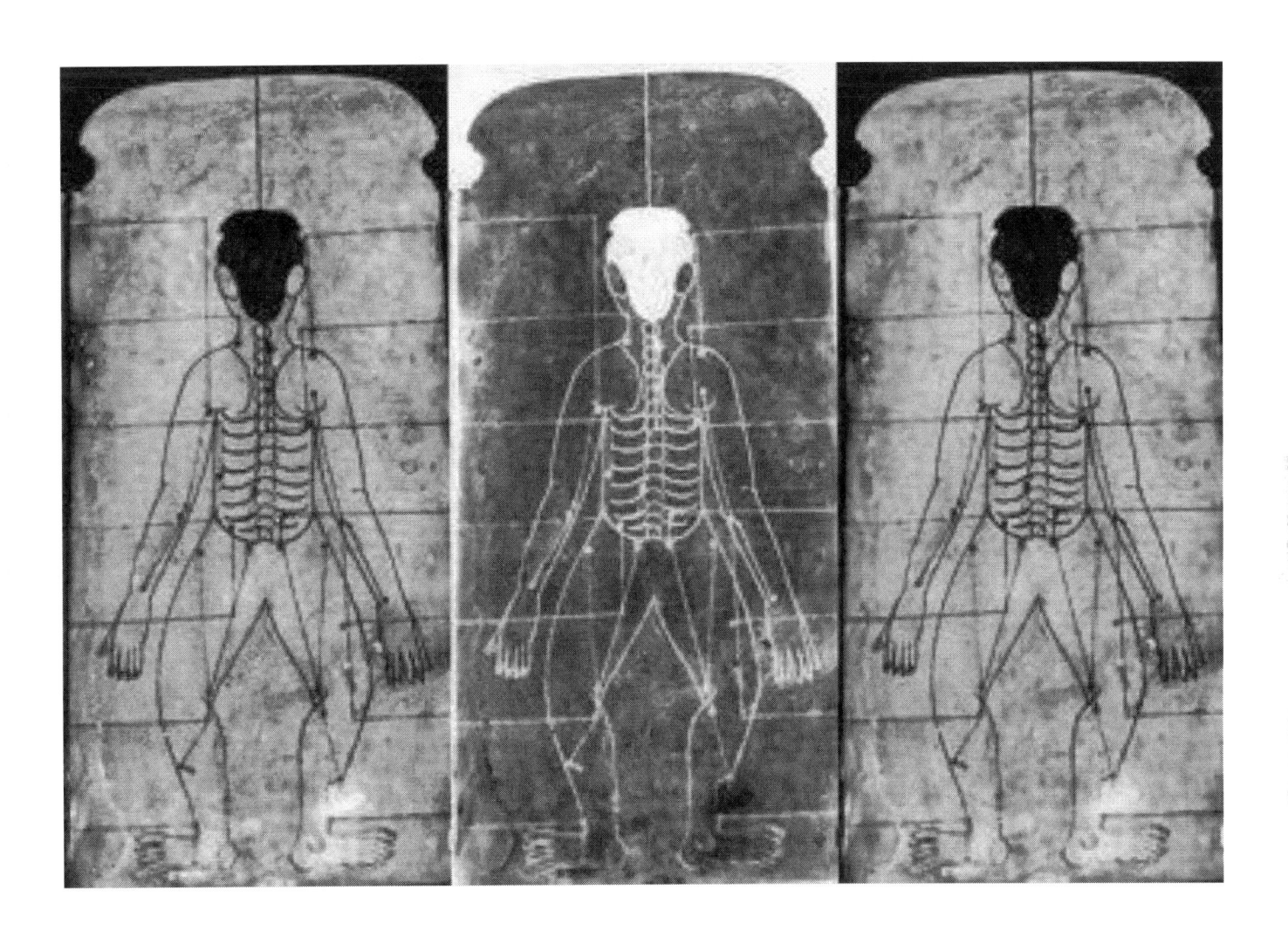

So let's get to what we 've been waiting for: the prone position!

Definetely, the prone position is the most relaxing massage position. In fact, most people have in mind the prone position when they hear the word "massage" – it is something like a synonym.

Prone position is of course, great for back and legs massage. You may need some pillows in order to support the receiver's body properly. You may have to place one pillow under the receiver's belly, in case of lumbar lordosis. Also, a headrest is always handy, because it supports properly the head and the neck, and facilitates work on the upper back.

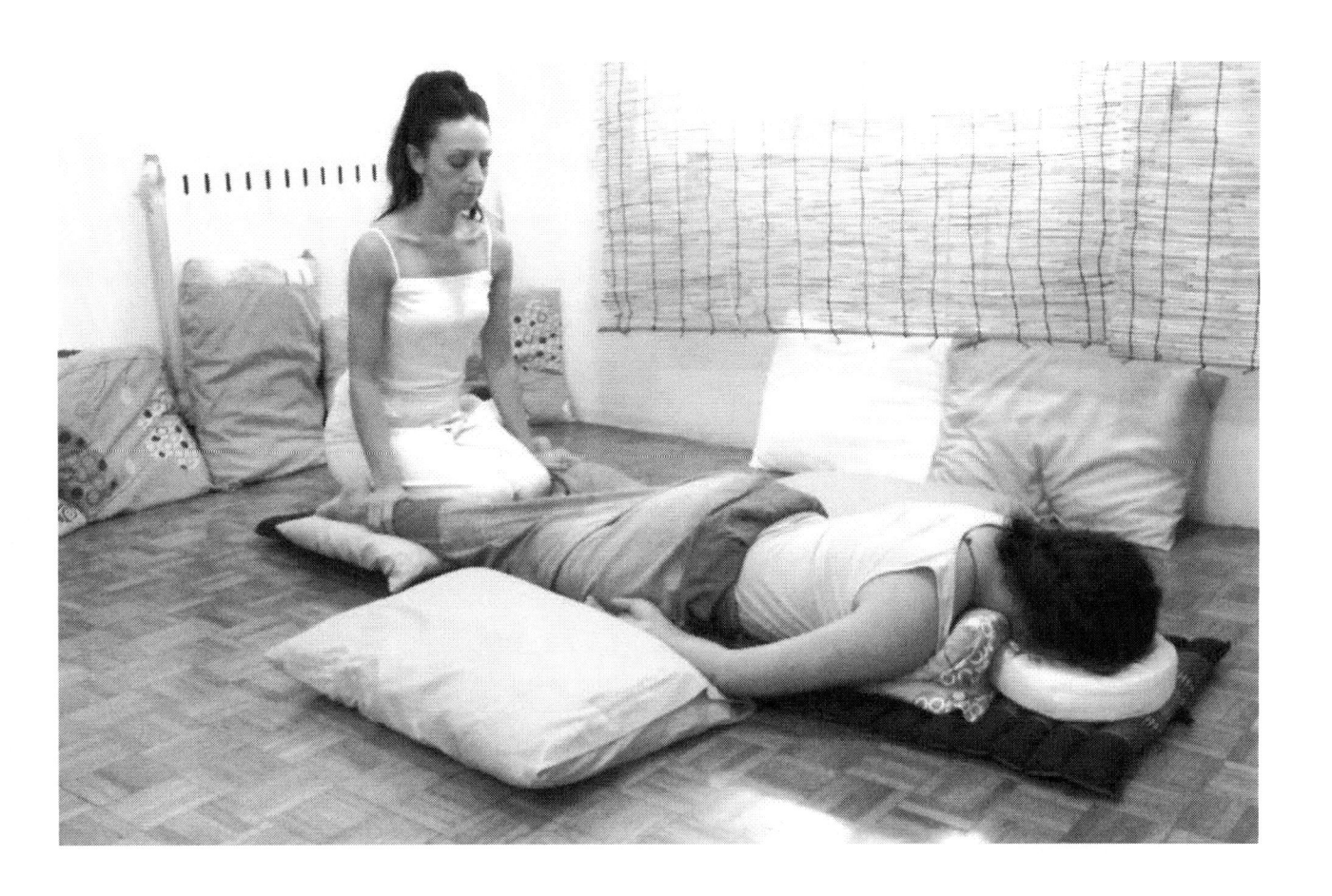

This is the proper setting for the prone position.

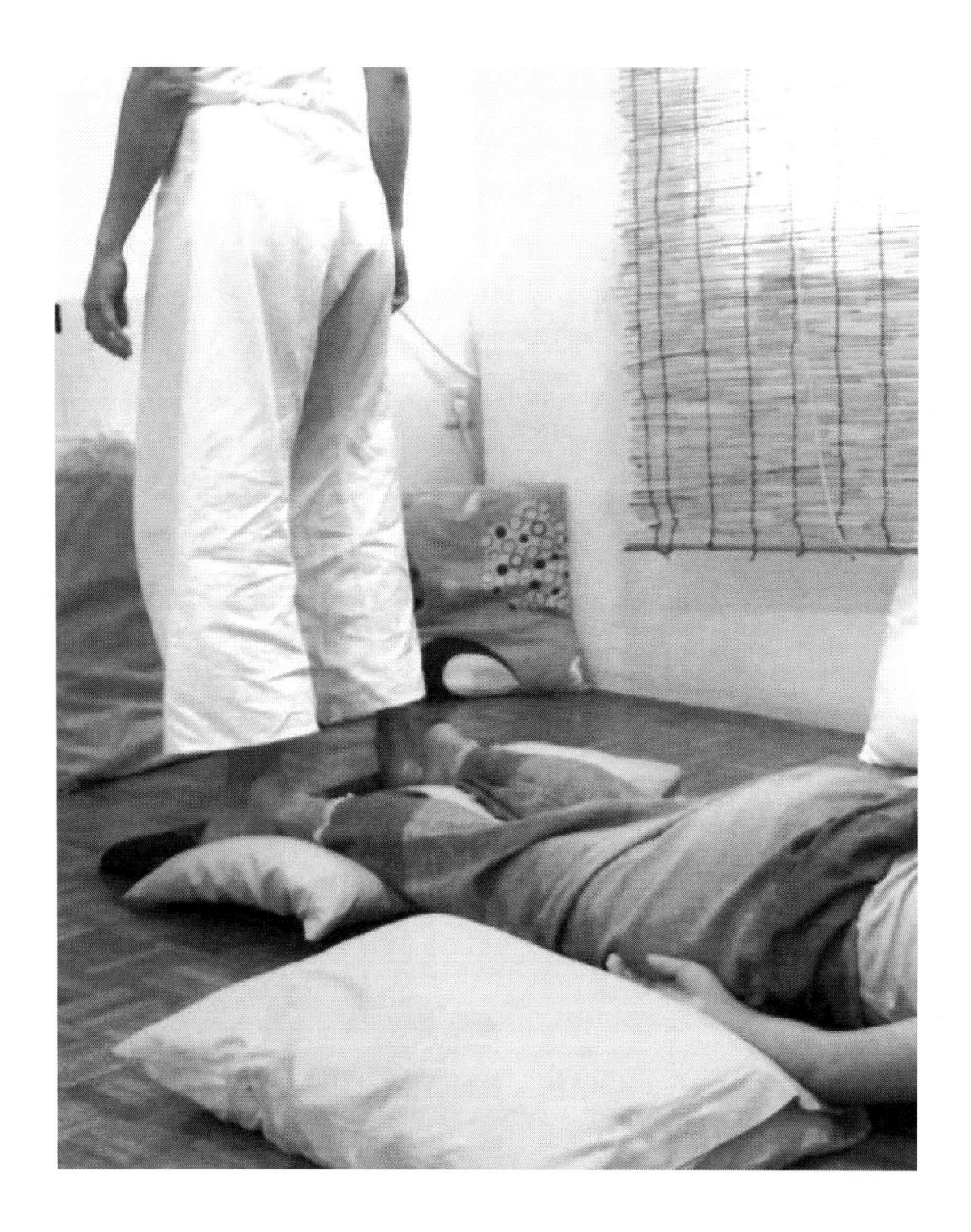

1. Begin by walking with your feet on the receiver's feet. Place the transverse arch of your foot to the receiver's transverse arch.

Walk slowly and smoothly. Repeat about 10 times.

Skip this technique if the client is an osteoporotic woman.

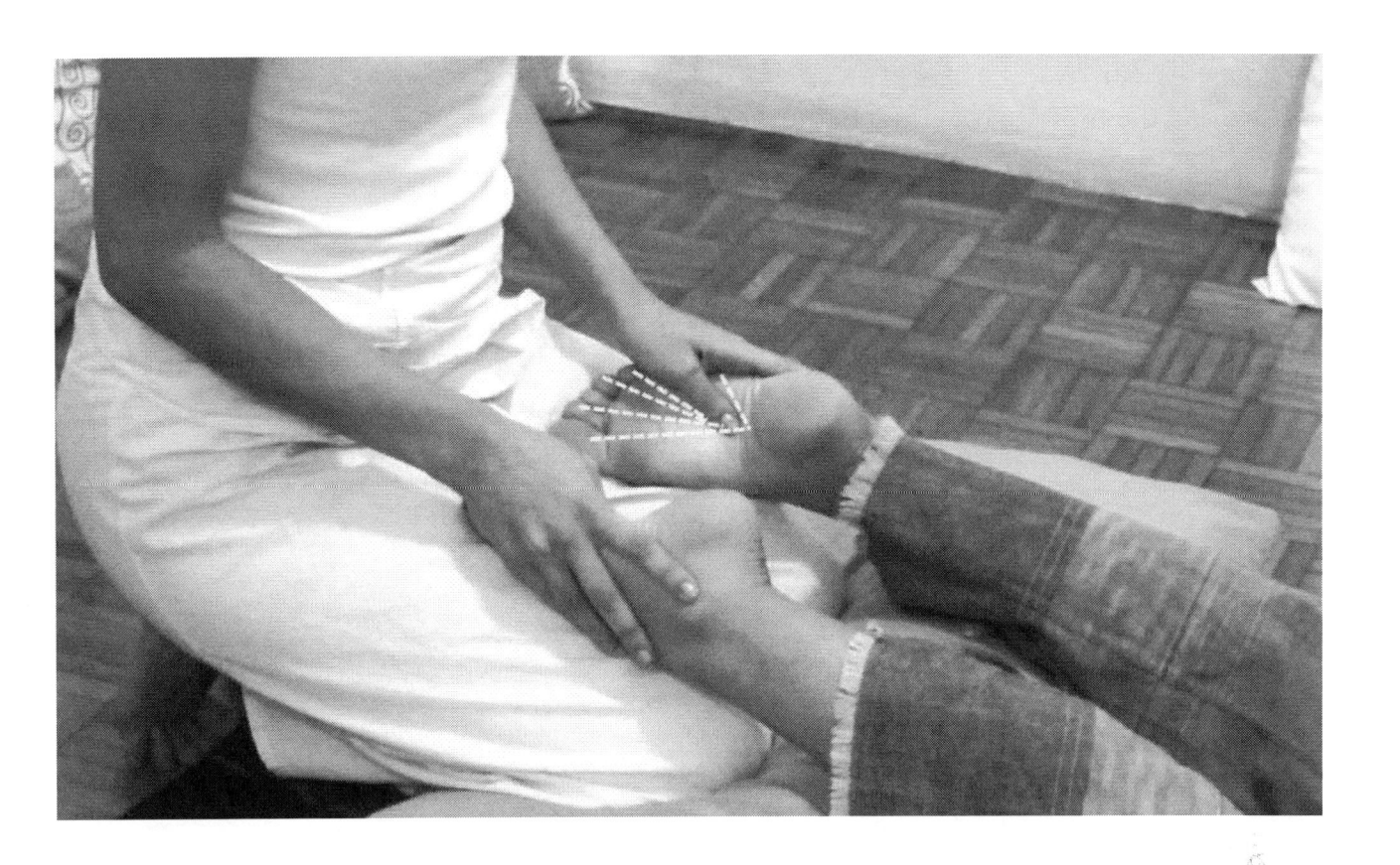

2. Then, place the receiver's feet on your thighs and press the Kalatharee sen lines.

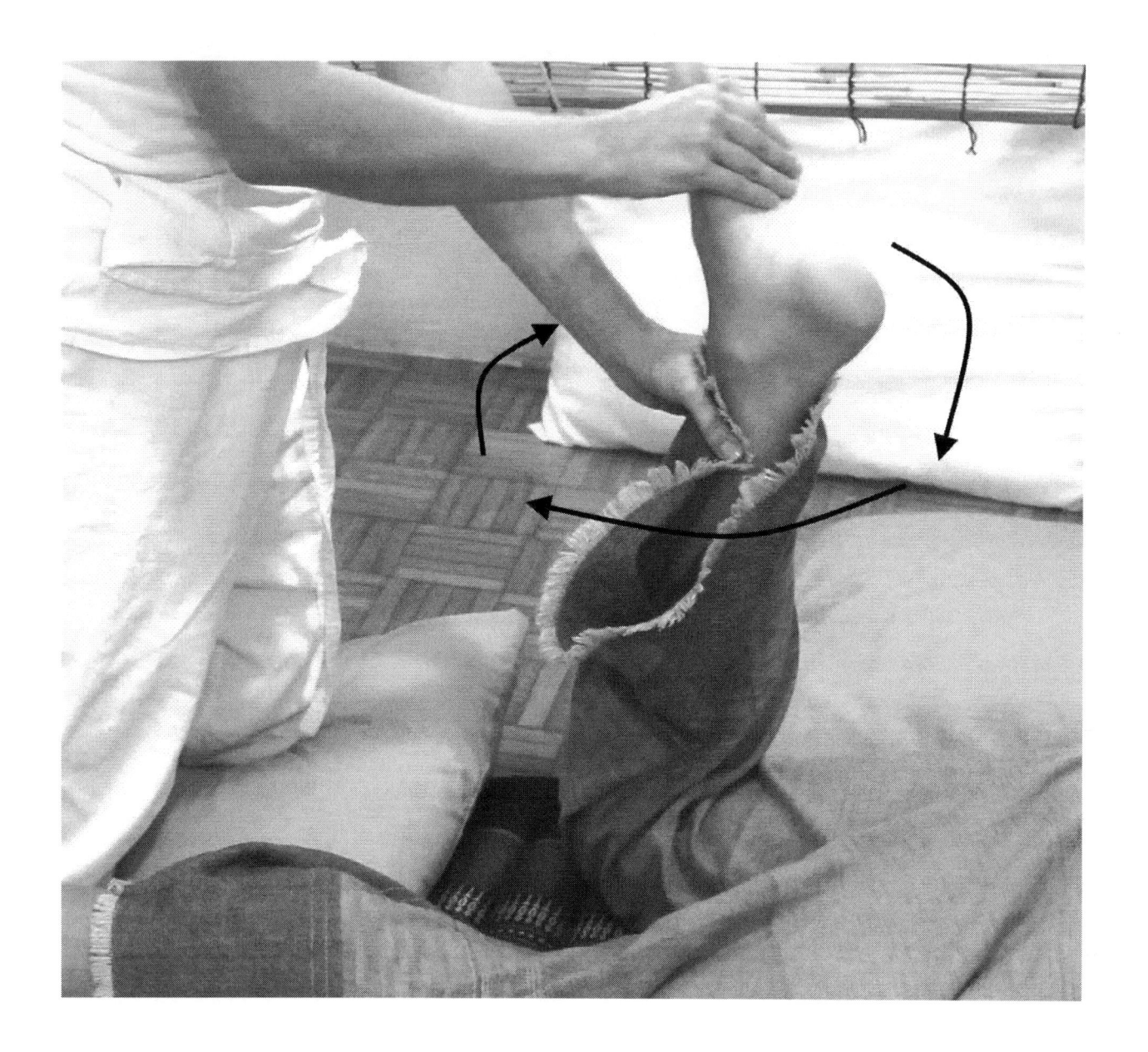

3. You can also rotate the foot joint. Grasp it gently – your grip should be firm but not tense.

Rotate at both directions.

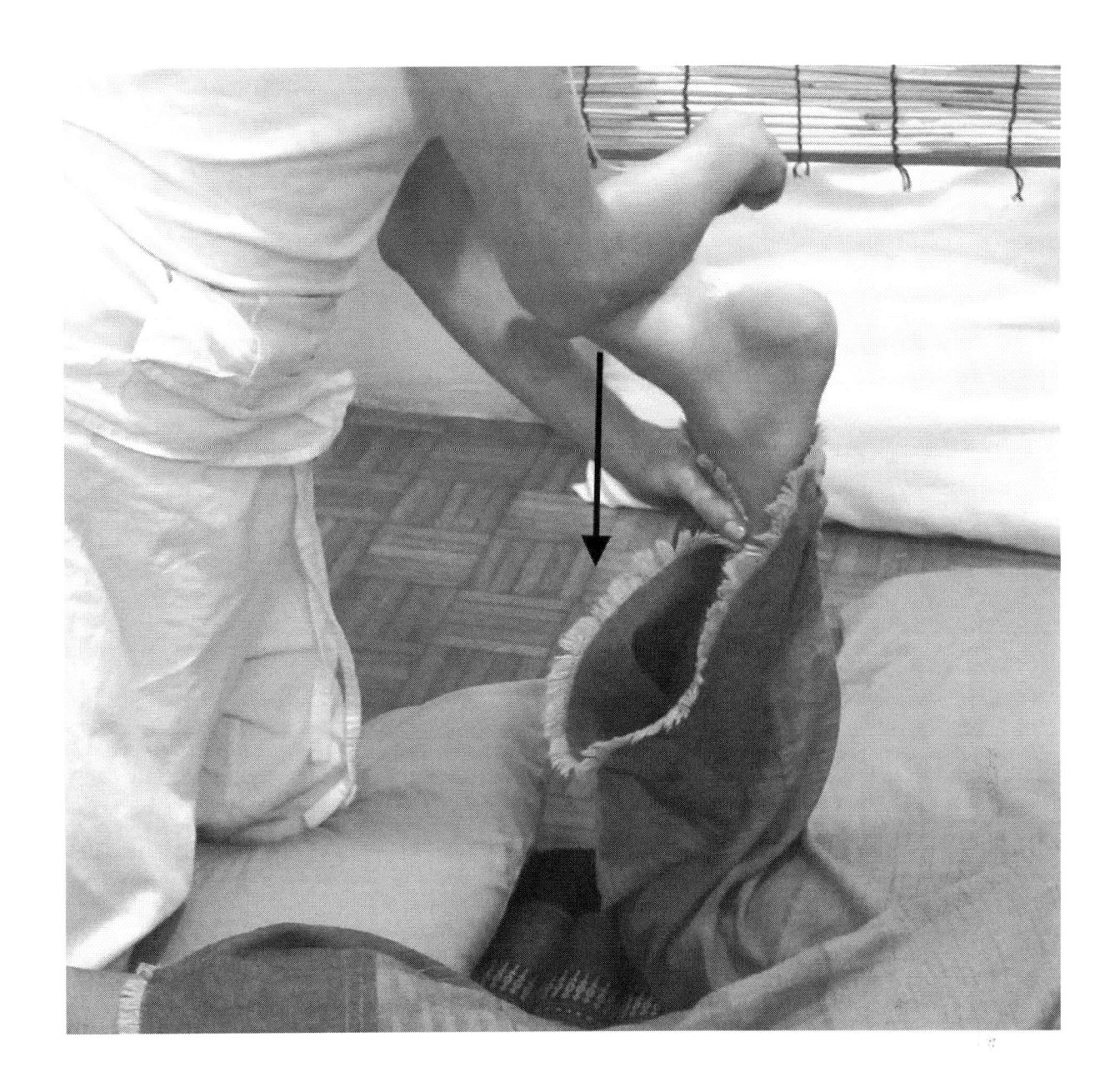

4. Then press the foot downwards with your forearm.

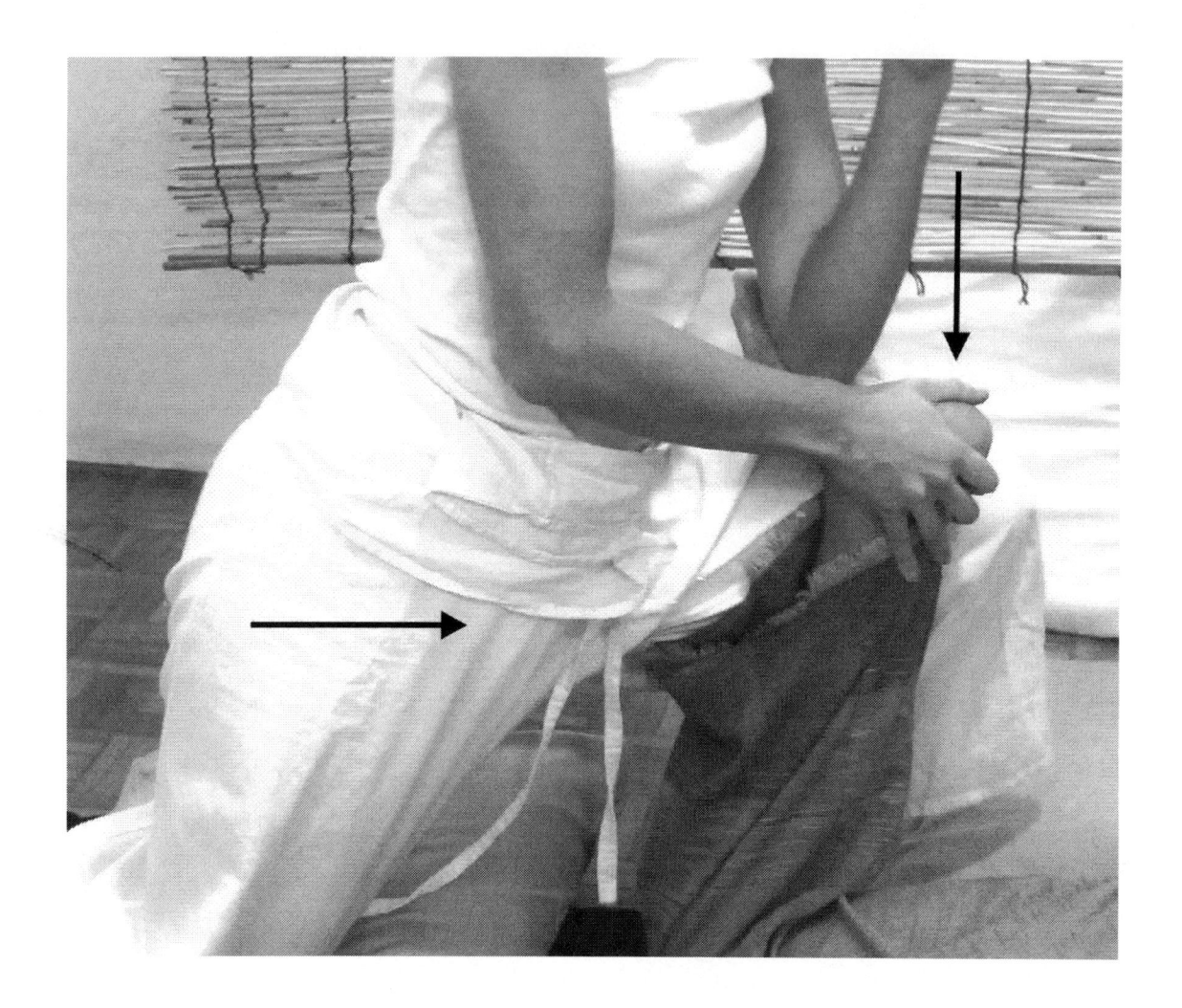

5. You can also place the foot on your thigh, and press it with your elbow. At each press, bring your body closer to the receiver's body (the movement should come from your pelvis).

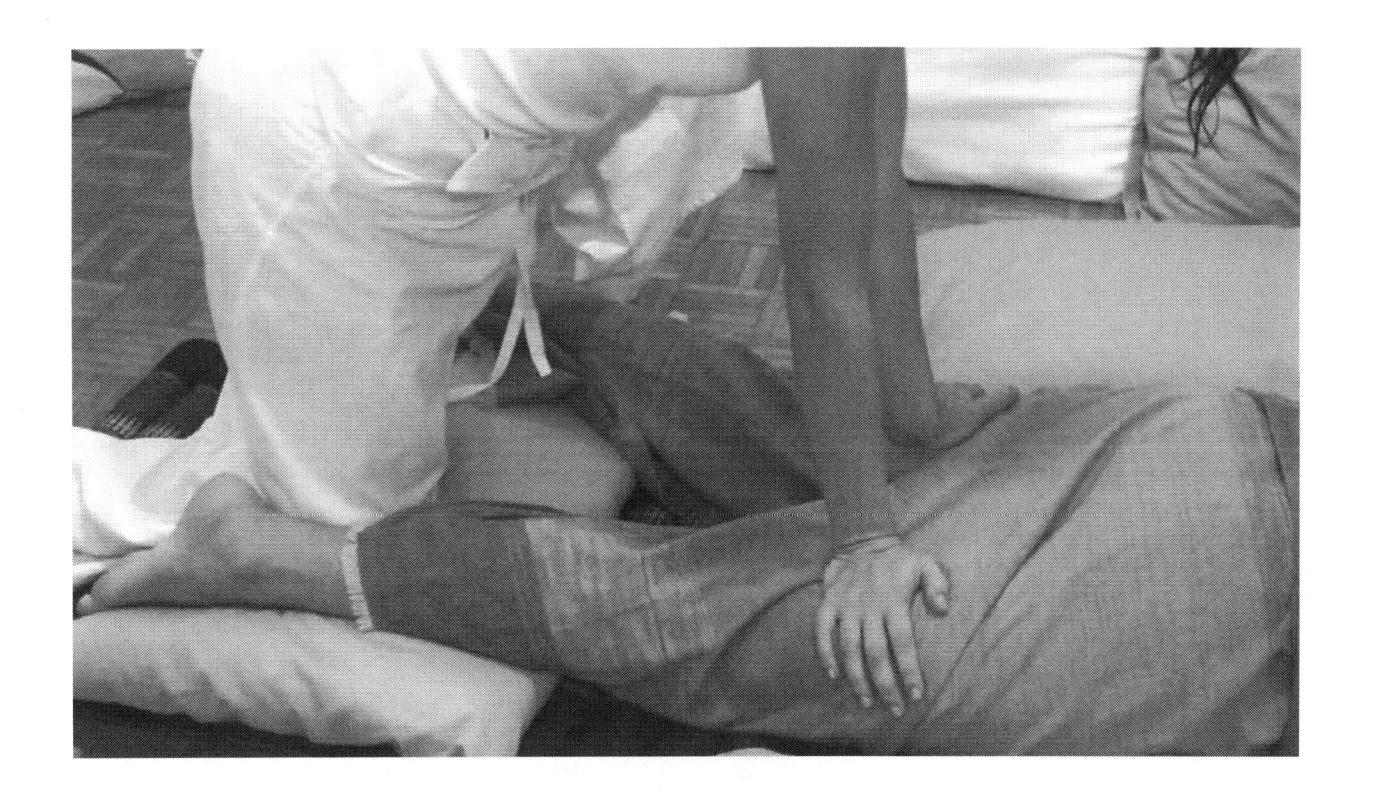

6. Walk with your palms on the Itha & Pingkala Sen line on the legs. Be sure to skip the knee joint. Then, walk on the lines with your thumbs, and again with your palms.

Start from the feet, move upwards and then return to the feet.

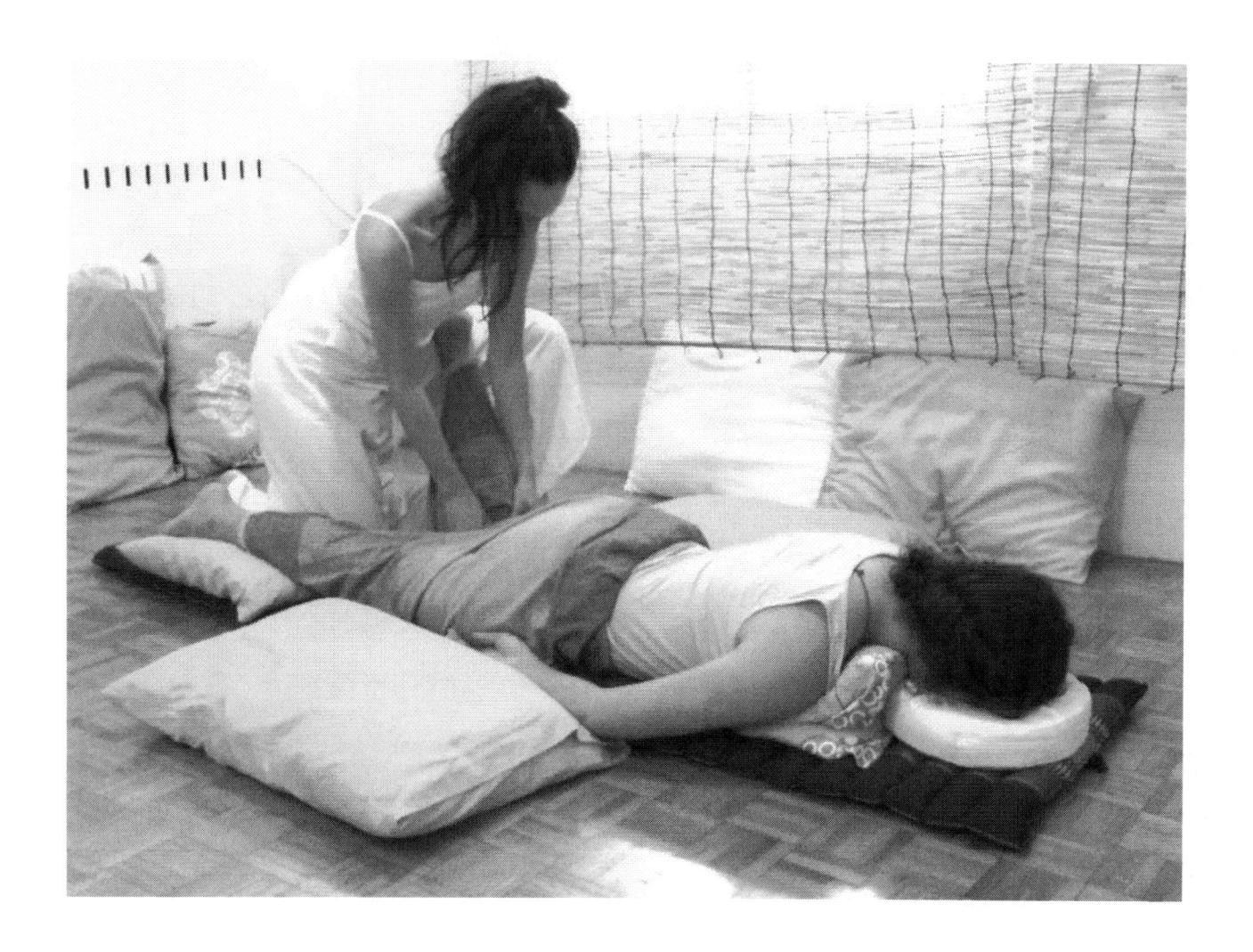

7. Then lift the lower leg and press gently into the popliteal fossa. This is good for lower back pain, and knee pain.

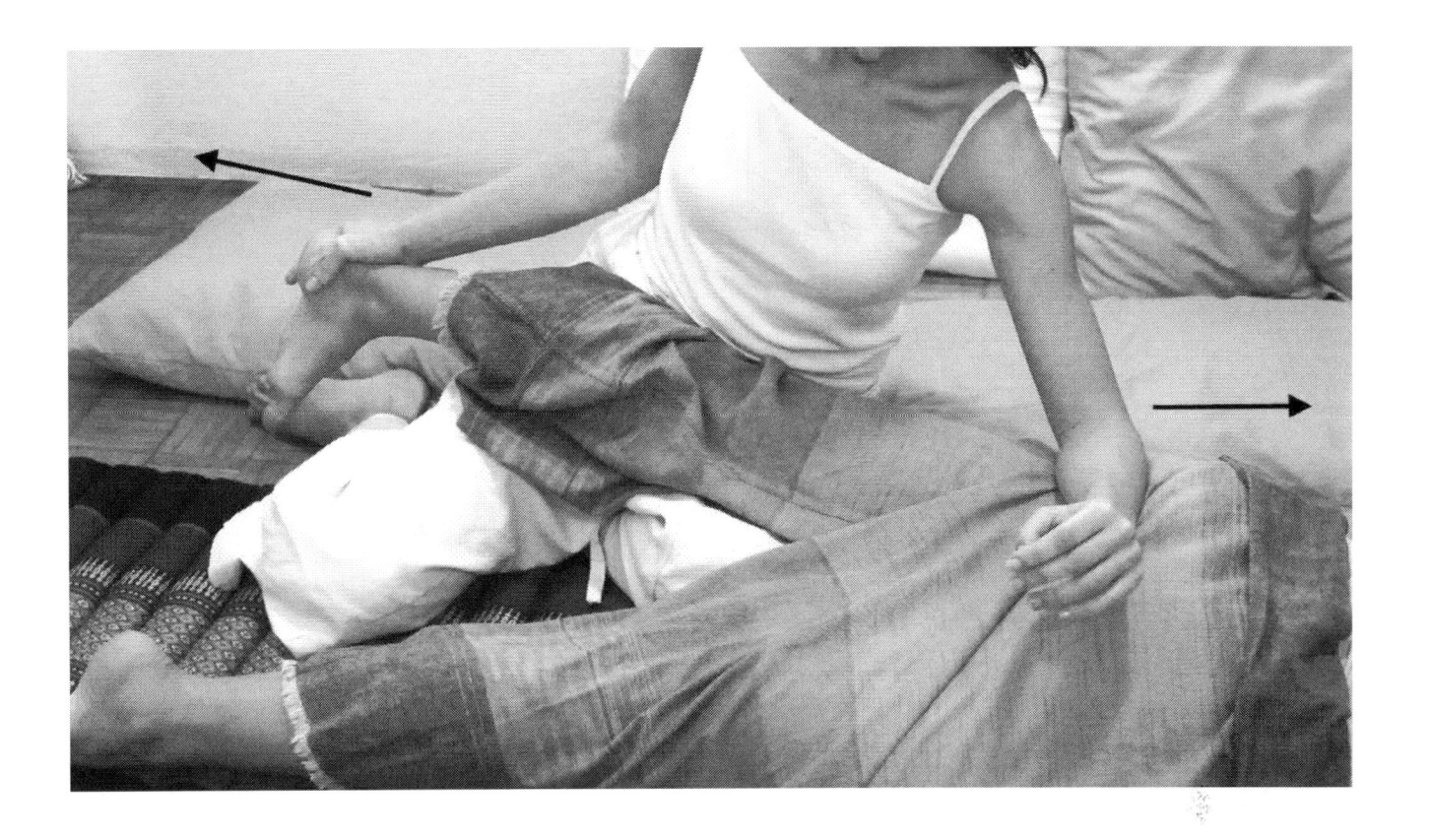

8. Sit down, and place the receiver's leg on your legs. The knee joint should not touch your legs, and should not be squeezed.

Begin by stretching the leg. Place one hand on the receiver's heel, and your forearm under the gluteus muscle. Maintain the stretch for at least 5 seconds.

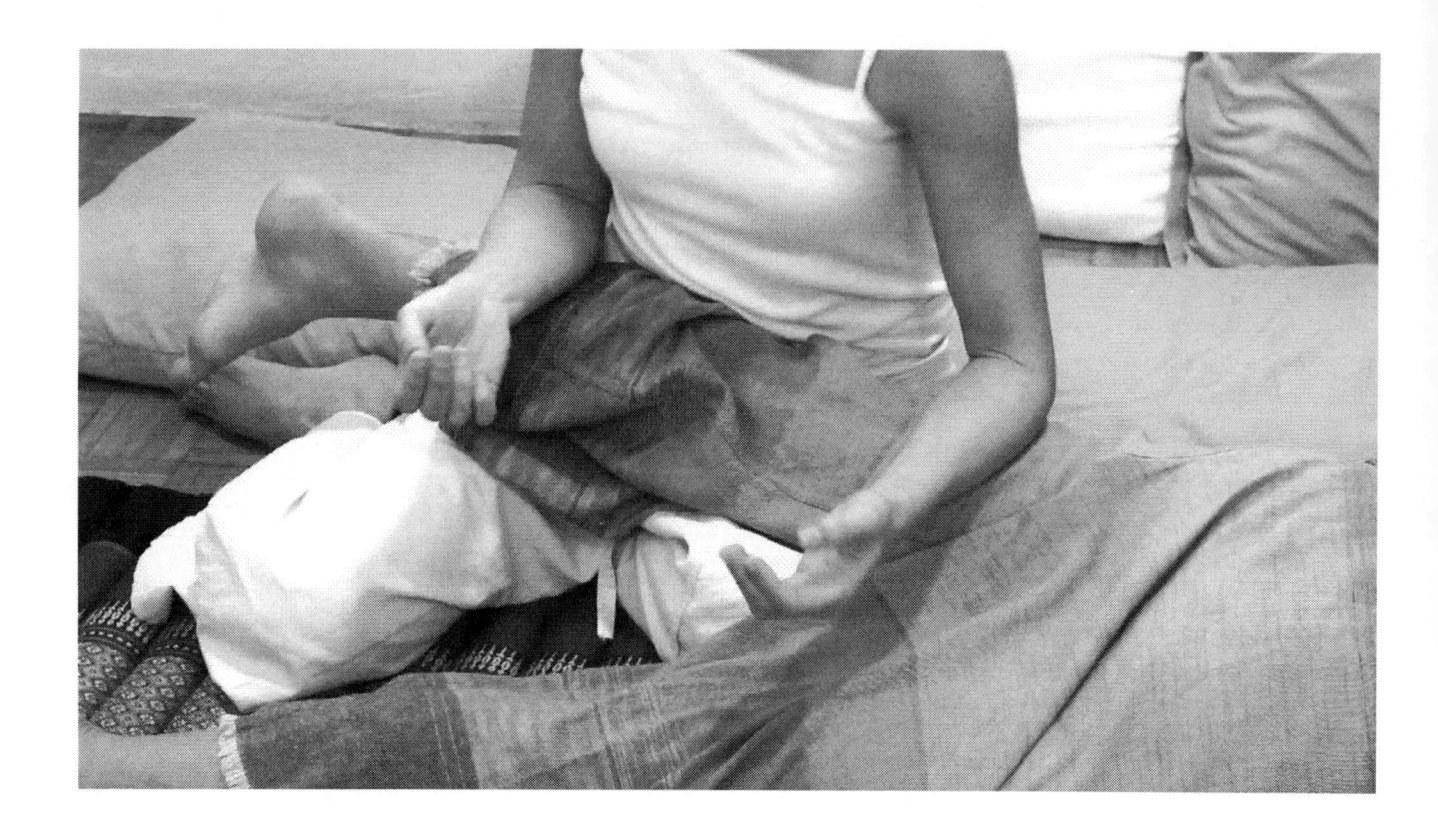

9. ...Then, roll your forearms on the legs. In order to make it easier, use your body weight each time you make a roll.

As always, skip the knee joint. This is a good technique for tight leg muscles and sciatica. Bonus: It can be applied easily in heavier clients, as there are no lifts or pulls.

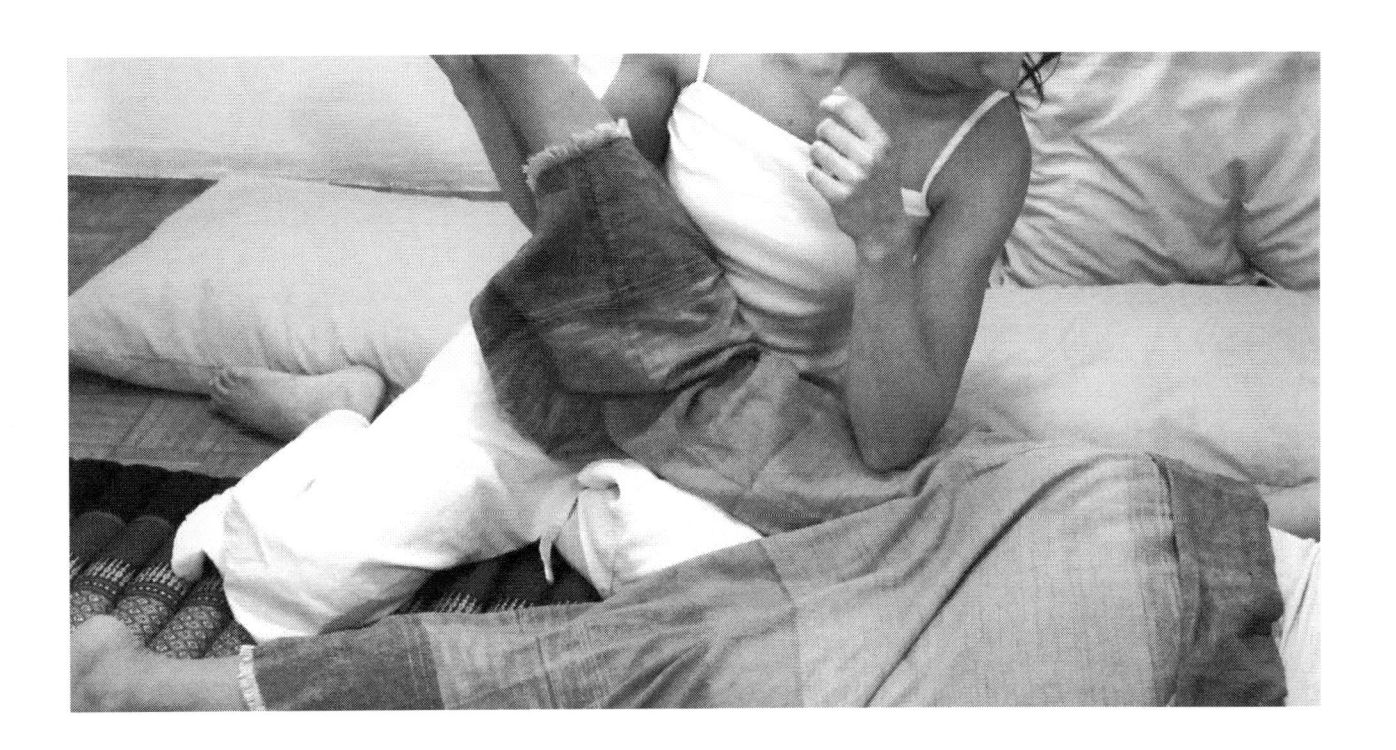

10. You can also lift the lower leg and work with your elbow. Do circular movements and presses. Do not apply too much pressure – remember that the elbow is a strong tool!

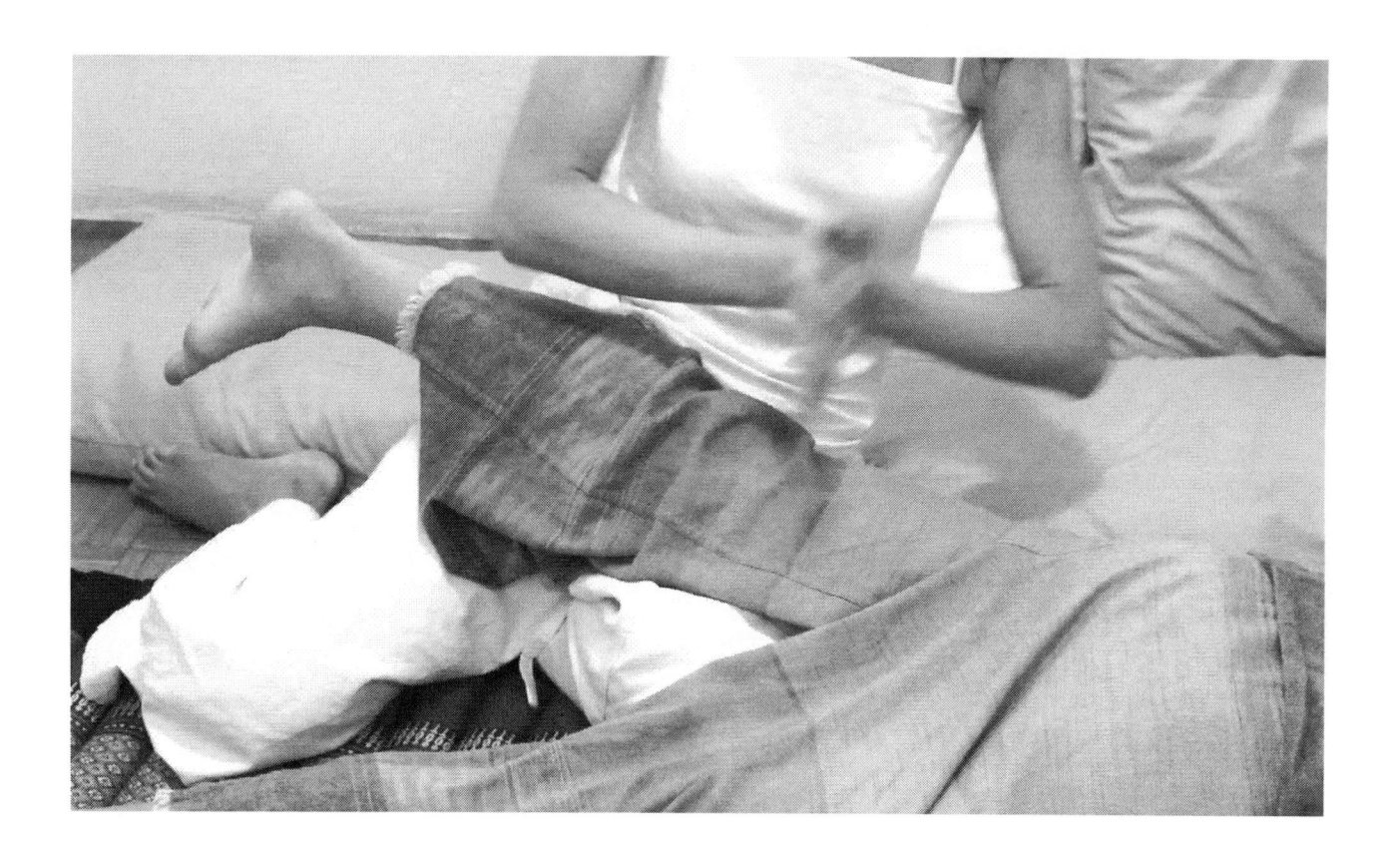

11. Tapping techniques like this one, are also helpful for muscular tension. Do the Thai Slap and the typical Swedish massage tapotement.

How to do the Thai Slap Technique

*This is one of the most characteristic tapotement techniques of Traditional Thai Massage.
In order to perform it properly:*

*1. Join palms.
2. Keep fingers apart.
3. Maintain loose wrists - Release all tension from your wrists.
4. Join the heels of your hands - however, do not join the wrist joints.
5. Then, let your hands fall, performing the slap. You should hear the typical clapping sound.*

It is important to let go of all tension throughout the technique.

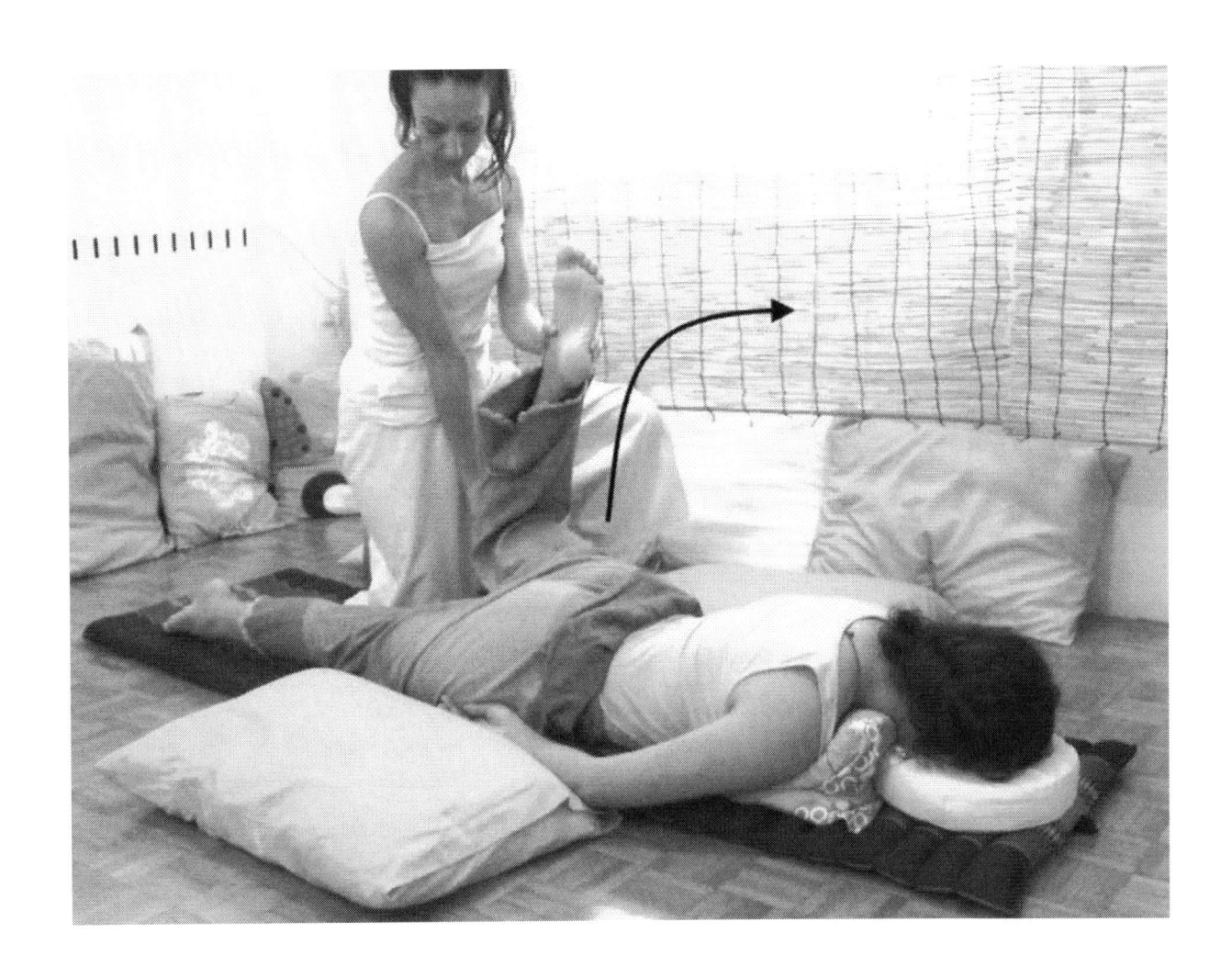

12. Grasp the receiver's leg from her knee, and lift it upwards.

Skip this and the following technique if the receiver has any degenerative knee problem, spinal stenosis and / or lordosis.

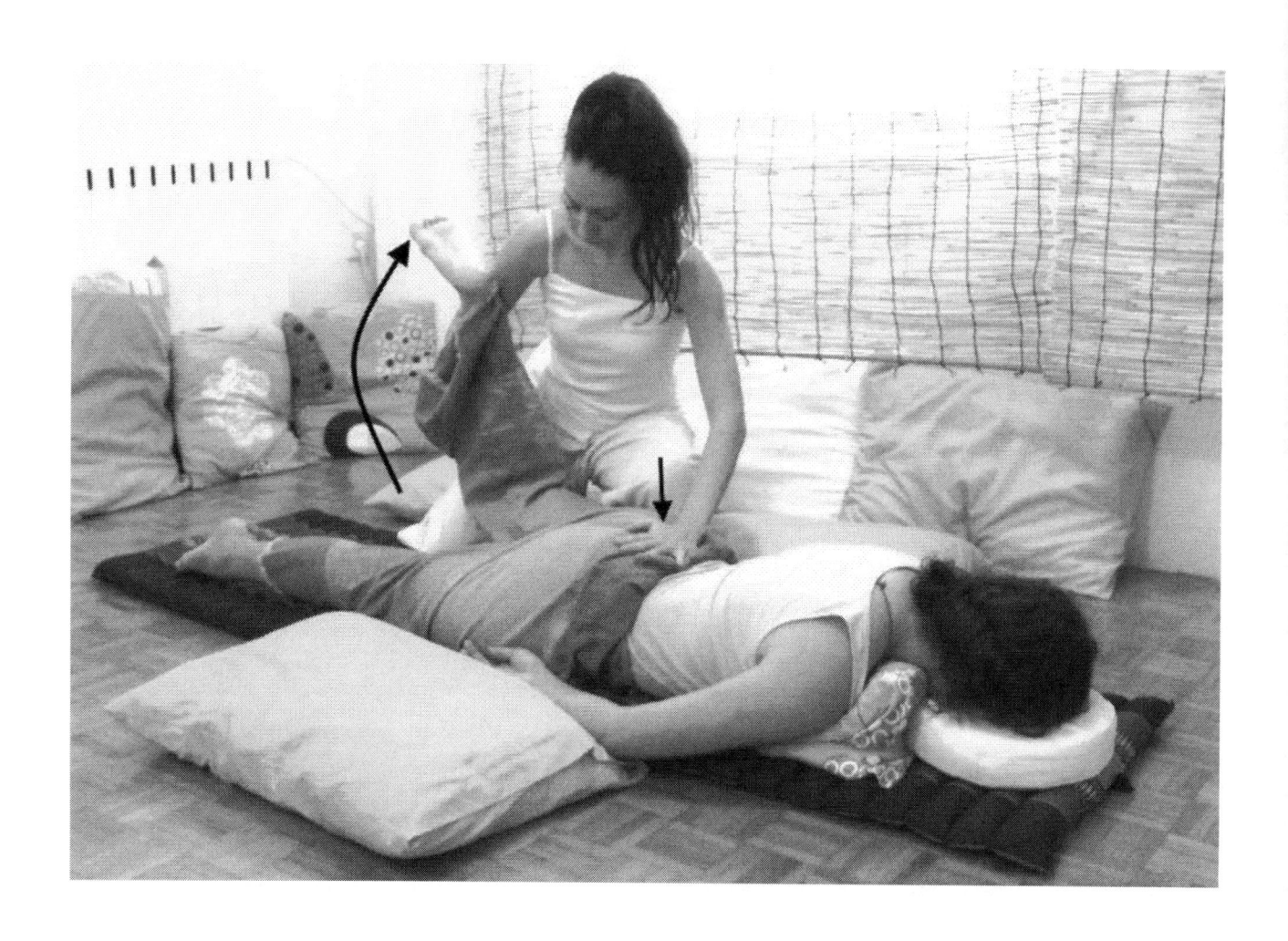

13. Then repeat the technique, with your hand placed on the receiver's sacrum.

This technique has similarities with the typical orthopedic Femoral Nerve Stretch test or Mackiewicz sign – if it is positive (that is, if the receiver experiences pain in the lumbar spine) it may mean that the nerves in the 3rd – 4th lumbar vertebrae are compressed.

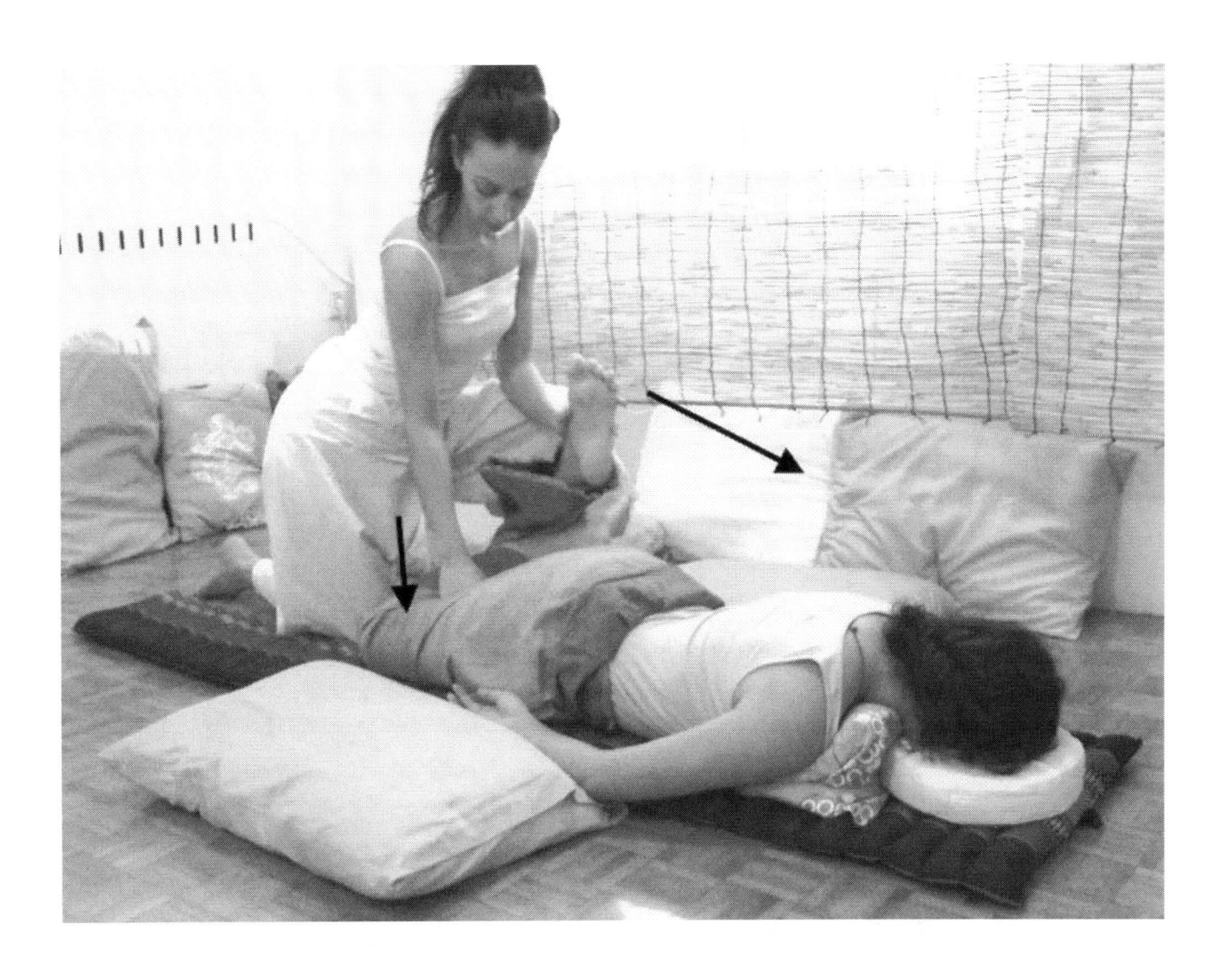

14. Now lock the receiver's leg in her knee joint, grasp her foot, and simultaneously press the posterior thigh muscles with your fist. Each time you press the thigh, bring her other leg and your body towards her head – move from your pelvis.

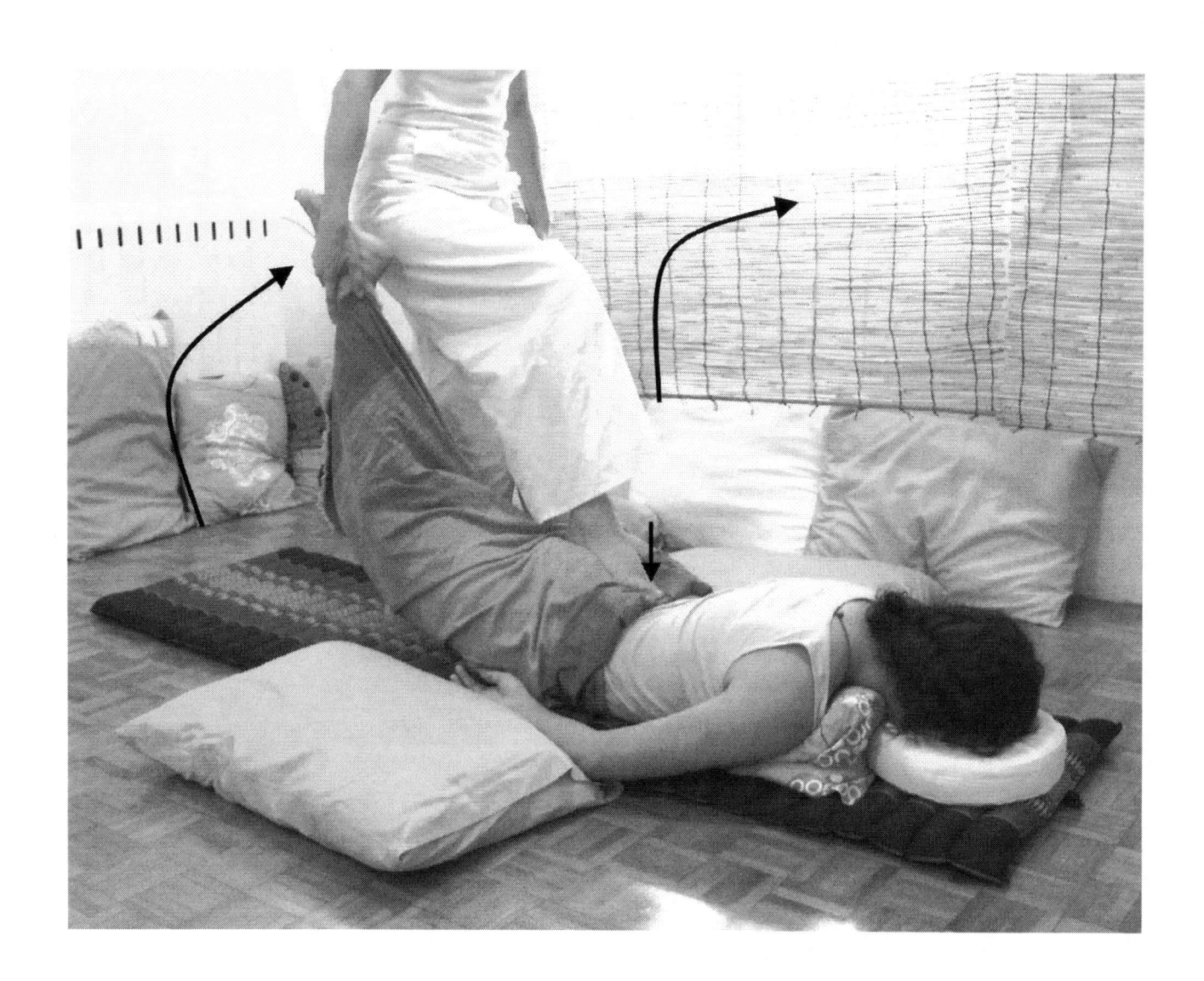

15. Lift the receiver's legs from the mat, and place your foot gently on her sacrum. Then bring her legs upwards, always respecting the body's limits.

This technique is a passive application of the yogic asana *Salabhasana*.

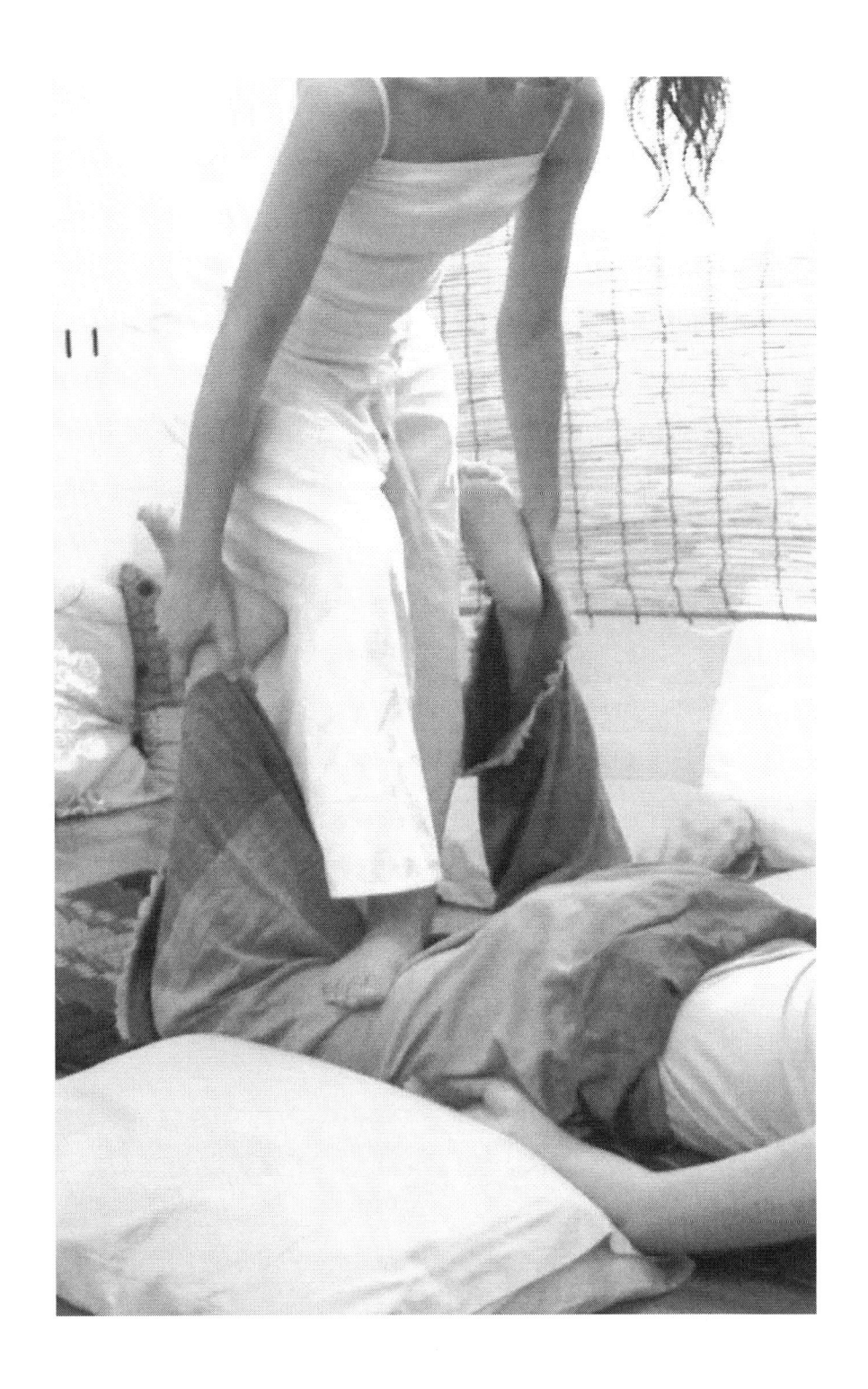

16. You can also press the receiver's posterior thigh muscles with your feet. Then let the receiver's legs down gently.

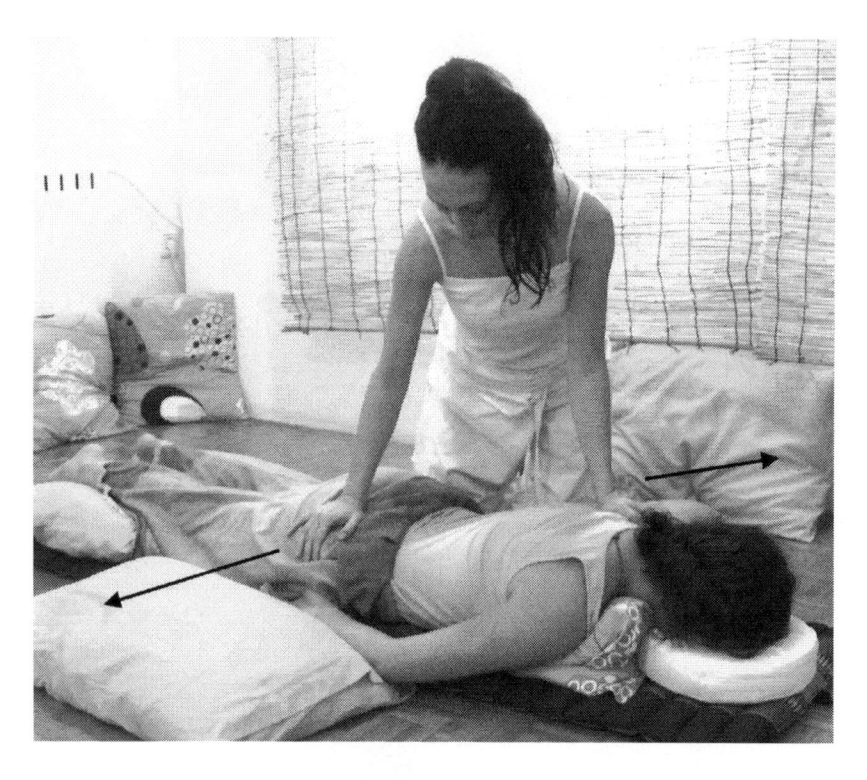

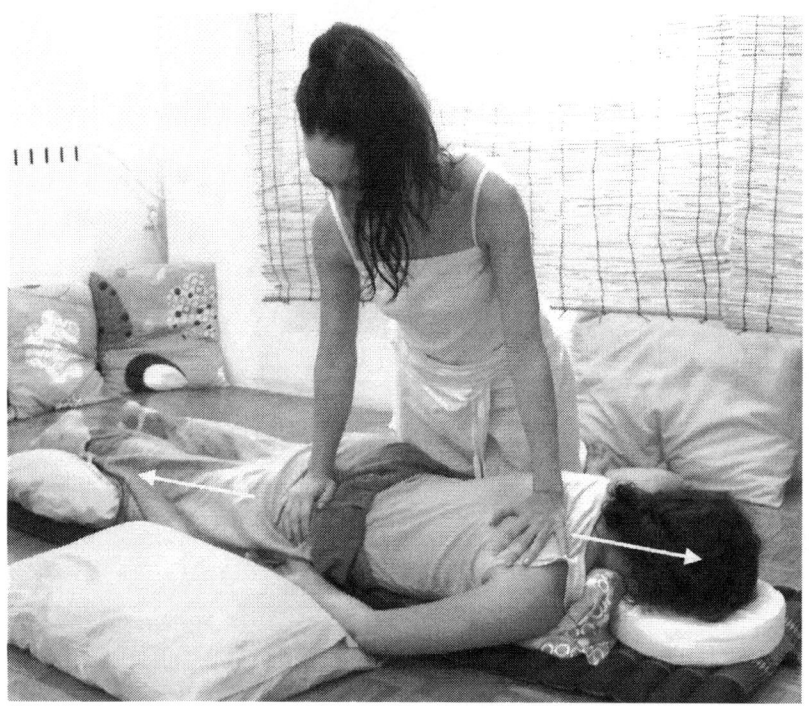

17. It is time to start working on the back! Begin by stretching the back. Place one hand next to the shoulder blade, and one hand on the gluteus muscle. Upon exhalation, use your body weight in order to apply the stretch.

Do four stretches on the back – two one the same side, and two on opposite sides. This is Step 1 (and 5) of *Jap Sen*.

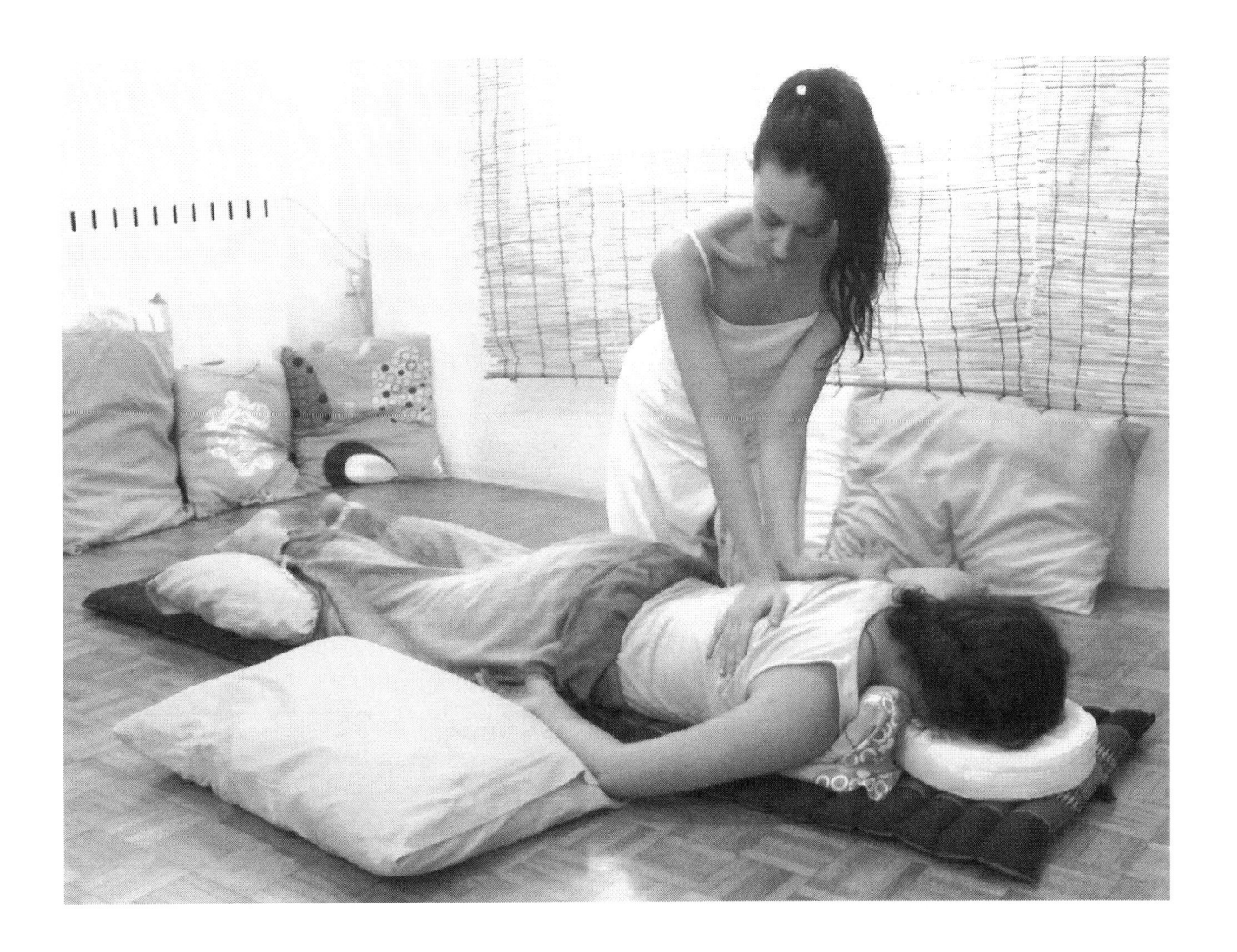

18. Then, start working on the Itha and Pingkala sen lines on the back. Do palm presses next to the spine. Start from the lower back, proceed towards the thoracic spine, and return all the way down.

This is Step 2 (and 4) of Jap Sen.

Never press on the scapula. Work 1.5 cm away from the spine.

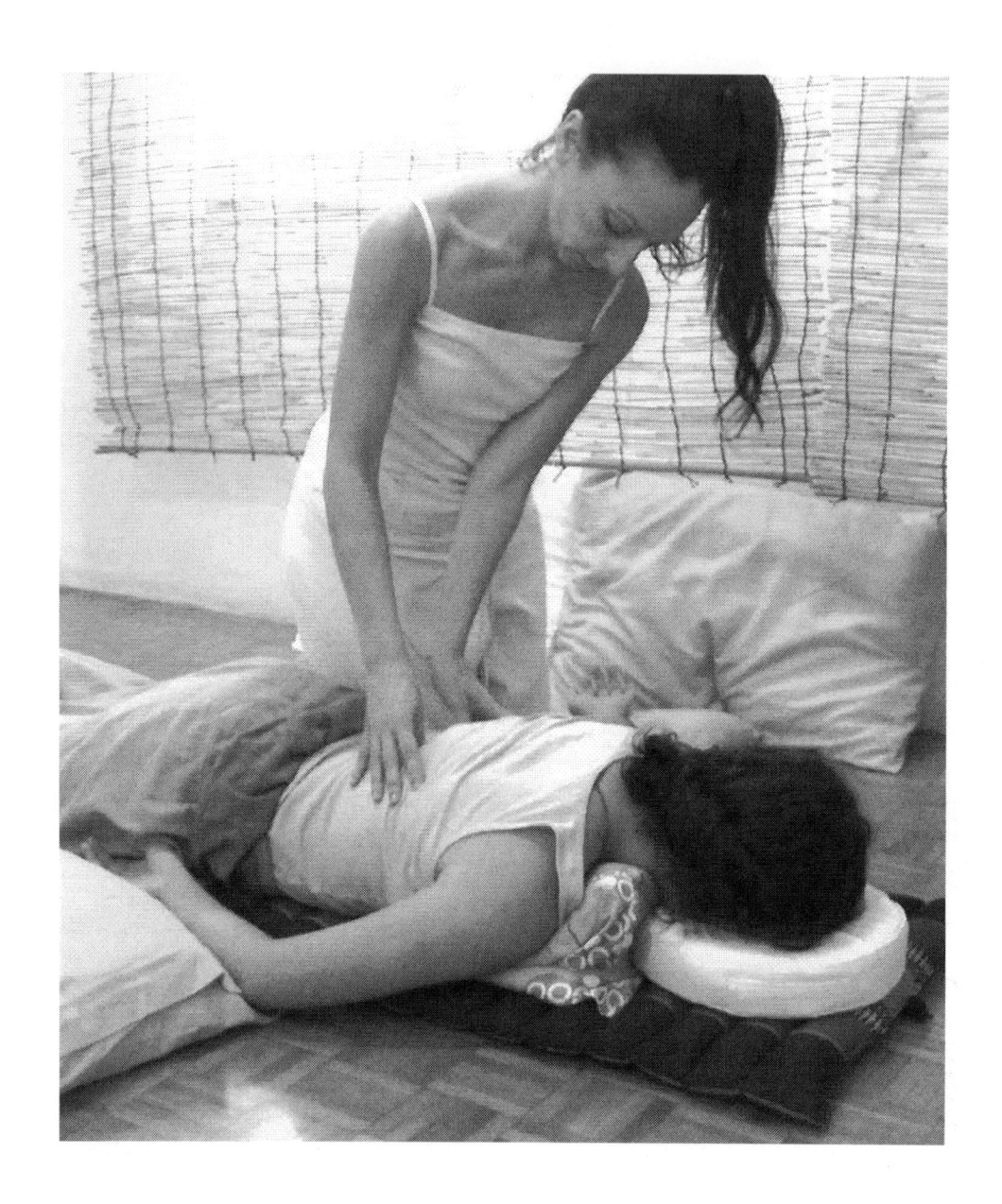

Then do thumb presses on the *Itha & Pingkala Sen* lines on the back. Work your way up the 7th cervical vertebra.

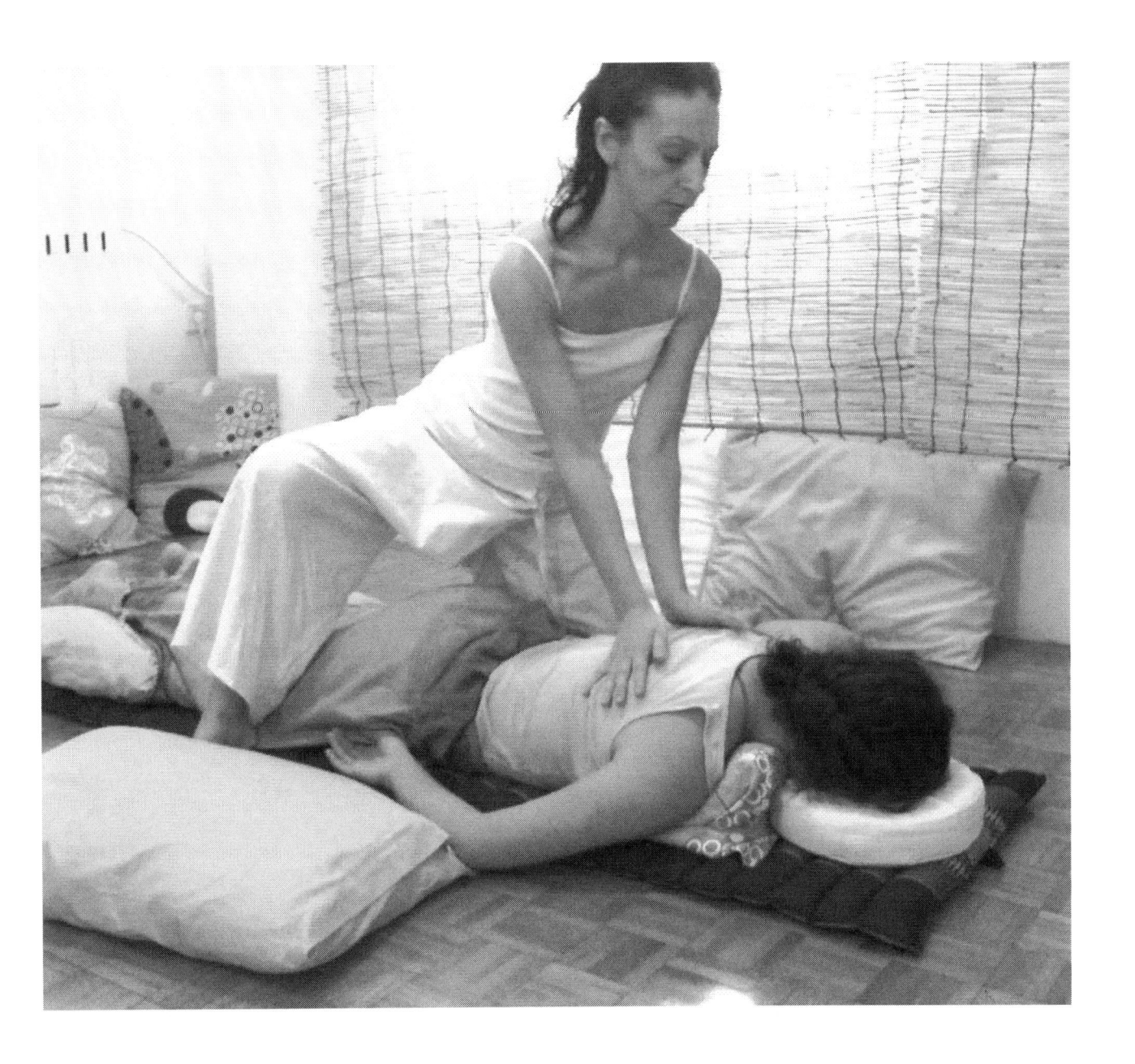

19. You can also work on the back from this position – actually, this allows you to use your body weight more efficiently.

Note: Your pelvis should maintain a professional distance from the body of your client!

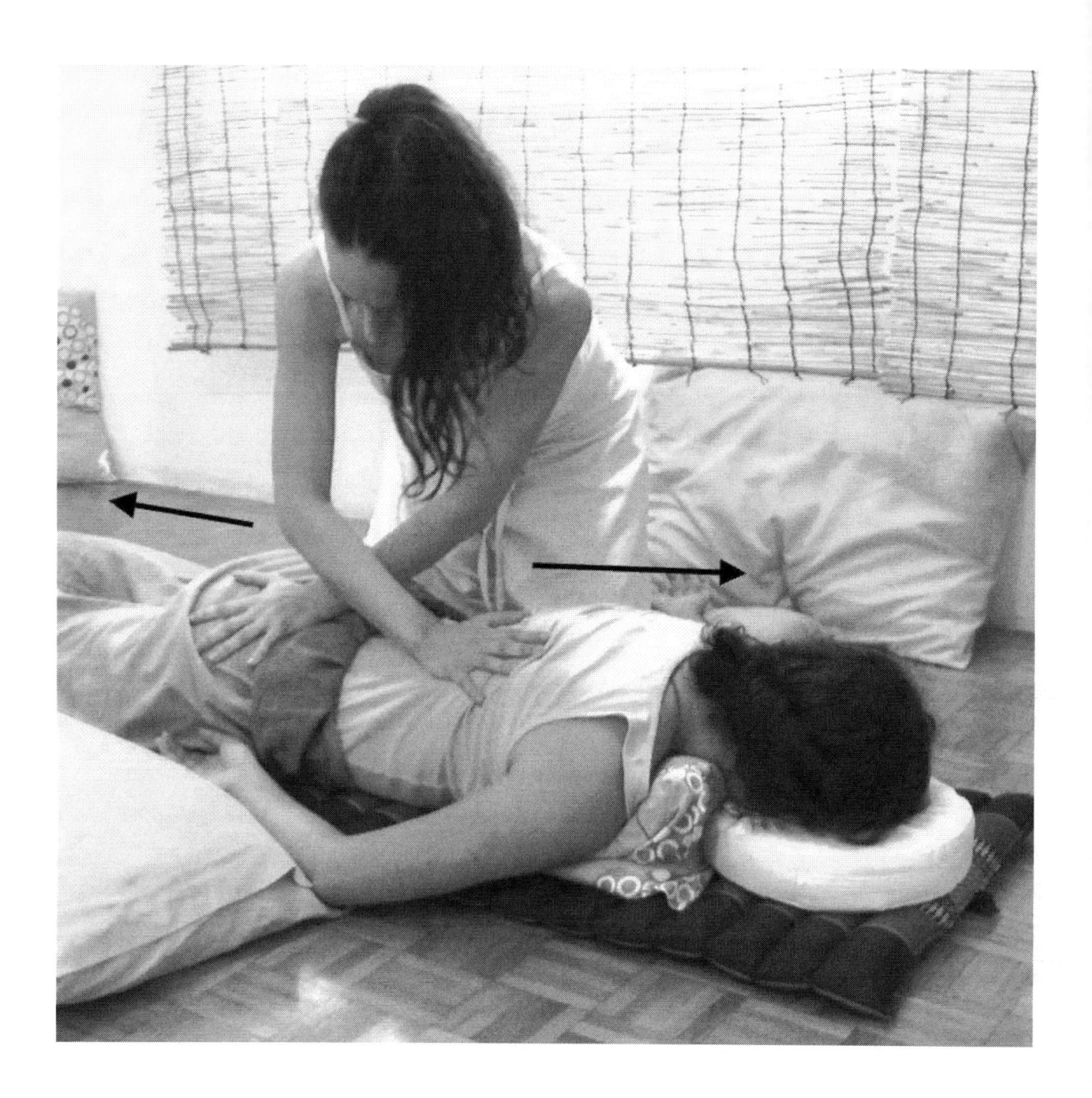

20. This is a good technique for the lumbar spine. Just cross your arms, and place one hand on the sacrum and one on the end of the thoracic spine. Breathe out and stretch gently.

Discs like decompression, and this technique gives them space!

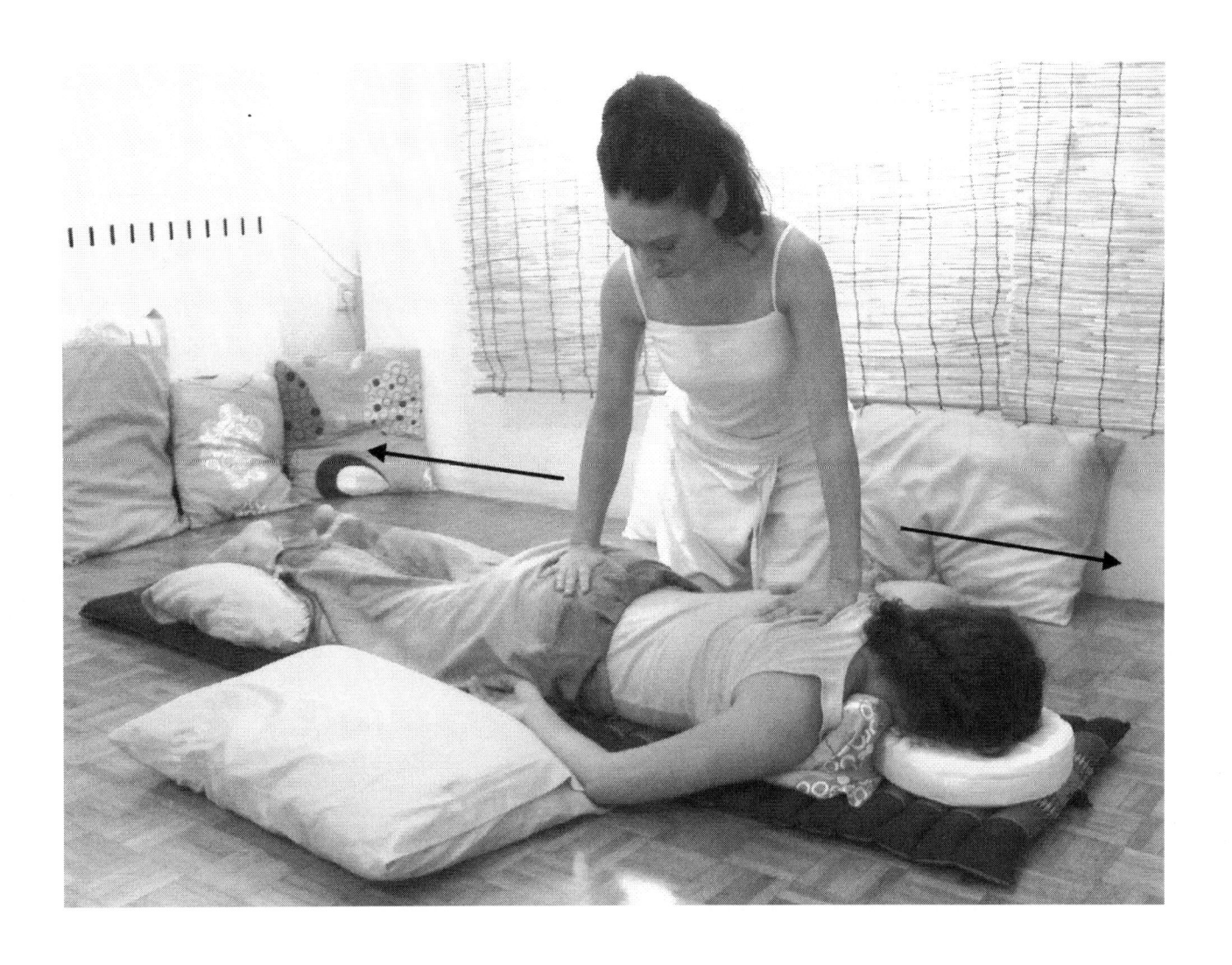

21. You can also perform the same technique without crossing your arms – however, this stretch is not as efficient as the one with crossed arms, because crossing your arms allows more leverage.

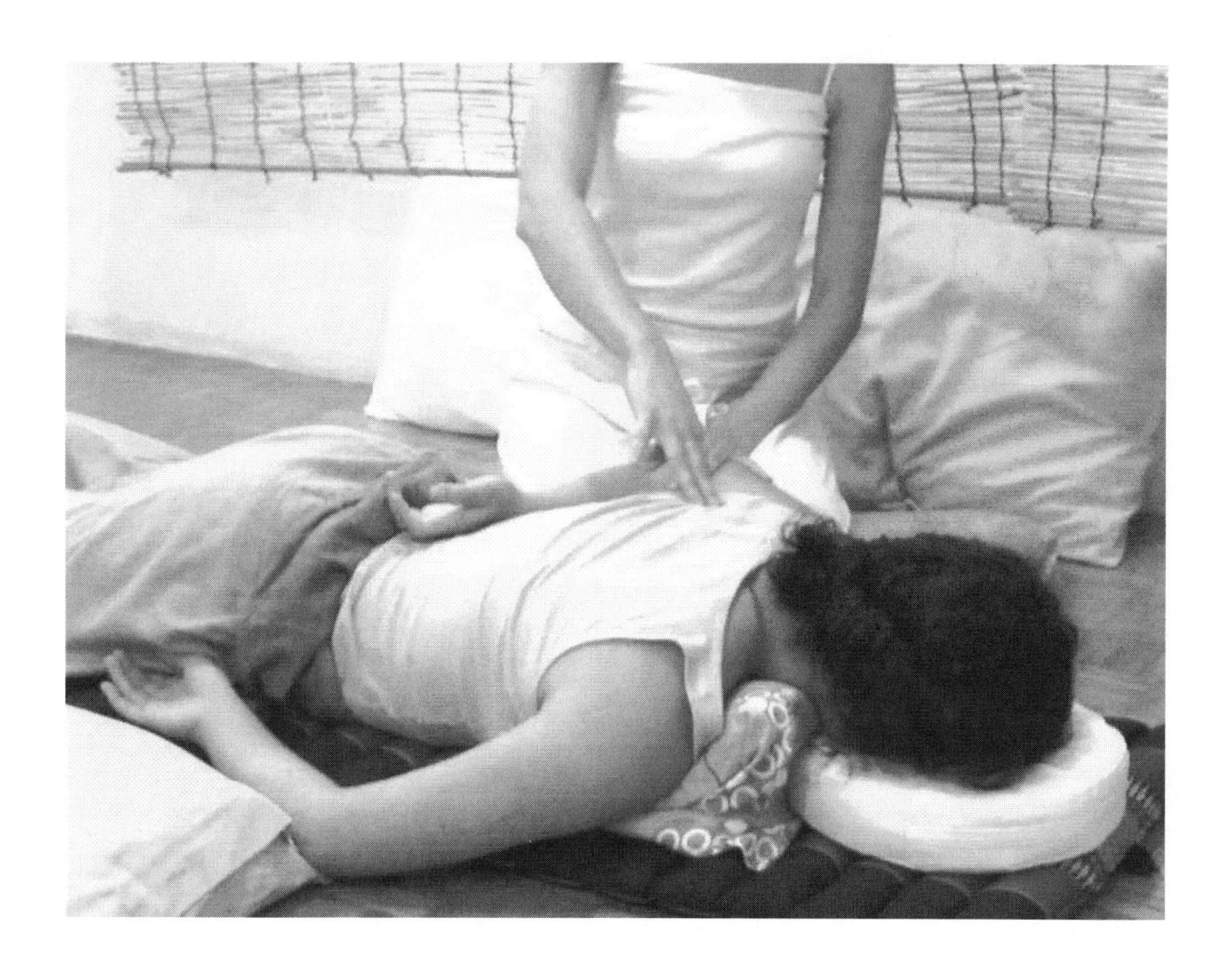

22. Then kneel next to the receiver, and do massage work next to her shoulder blade. Do circular friction and deep tissue (transverse friction).

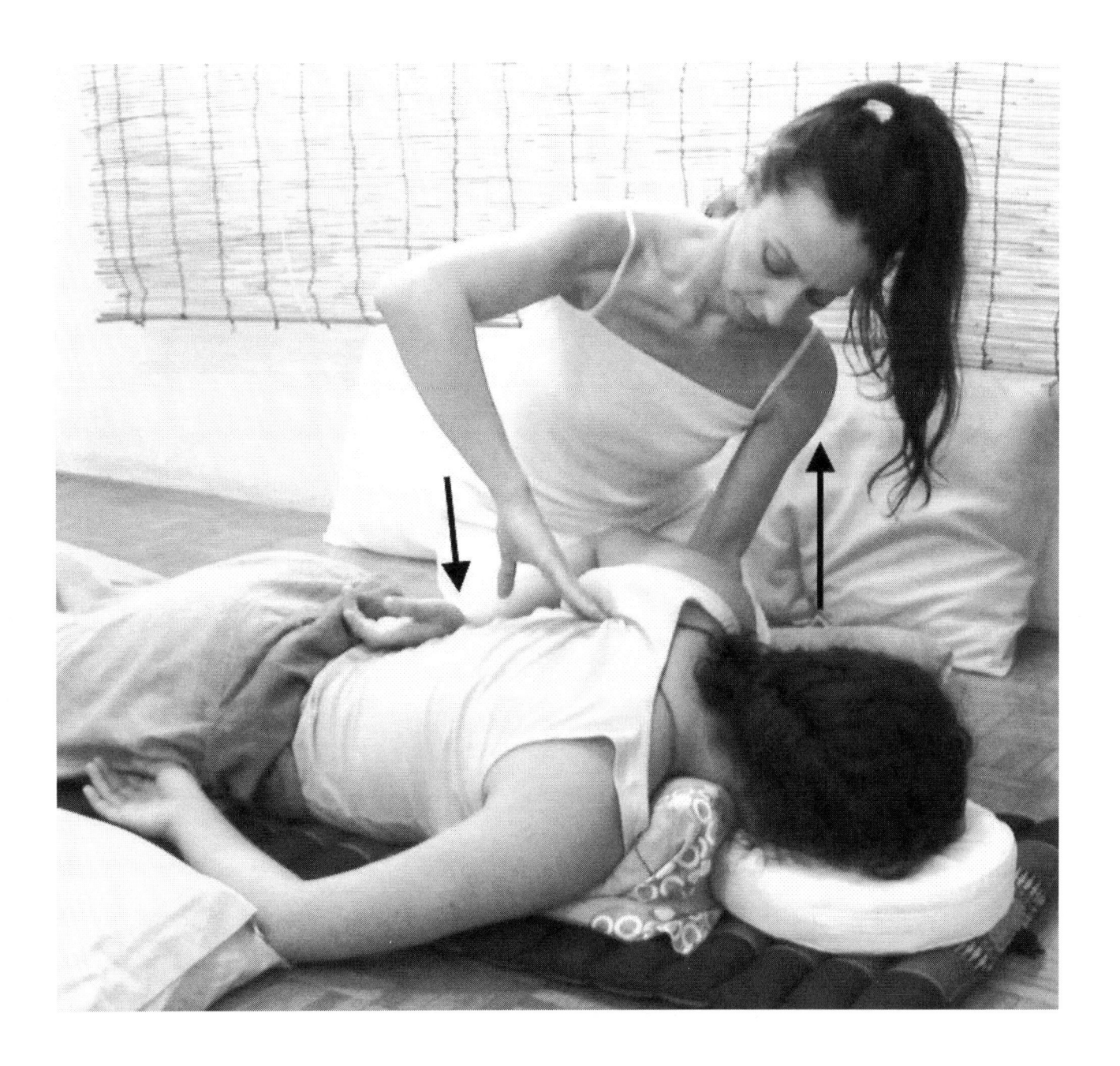

23. You can also place your fingers inside the shoulder blade, simultaneously lifting her shoulder. Do this on 3-4 spots around the scapula.

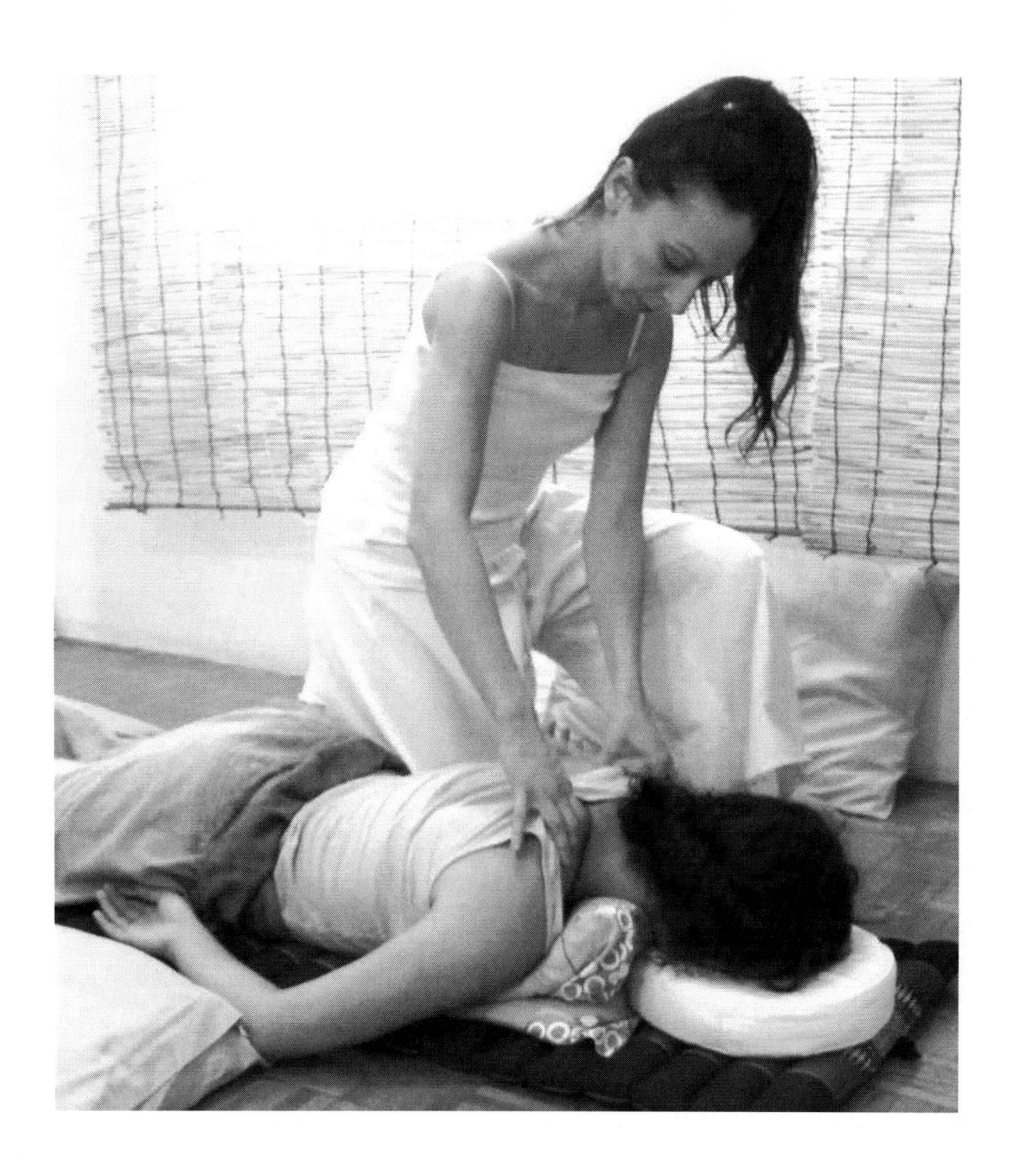

24. Then do some nice kneading on the shoulders. This is the typical Swedish massage kneading, and works very well as a dry massage technique as well.

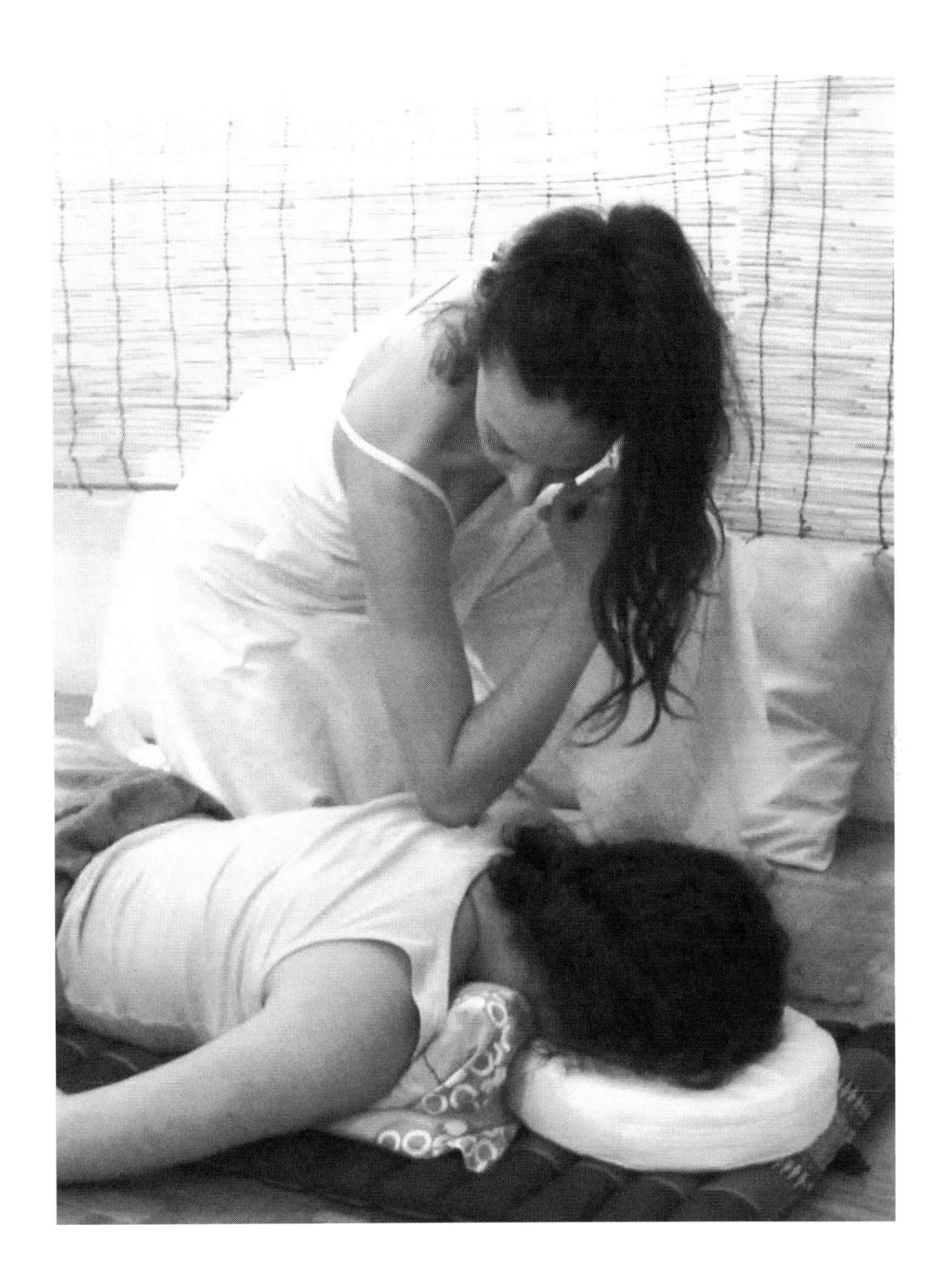

25. You can also use your elbow, but be careful not to press too strongly. Actually, the elbow can be a quite precise tool, and is always valuable in dry massage.

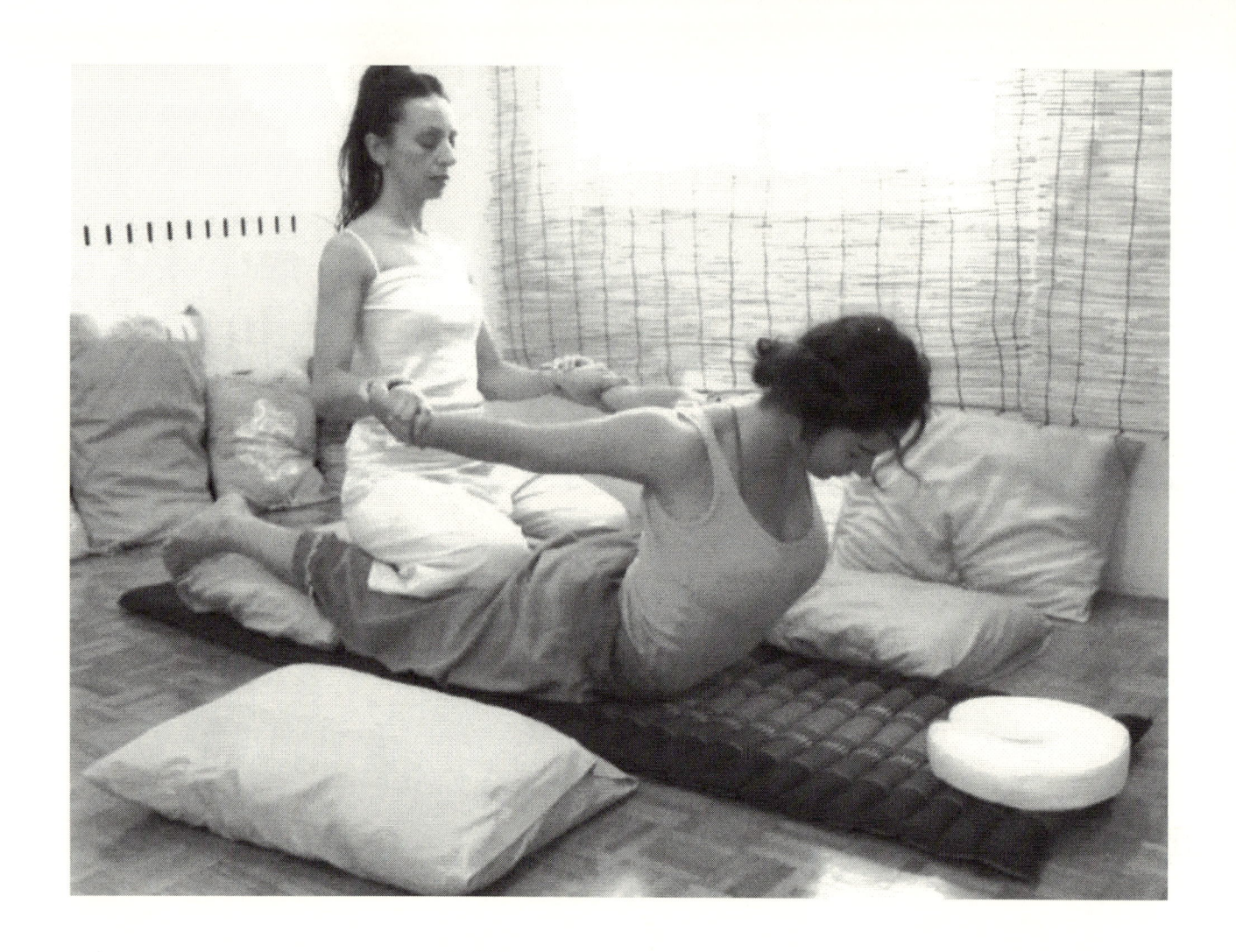

26. Now we will see some typical Thai Massage stretches. In order to do the "cobra", kneel on the receiver's thighs, grasp her arms, and lift her torso as she exhales.

This is a passive application of the yogic asana *Bhujaungasana*.

It "opens" the thorax, and thus is great for breathing disorders and kyphosis. However, it should not be applied to clients who have spinal stenosis.

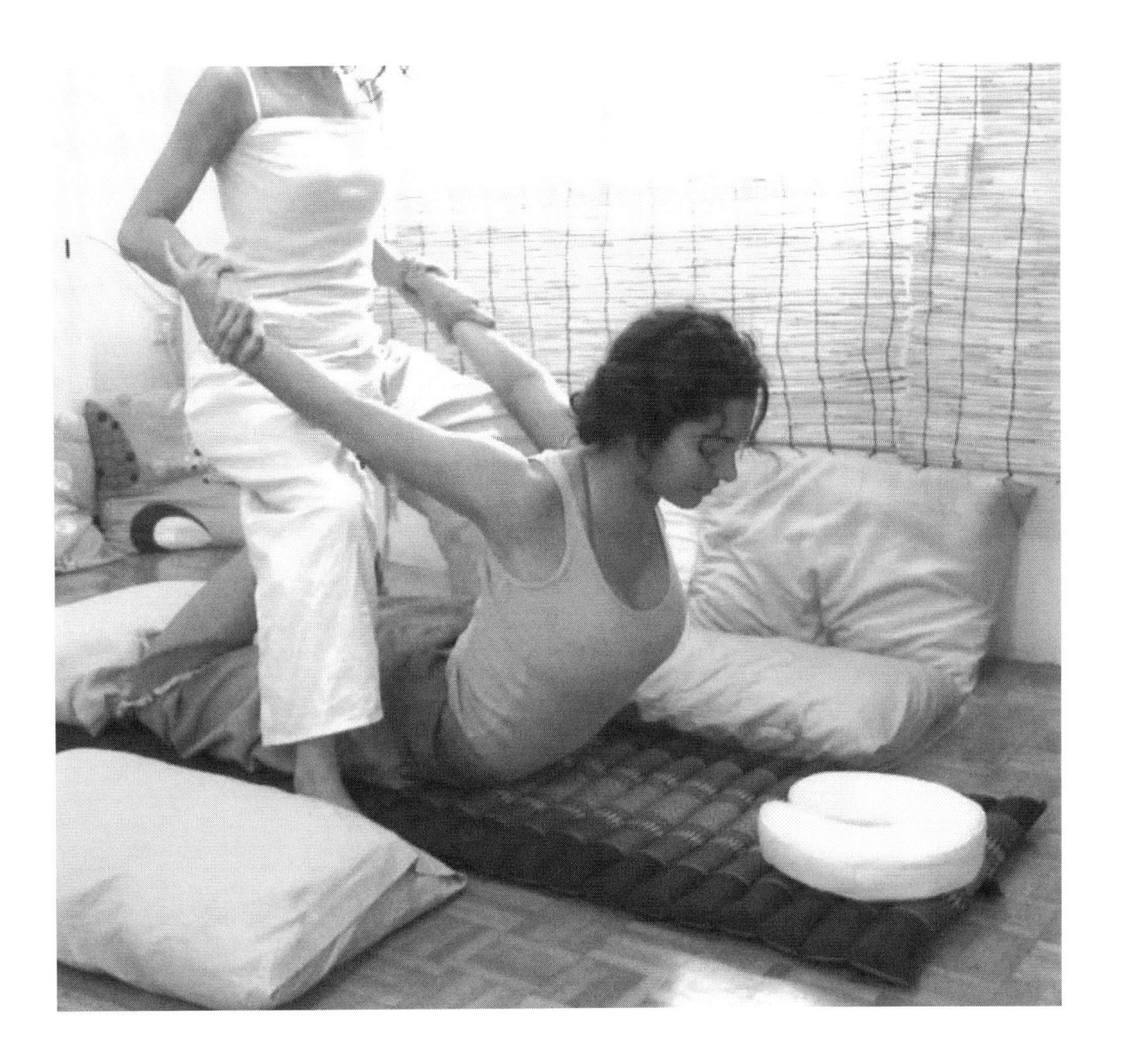

27. Then perform the Bow stretch. Bend the receiver's legs, and sit on her feet! Grasp her arms, and pull her torso, as she exhales. This is a passive application of the yogic asana *Dhanurasana*.

Have in mind the same contraindications that apply for Cobra, the previous technique, as this is a similar spinal bend.

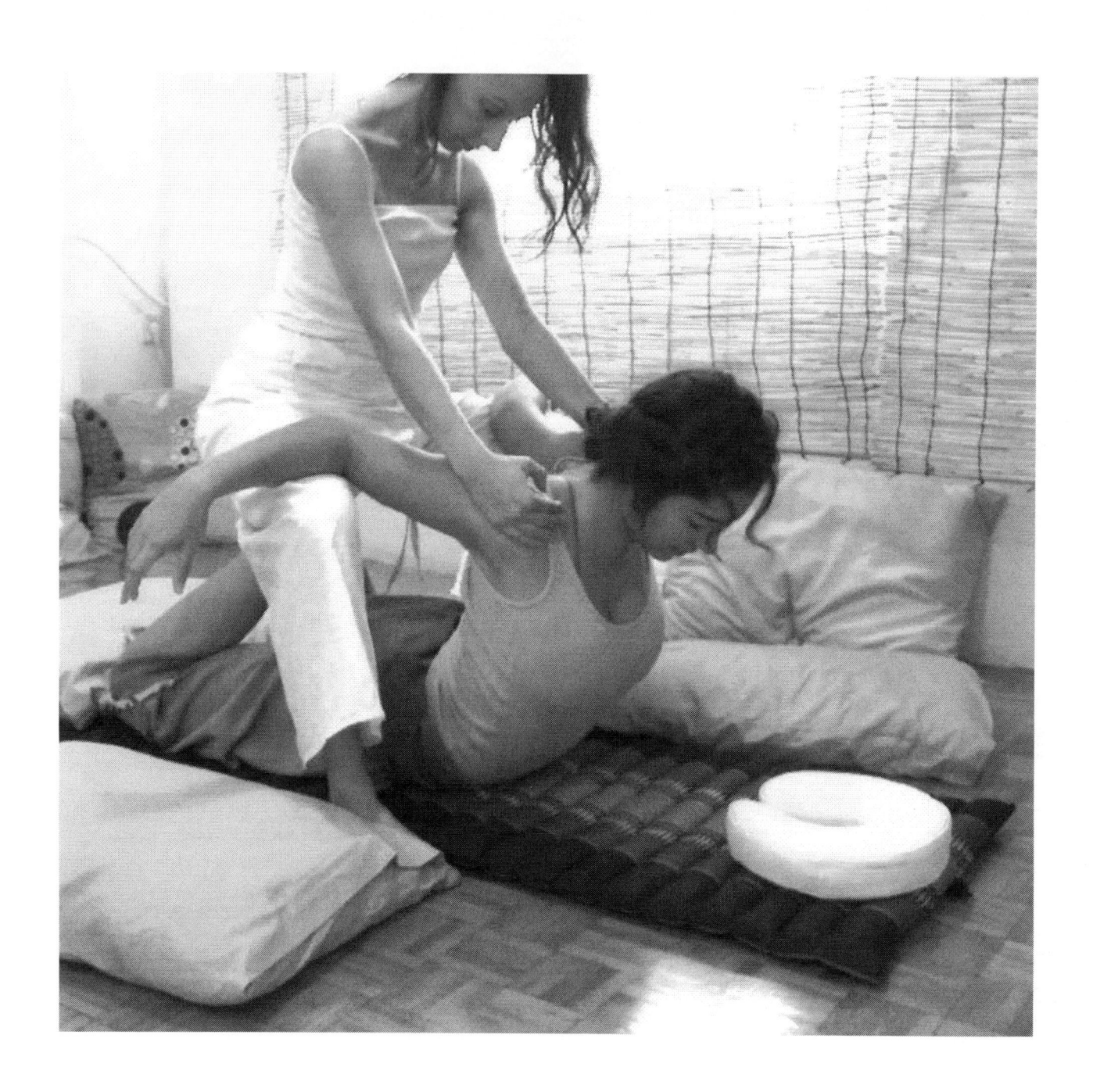

28. As a variation, the receiver's arms lie on your thighs, and you pull her torso from her shoulders.

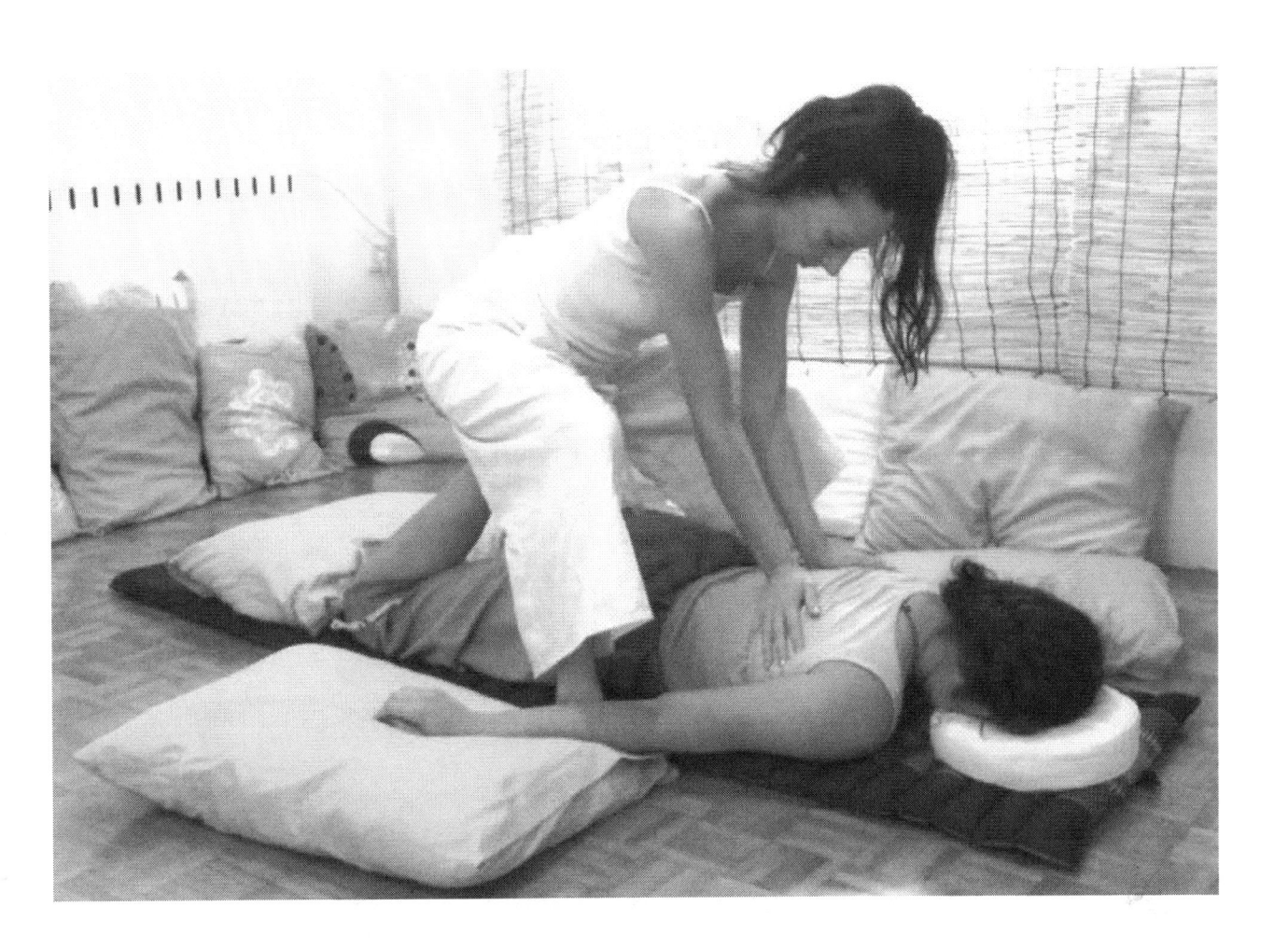

Then lay the receiver down gently, and press her back with your palms, in order to "ground" her and complete the session.

what lies underneath

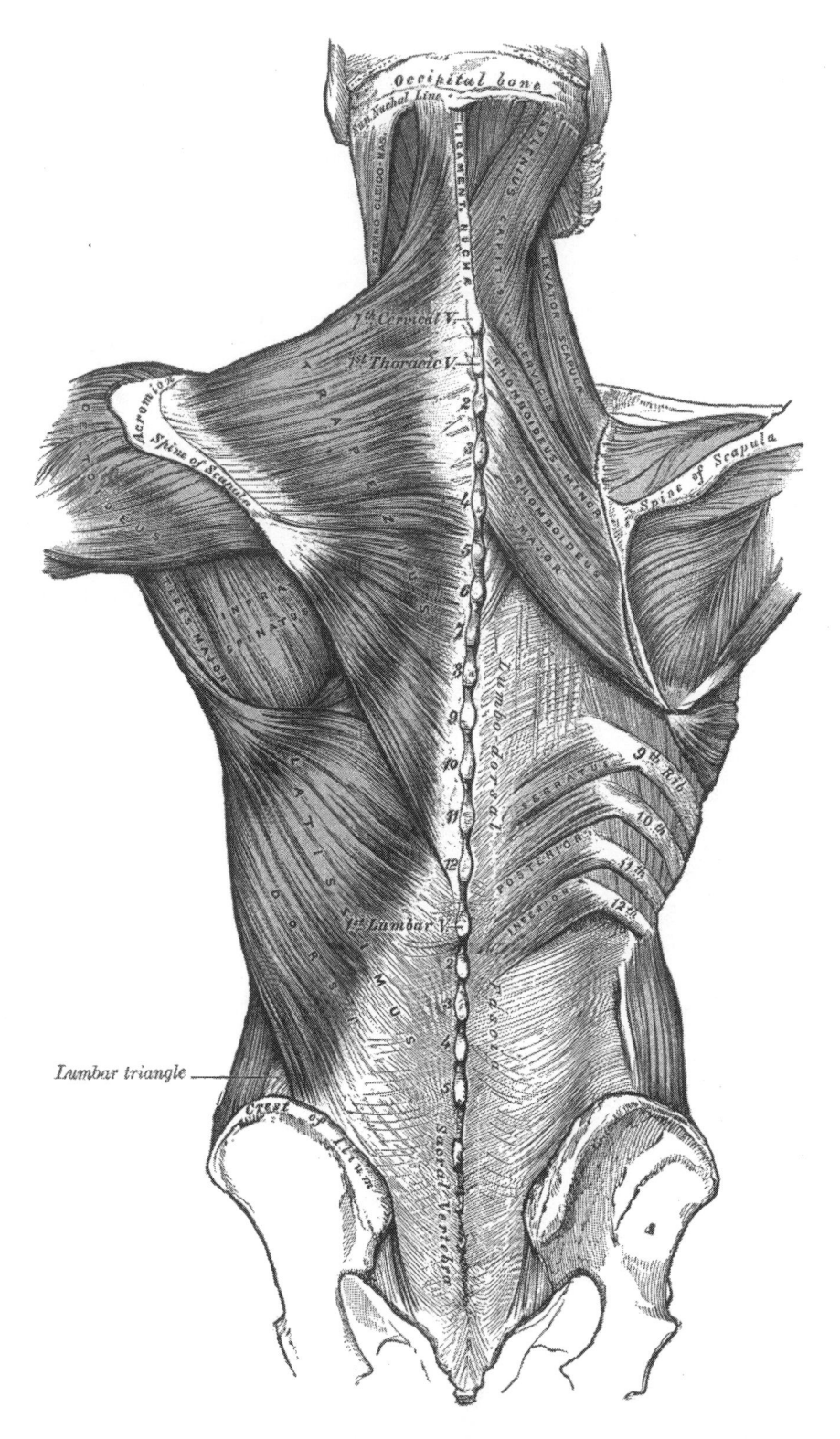

Back muscles

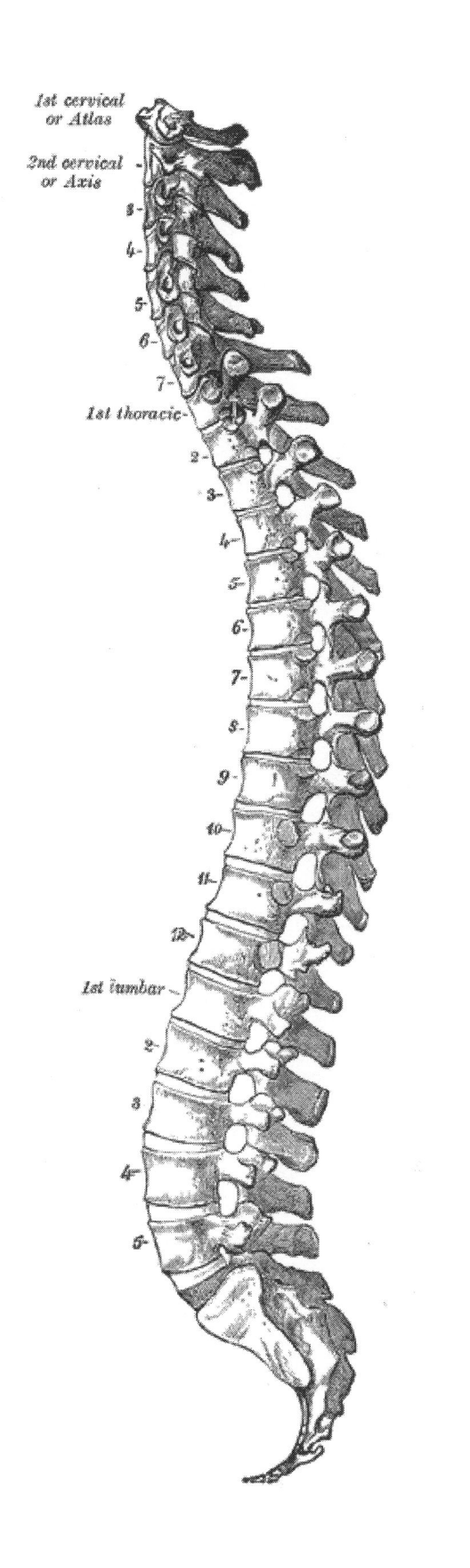

The spine

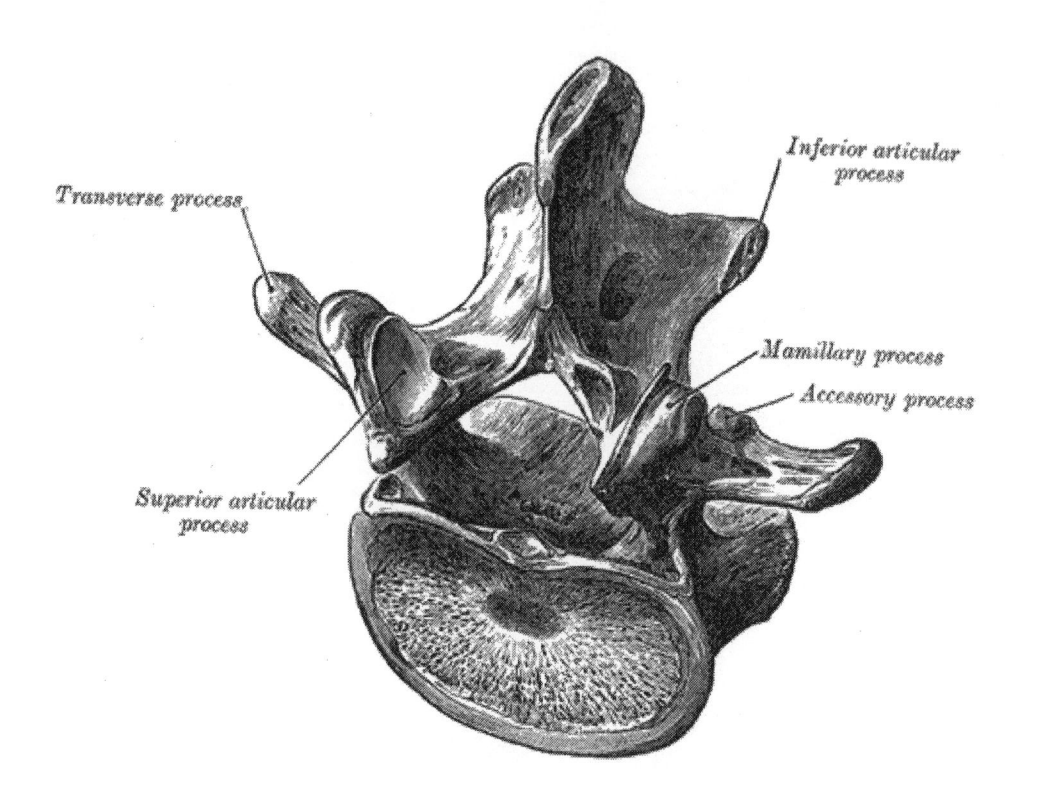

A lumbar vertebra

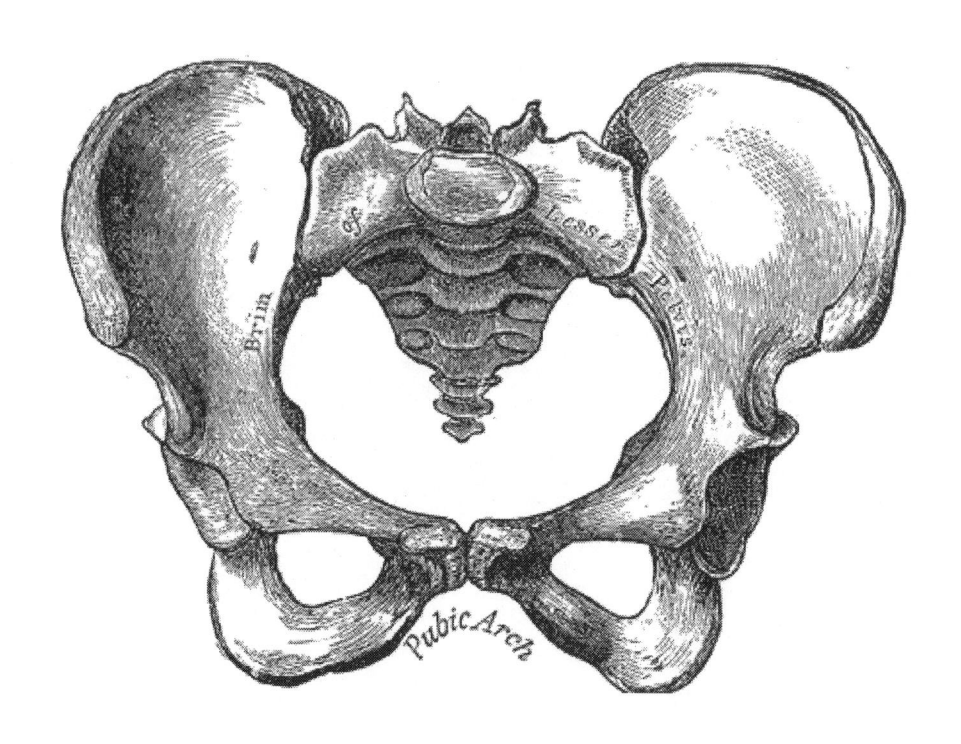

The pelvis

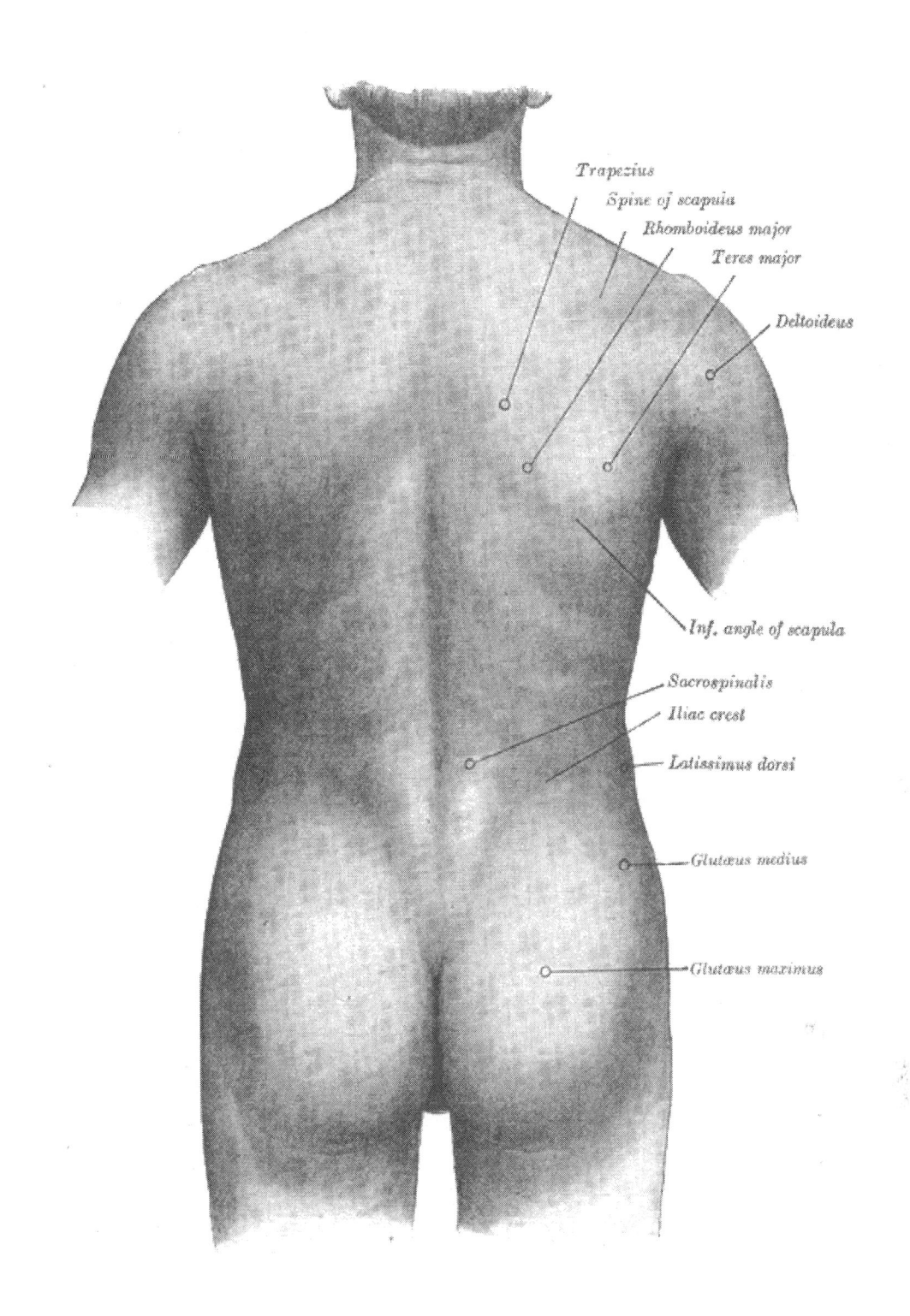

Surface anatomy

Thai massage and lumbar disc degeneration

Disc degeneration is a very common problem, especially for people aged over 30. While conventional physiotherapy can help, many patients will seek a Thai therapist (usually after a recommendation), as Thai Massage stretches and balances the deepest muscle layers, and not merely the upper layer which is typically addressed in an oil massage.

However, Thai Massage is not a treatment in which the patient lies still on a massage table and does not "participate" – as is the case with the typical Swedish massage – as it contains many elements of kinesiotherapy. The bends and lifts of Thai massage can affect directly the lumbar spine and the discs, and the therapist should be aware of the (many!) aspects of this disorder.

Understanding disc degeneration

Disc degeneration may have many phases. In the beginning, the disc simply protrudes, then it prolapses (this is called "slipped disc"), then there may be disc extrusion, and in severe cases the disc may degenerate totally, to the point that it may actually become non-existent. Of course, there are different massage and treatment protocols, depending not only on the condition of the disc, but also on the phase of the disorder (acute, chronic, etc.).

Depending on the exact spot of the disorder (that is, the specific vertebra where the disc protrudes, possibly irritating / compressing a nerve), the patient may feel the pain on the outer or inner arch of the foot, or on the gastrocnemius muscle. The pain can also be localized on the lower back. E.g. the effect of the disorder will be different if the disc protrusion is located in L3-L4, L4-L5 or L5-S1.

Assessment
Many Thai Massage stretches have a definite resemblance with orthopedic tests, and may be applied gently and carefully for assessment, in the beginning of the session. Of course, it is best if the therapist is trained, apart from the Thai stretches, in the actual orthopedic tests. Ideally, the patient should show the therapist an MRI, and inform him/her about the MD's diagnosis.

Thai treatments
During the acute phase, no kind of massage is allowed, and the patient should rest.

However, Luk Pra Kob (steamed herbal compress / ball) may be very beneficial. Be sure to add lots of turmeric in the ball, as it is a potent anti-inflammatory herb. Apply thermal treatment for 15 minutes, 3 times daily, for 3 days.

After the initial phase of the recovery, some light stretches may be applied. I always recommend the combination of heated herbal packs with the Thai stretches. Apply them before and after the stretches.

In this phase, do not apply any technique that contains bends of the lumbar spine, and avoid altogether the sitting position of Thai Massage, as some of its techniques may apply pressure on the discs (anyway, most of the adjustments of the sitting position target other parts of the spine). Focus on the one-leg techniques of the supine position, and on the prone position.

You may need to place a pillow under the patient's belly, in order to support the waist and reduce the lumbar curve, especially if the patient also has lordosis. Work gently on the area of the lumbar spine, but efficiently enough as to relax the tension that is sure to exist there… Light back stretches (again, no bending!) will help. The Thai stretches increase the intervertebral disc space, thus decompressing the disc and decreasing the pain.

The therapist may start adding some stretches in the session, after the recovery. Some bends may be applied in this phase. Here is where the MRI can be useful. Generally, the disc protrudes backwards, but this is not the case always.

Before applying any dynamic bends, the therapist could place carefully the patient is some Thai Massage positions. As it can be seen in the McKenzie method as well, the gentle application of Bhujaungasana can be helpful. Of course, it should not be applied if the patient feels pain while in the position. Depending on the characteristics of the disorder, the patient may also benefit from forward bends. I have seen people with totally degenerated discs who can do comfortably any spinal bend, especially devoted Yoga and Pilates practitioners.

Finally, the Thai Massage therapist should remember that a disc herniation may be asymptomatic. Thus, we should never press the patient's body far beyond its limits. The goal is not to apply an impressive, exotic therapy, but to really benefit and balance the body and the spirit.

seated position

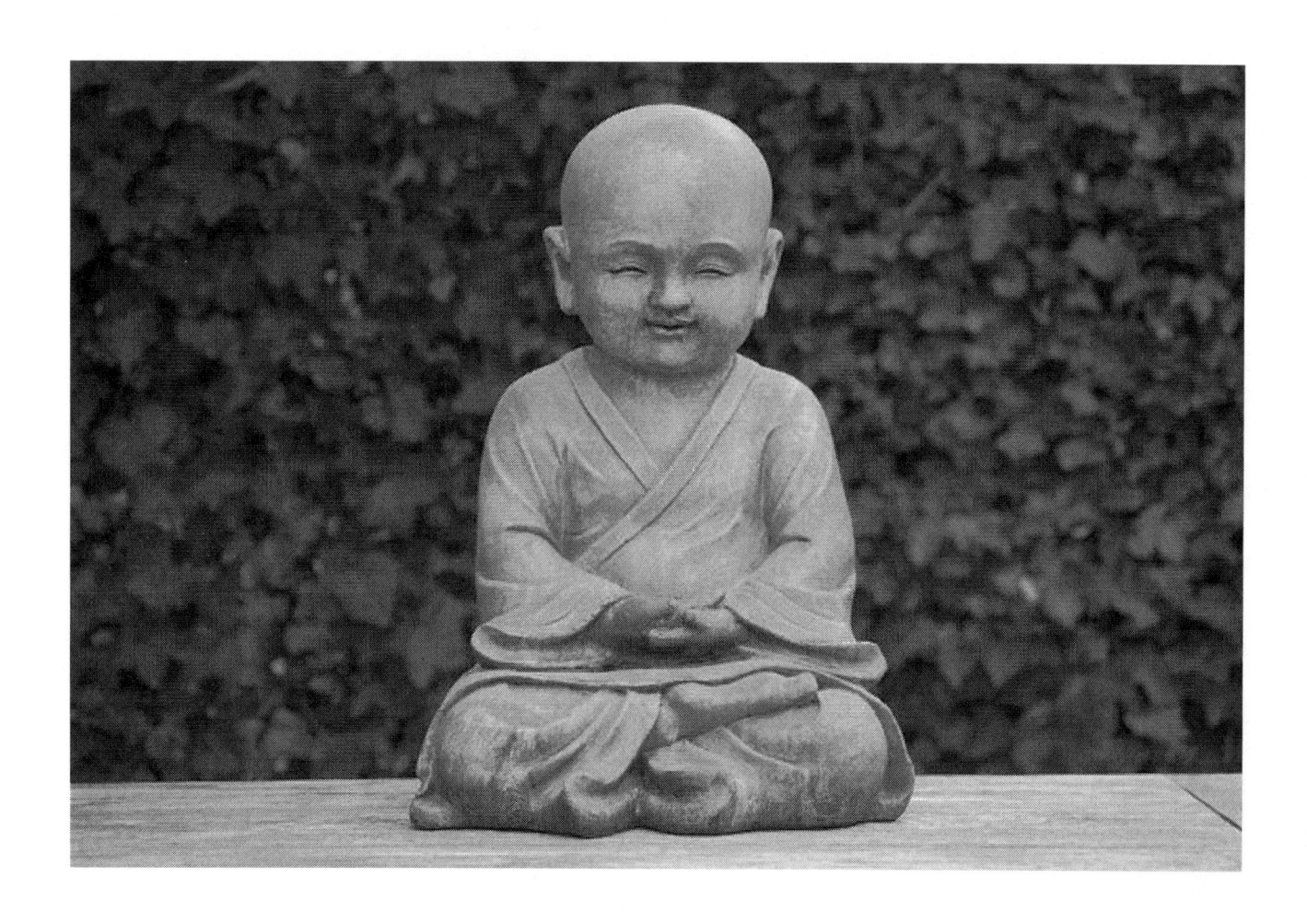

Seated position techniques are very effective for neck and shoulder pain. Since most of them target the skeleton and not the soft tissues, it is important to apply them only if the muscles have been warmed properly. As always, they are more efficient when combined with warm herbal packs and heat rubs.

The recipient should be seated with his or her legs crossed. If this is not possible, he or she may sit on the mat with spread legs. However, this does not allow us to apply all the techniques.

Many of these techniques target the spine. Therefore, the soft tissues should have been warmed properly before.

It is best to skip the seated position if the client has had a recent lower back pain crisis, since some of these techniques may put pressure on the spine.

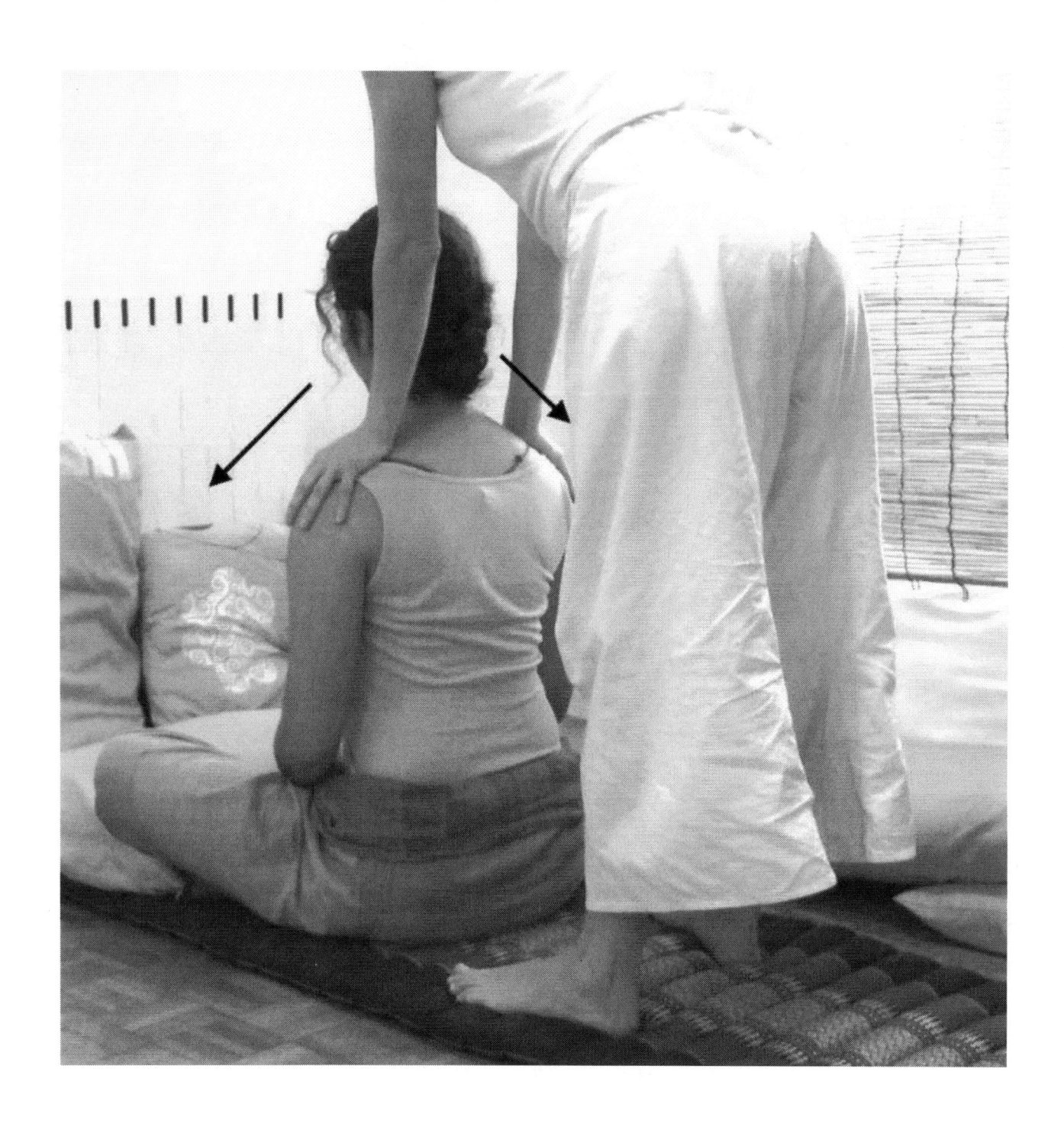

1. Press your palms on the receiver's shoulders. Apply diagonal pressure, in order to avoid pressing the spine.

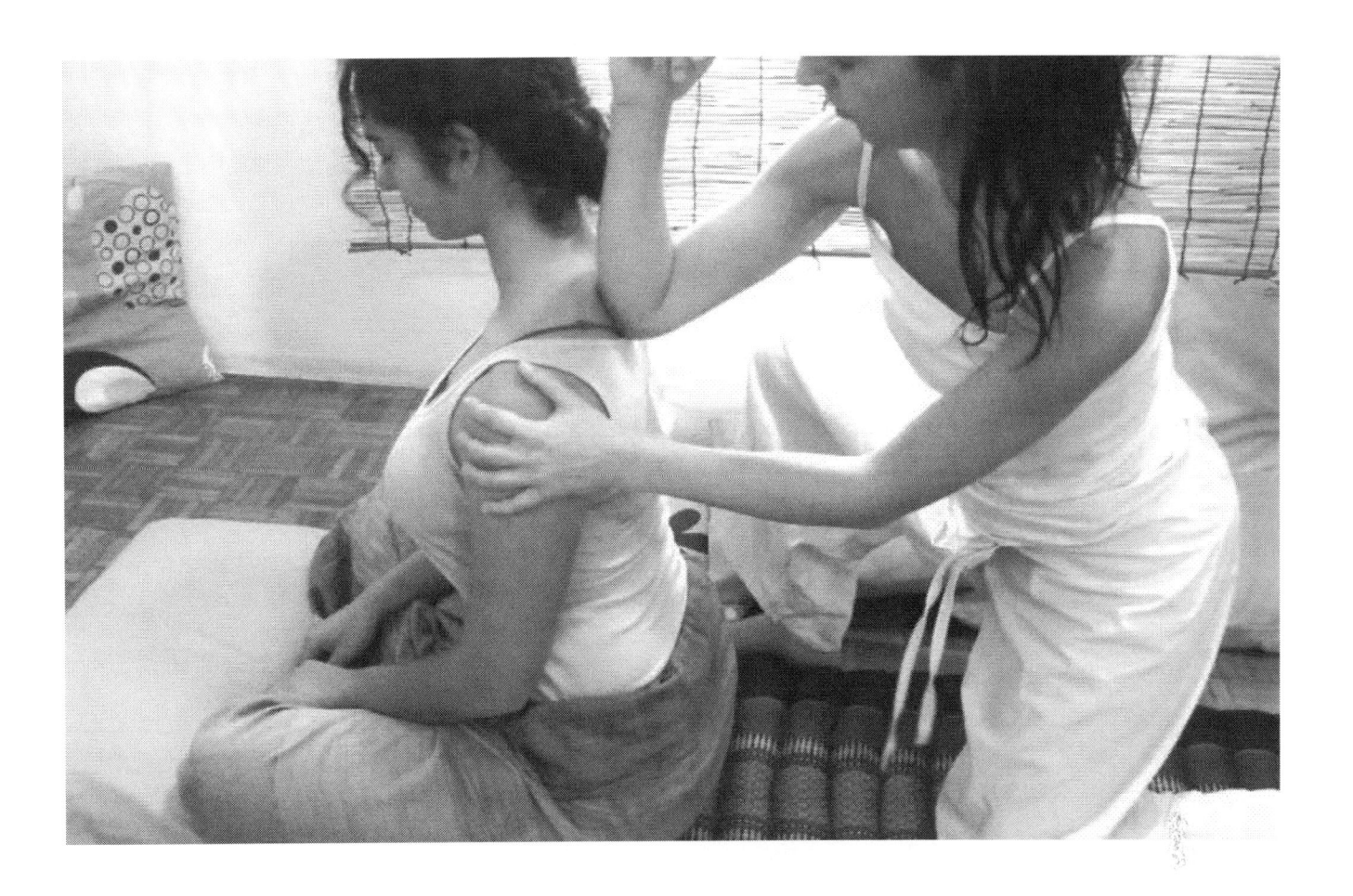

2. Then work with your elbow next to the shoulder blade.

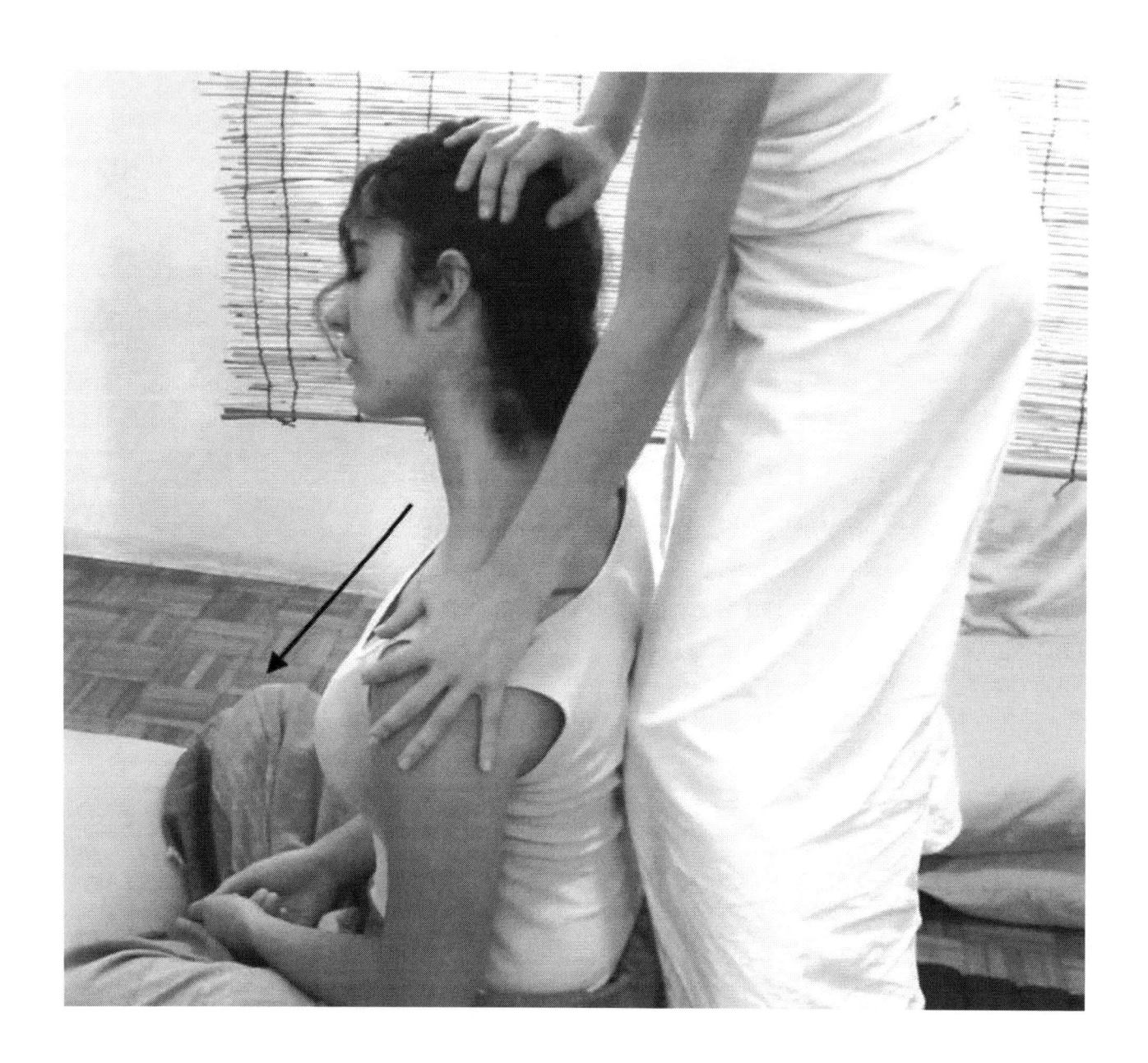

3. Now stand up, and place one palm above the receiver's ear, and one palm on her shoulder. As she exhales, push down gently only the hand that is on the shoulder.

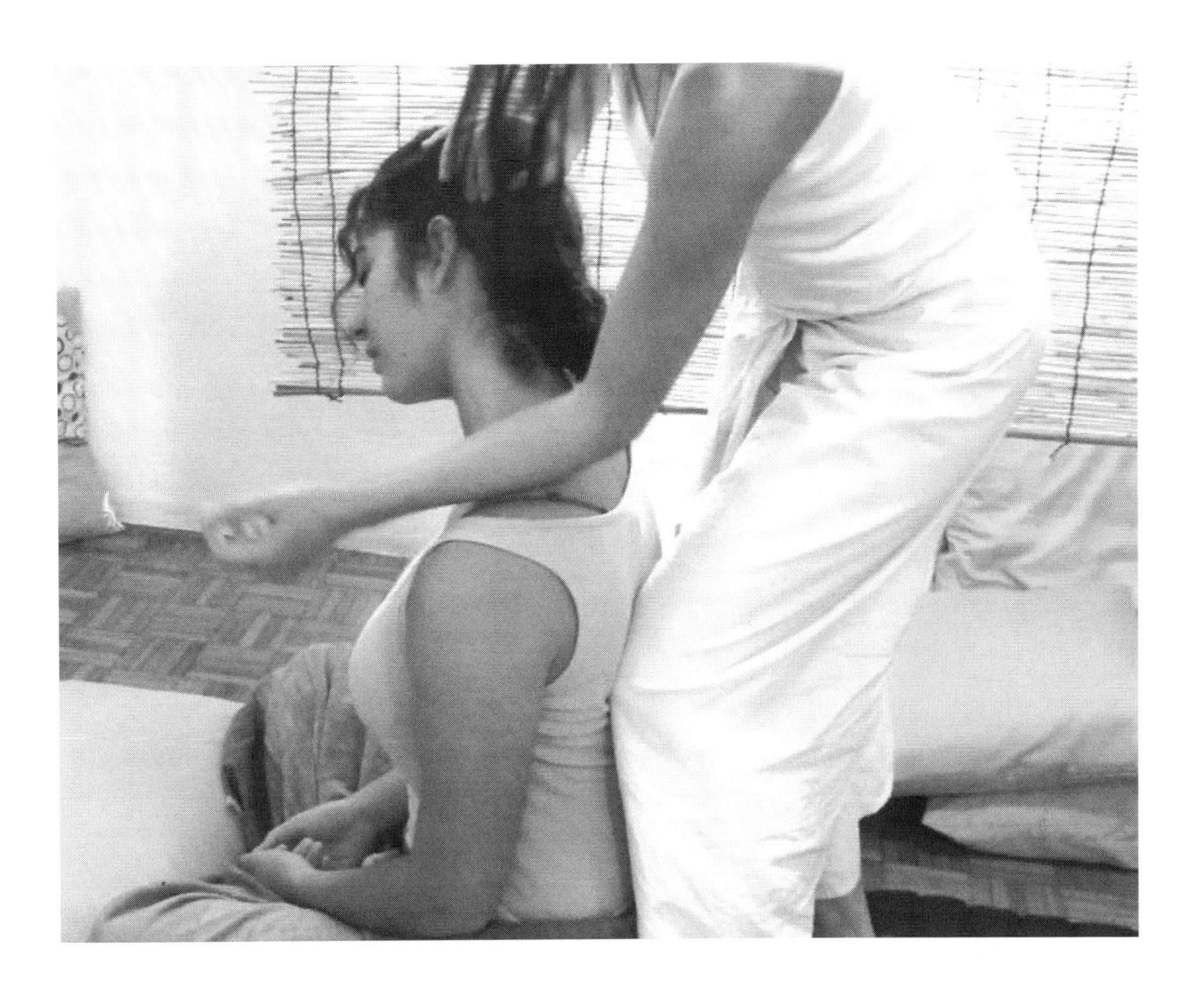

4. Then roll your forearm on the upper part of the trapezoid muscle.

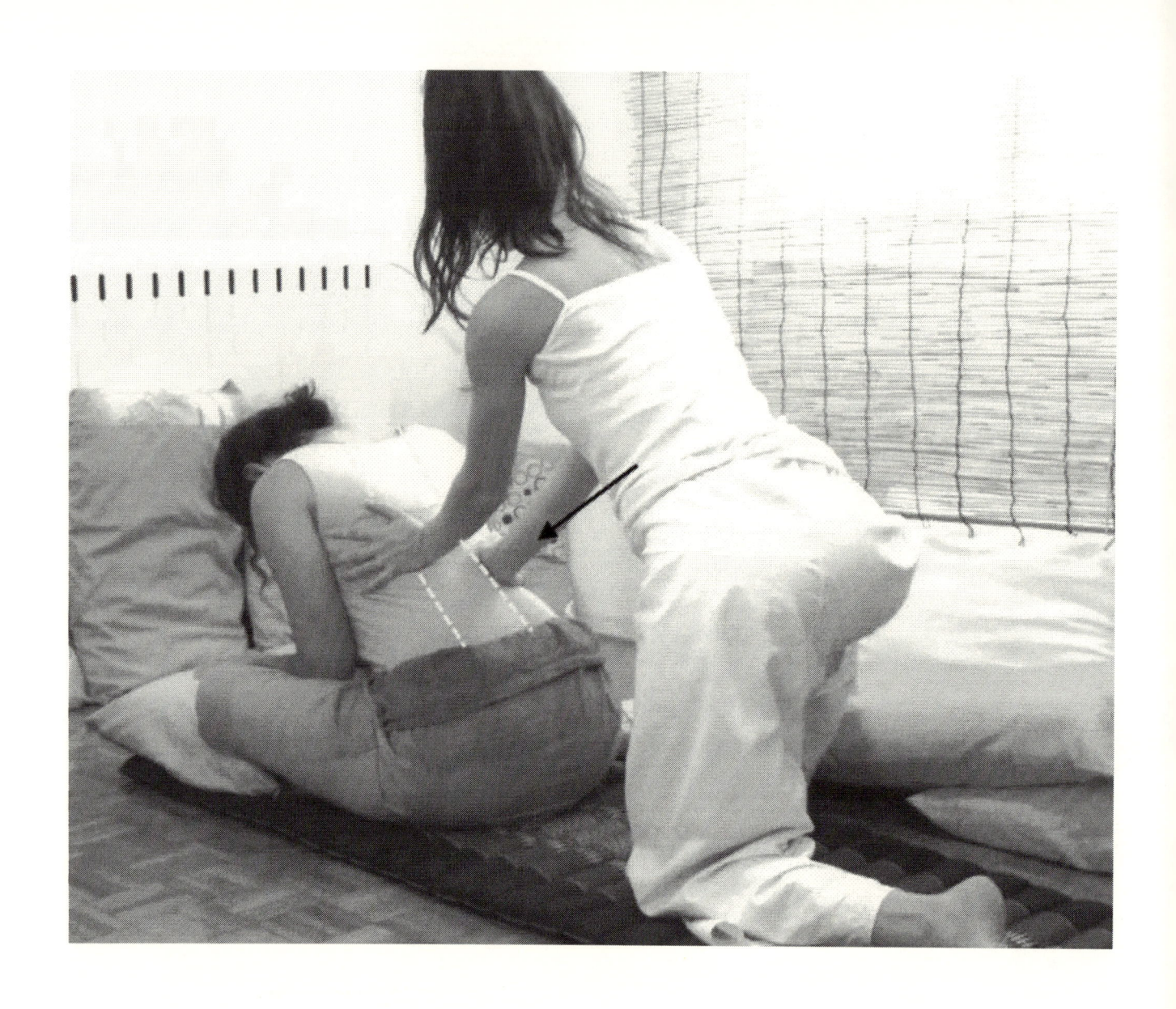

5. Ask from the receiver to place her palms on the mat, and work on the *Itha & Pingkala Sen*. Apply Steps 2, 3 and 4: Do palm walking, thumb presses and again palm walking.

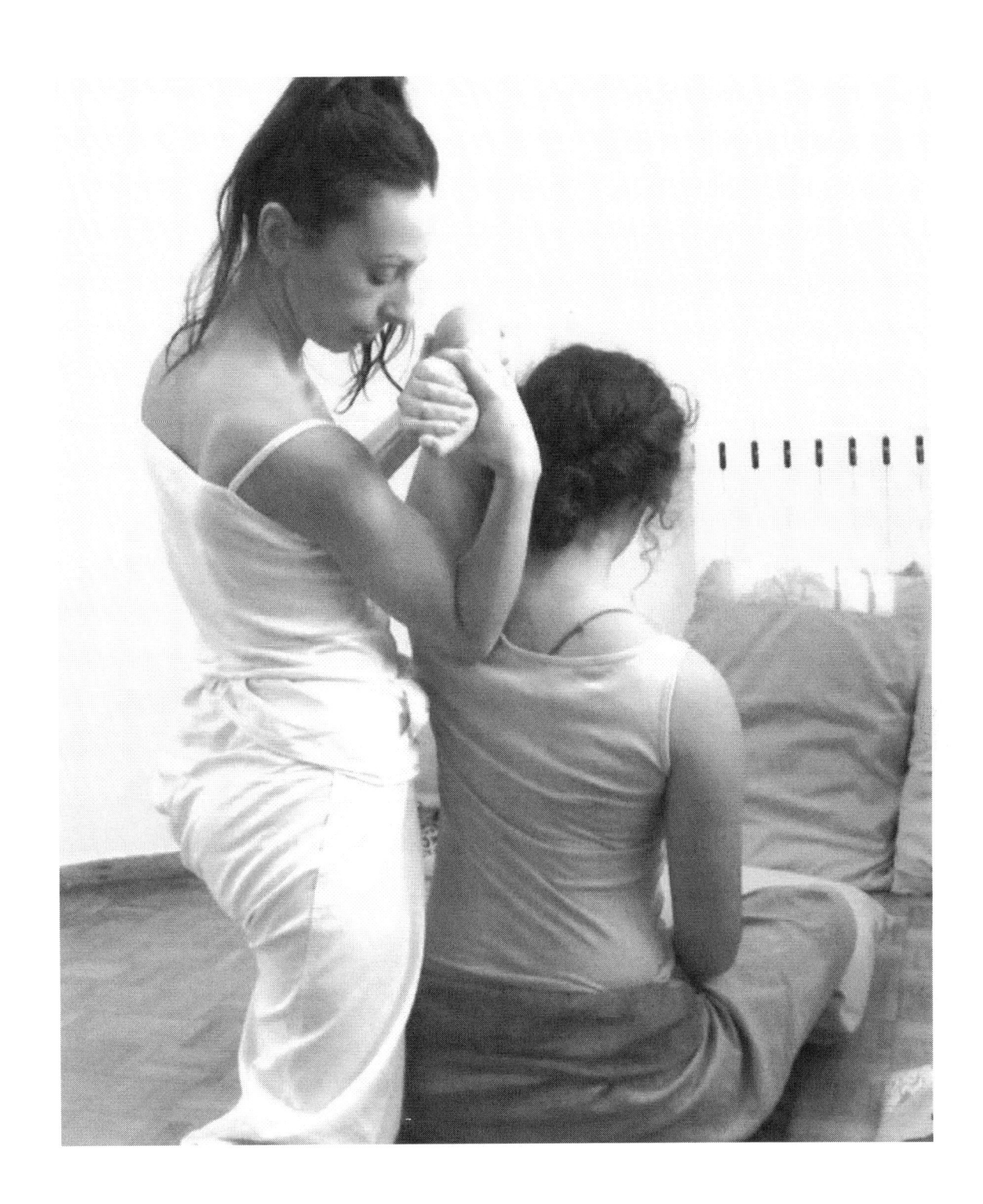

6. Kneel beside the receiver's body. Grasp her wrist with your inner hand, and her elbow with your outer hand. As she exhales, push her elbow backwards. It is also possible to work on the triceps muscle from this position.

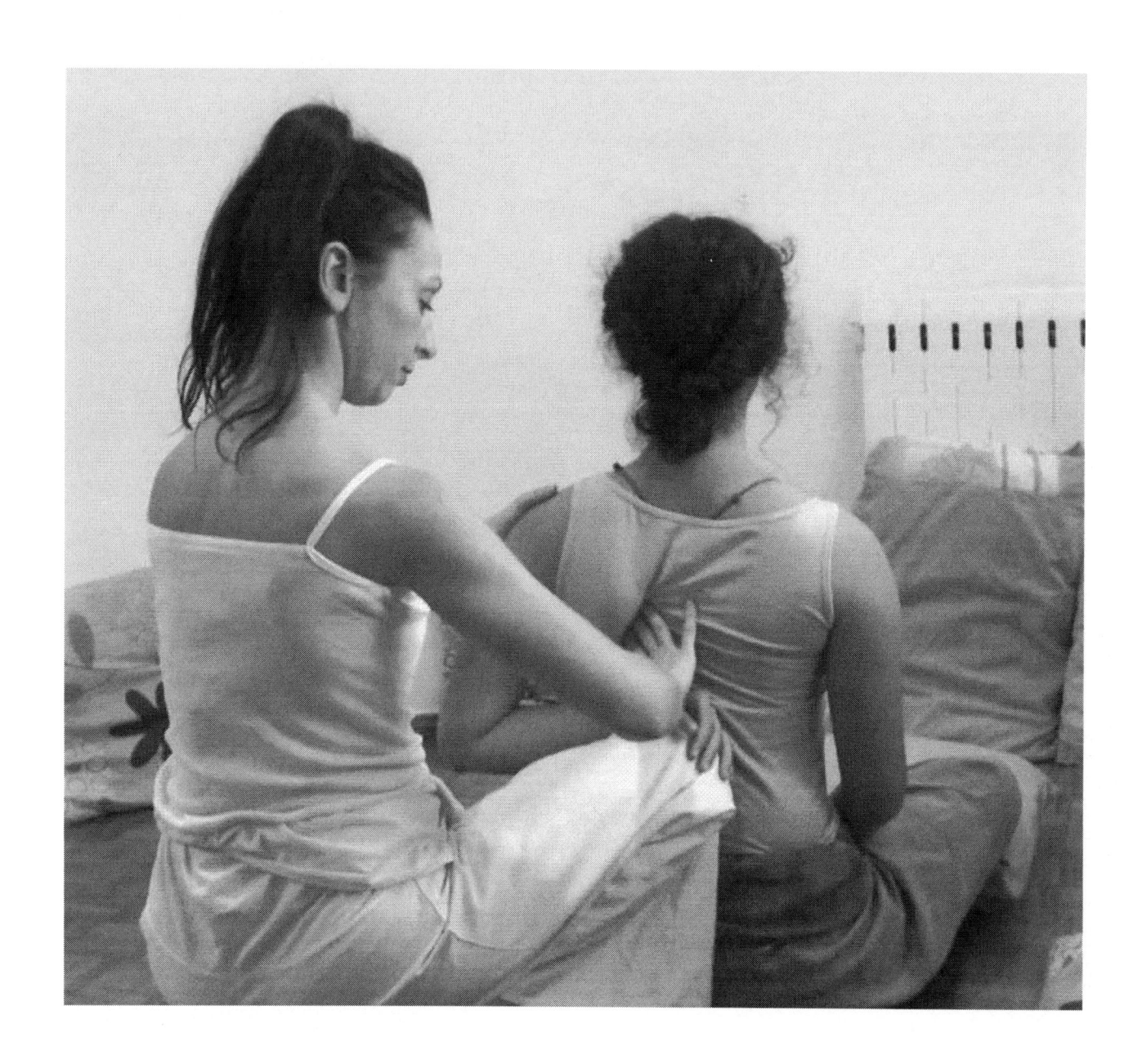

7. Now place one hand in front of the receiver's clavicle, and one hand inside the receiver's scapula. Stabilize the receiver's palm by placing it on your patella. As you pull the scapula towards you, push your fingers inside the scapula.

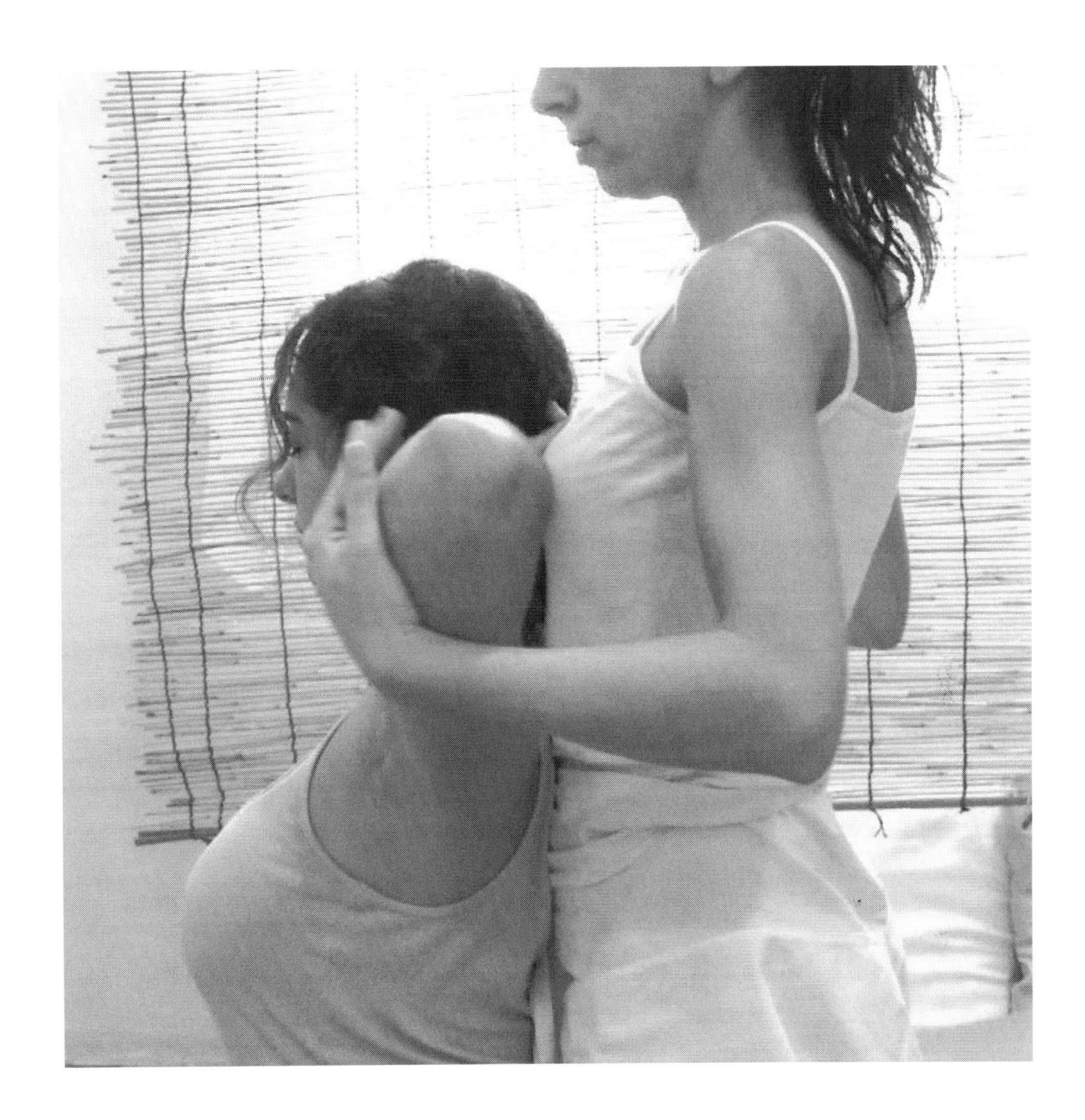

8. Tell the receiver to interlock her fingers behind her head. Place your palms on her elbow joints, and as she exhales, pull her arms backwards.

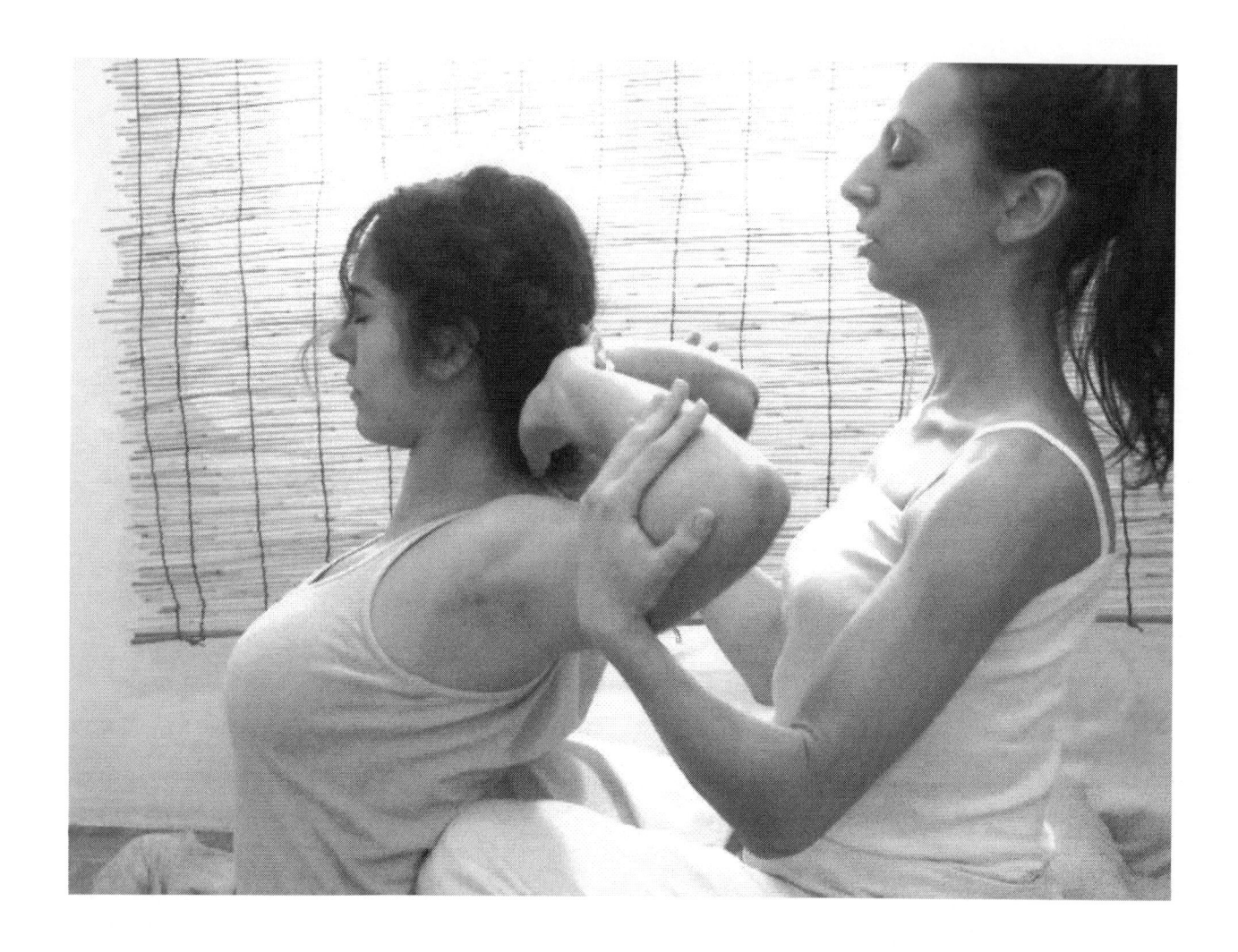

9. Then place your knees on the receiver's lower back, under the scapula, and pull her arms backwards.

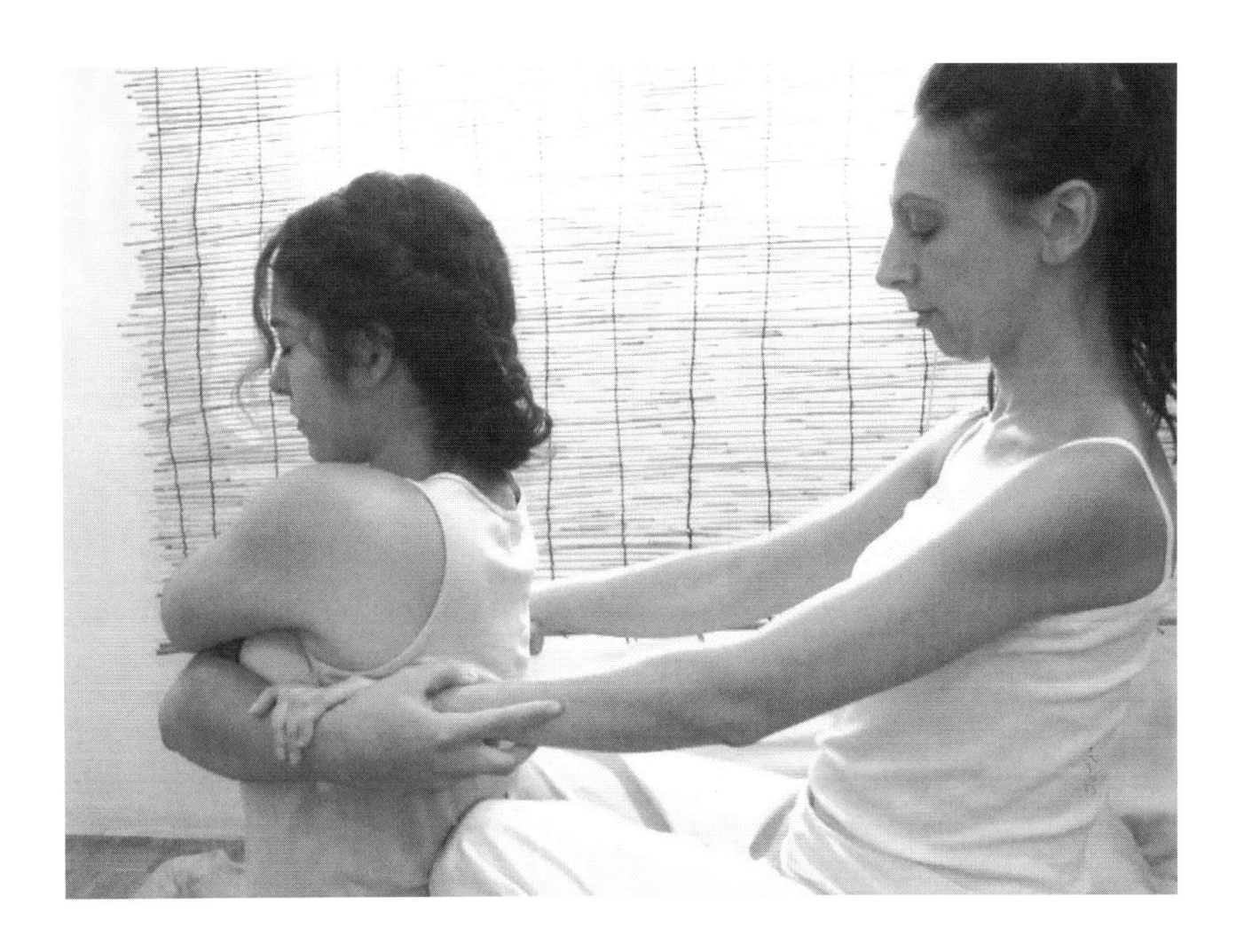

10. Now repeat the previous technique, but grasp the receiver's forearms. Pull back her arms as she exhales, and simultaneously push your knees gently forward.

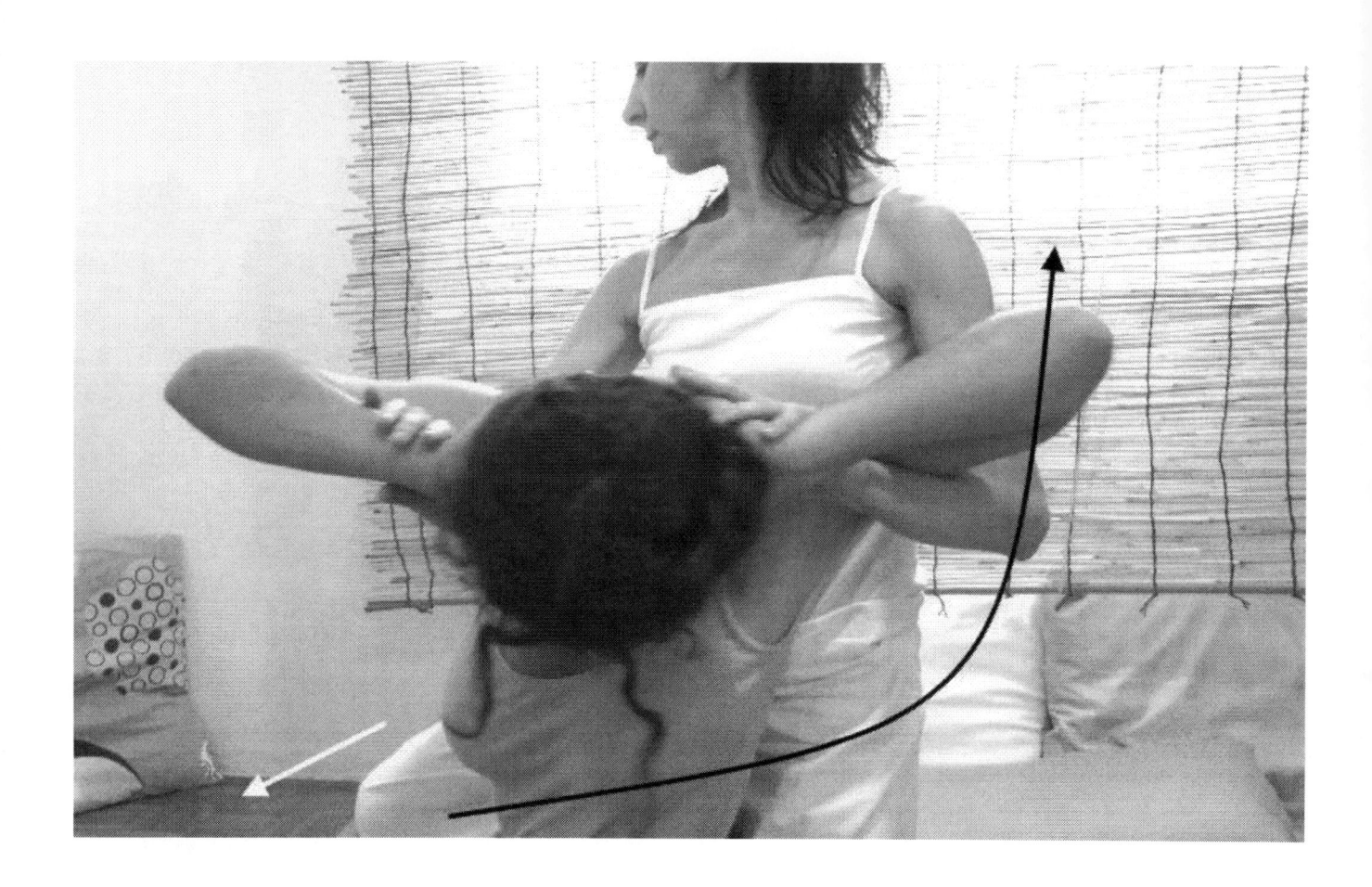

11. Tell the receiver to interlock her fingers behind her head, and interlock your arms in hers. Grasp her from her wrists, and bring her torso forwards. Place your knee on her thigh and twist her body sideways and upwards. Repeat on the other side of the body.

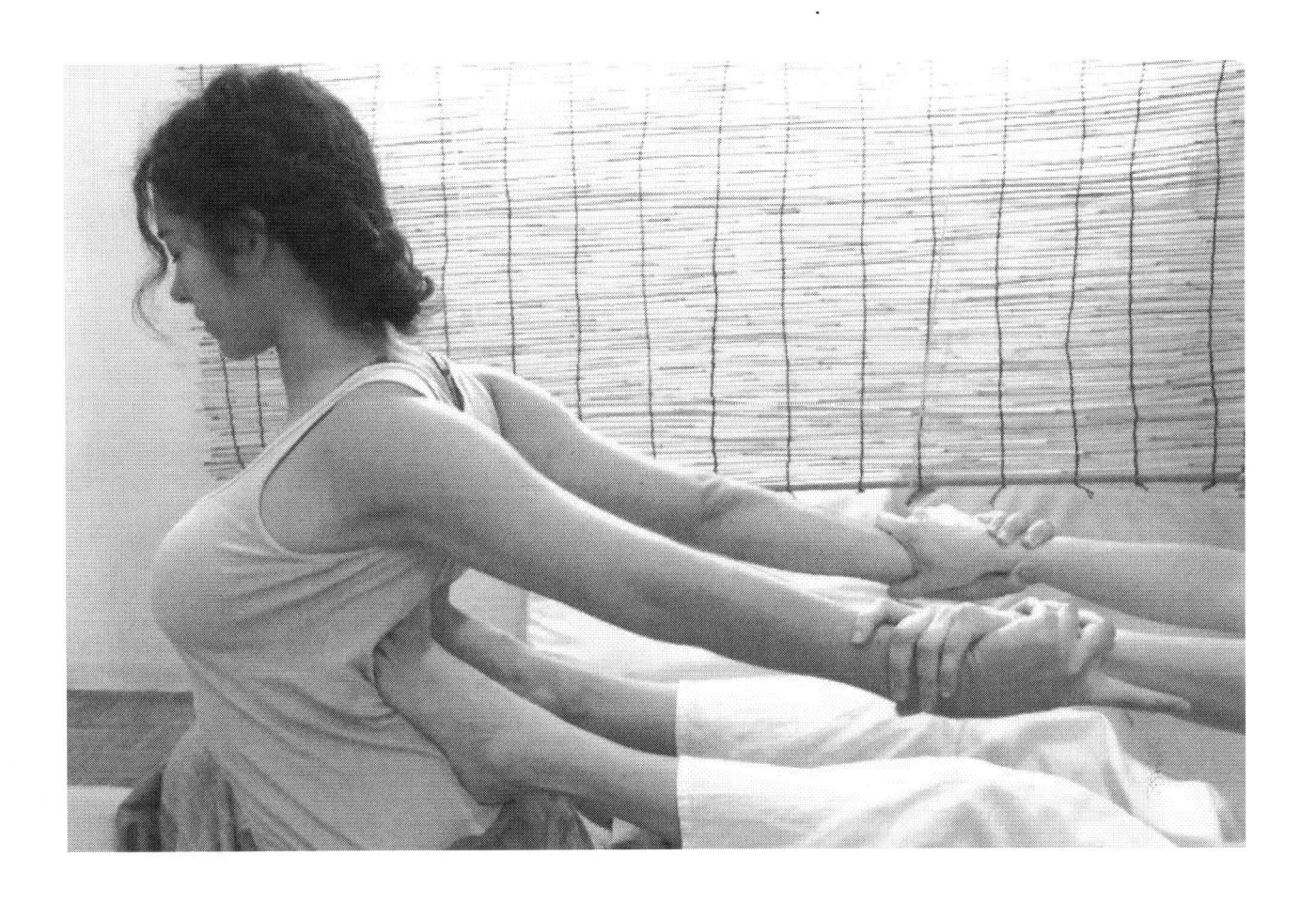

12. Then grasp the receiver's wrists and place your feet on her back, under the scapula. As you pull her arms, push your feet. Move your feet on 2-3 spots on her back.

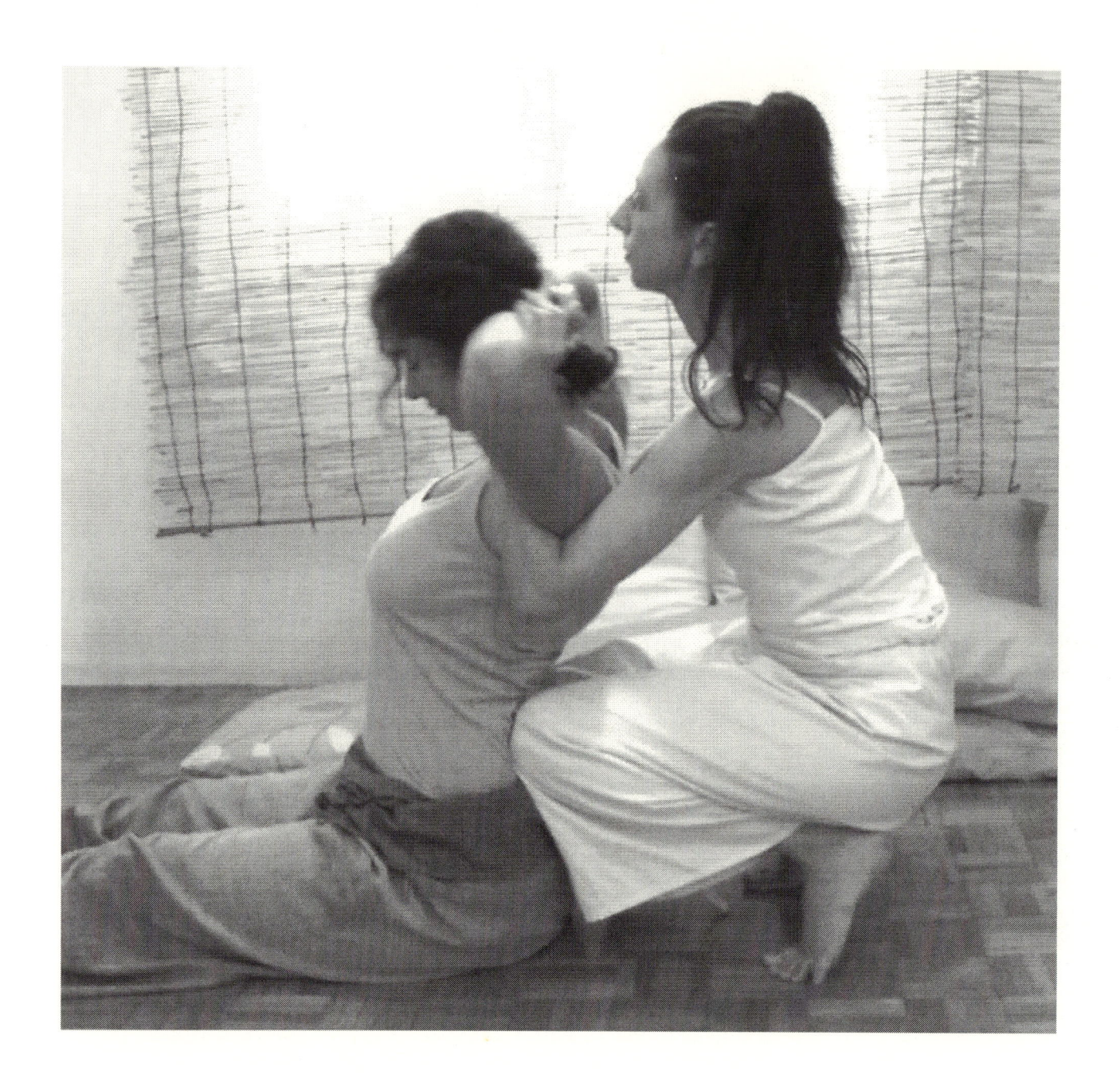

13. Stand on your toes, and interlock your arms in the receiver's arms. Place your knees above the pelvis, and fall back.

This creates a wonderful stretch on the back muscles and the spine.

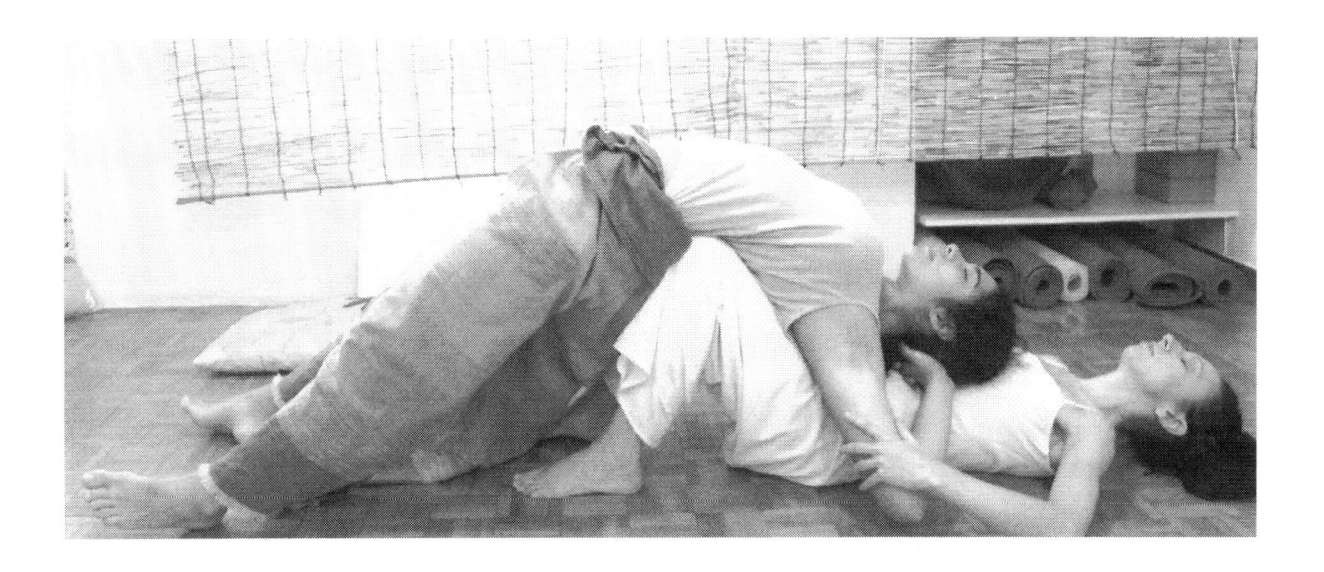

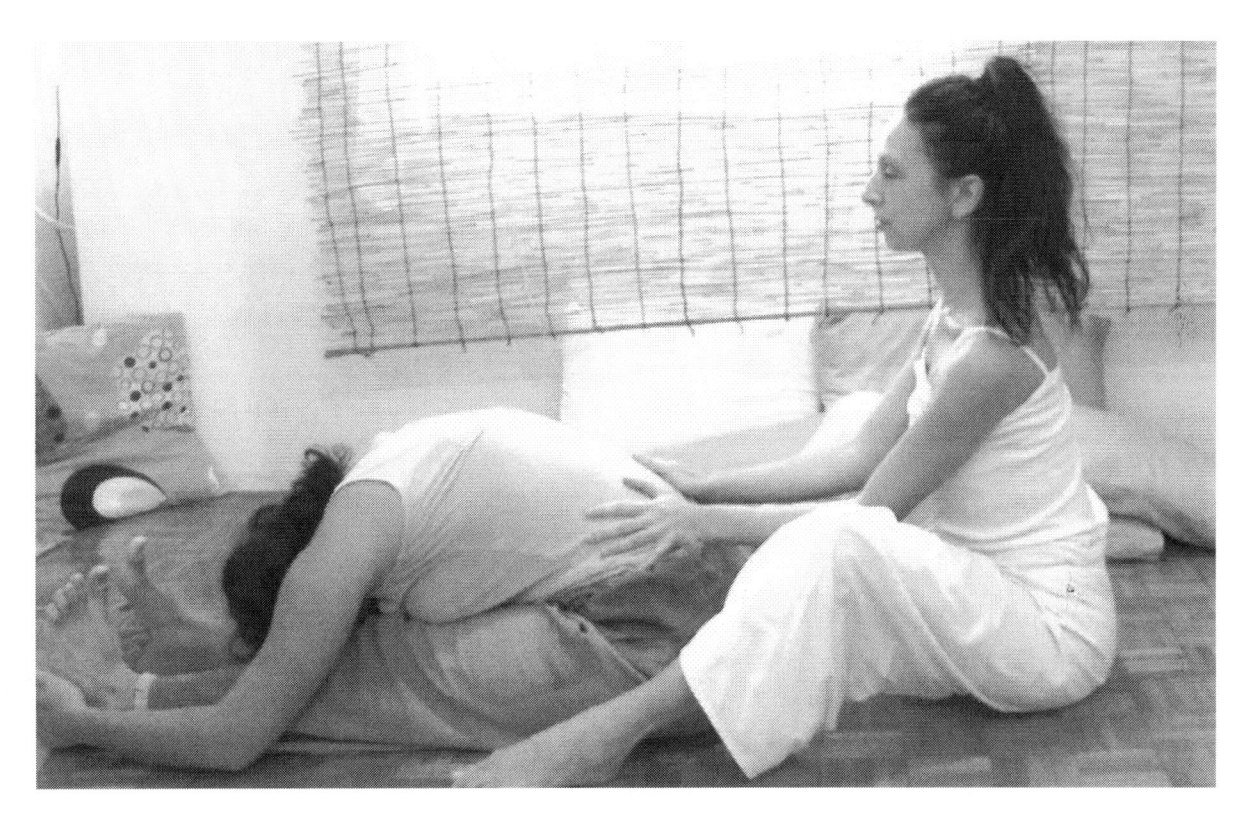

In order to step out of the position, push gently the receiver's back in order to lift it.

Never do this technique if the client is heavier than you.

what lies underneath

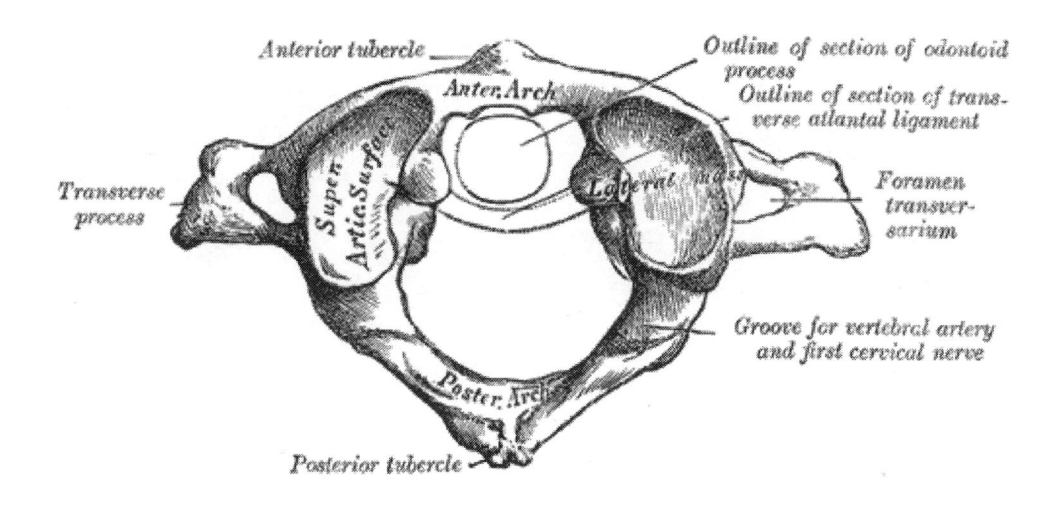

The first cervical vertebra (atlas)

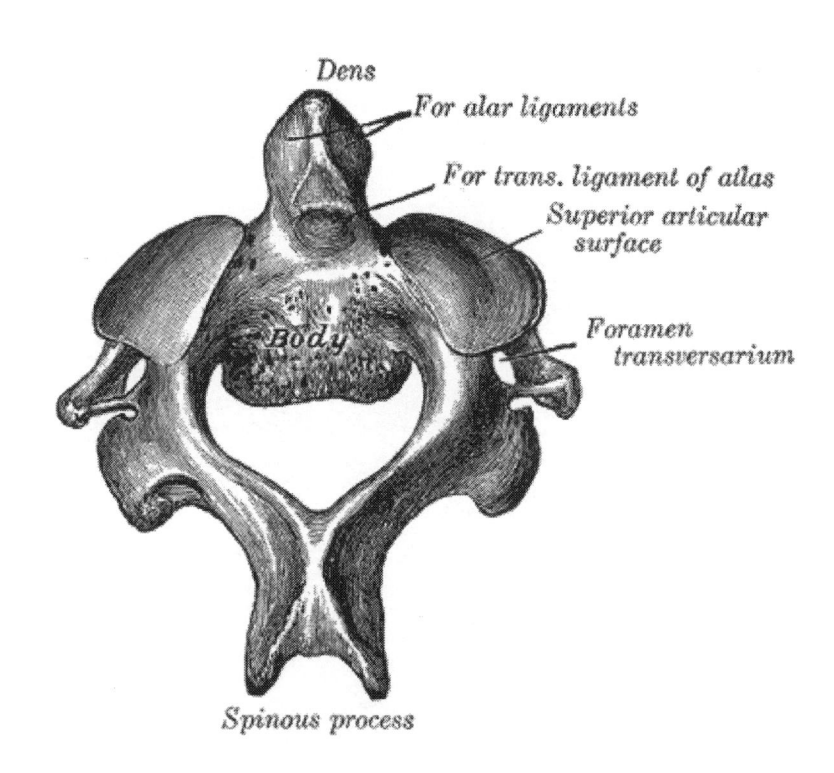

The second cervical vertebra (axis)

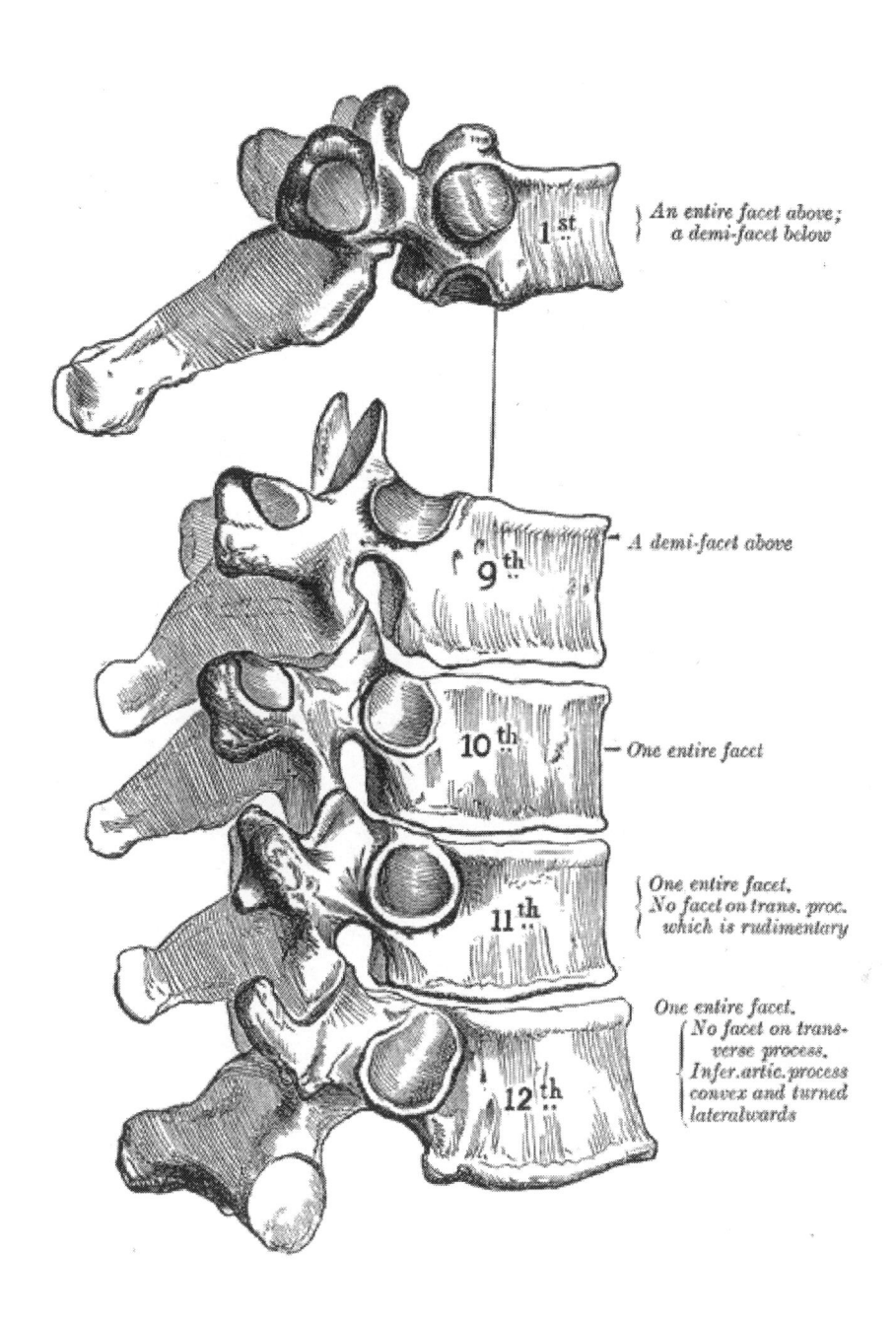

The thoracic vertebrae

face & scalp

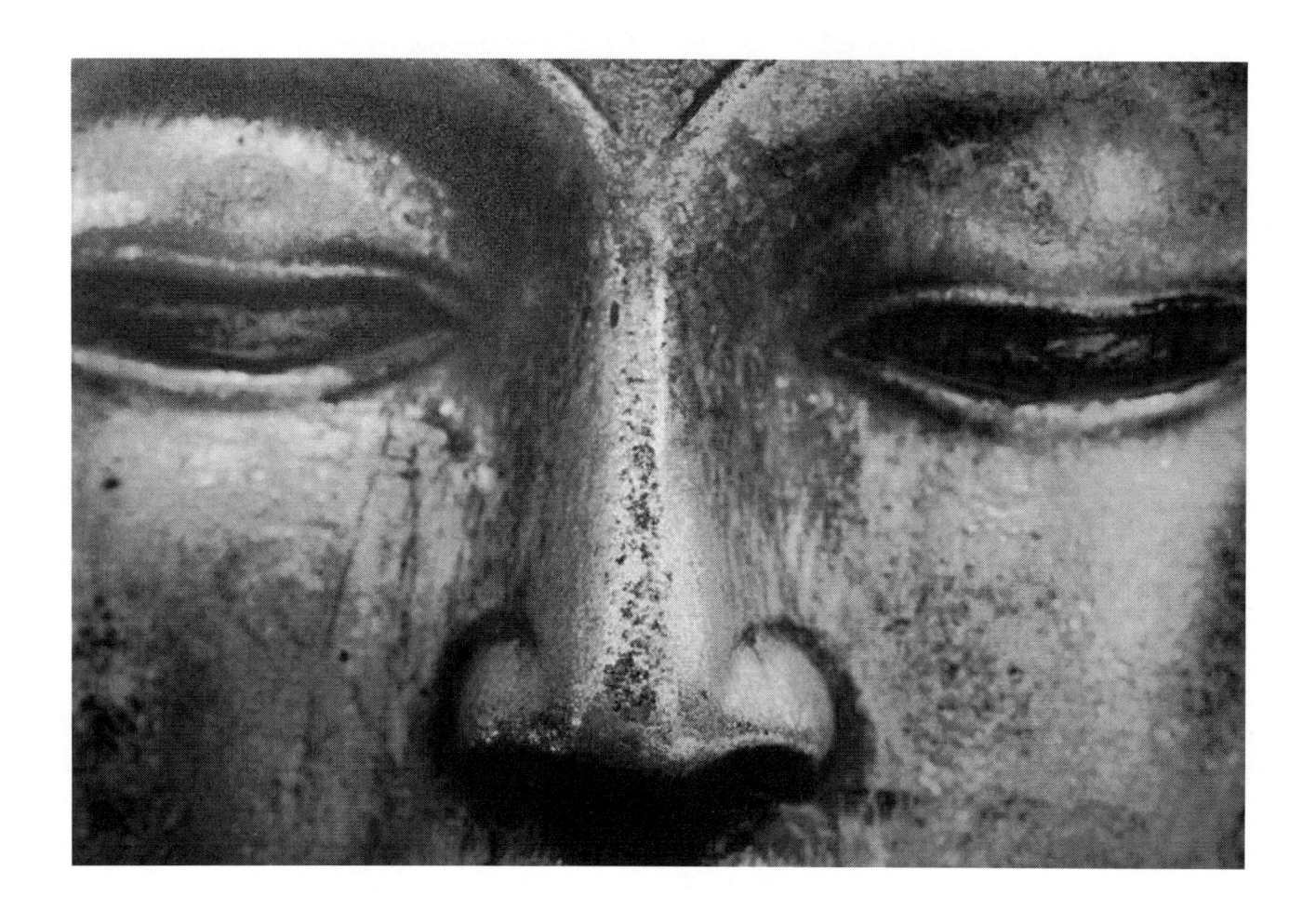

A Thai Massage session is concluded with face and scalp massage. These techniques are indicated for headaches, stress and neck pain.

It is recommended to apply them in the end of each and every treatment, since they help the receiver to calm down after the mobilizations. Moreover, many Sen lines cross these areas – these include *Itha & Pingkala Sen, Sahatsarangsi & Tawaree Sen, Lawusang & Ulanga Sen.*

There are also many acupressure points on the head. Ideally, the adequately trained therapist should apply warm herbal packs on the forehead and the temples.

Before starting, cover the receiver with a warm blanket, and place a large pillow under his head, and one under his knees – this promotes the total relaxation of the spine.

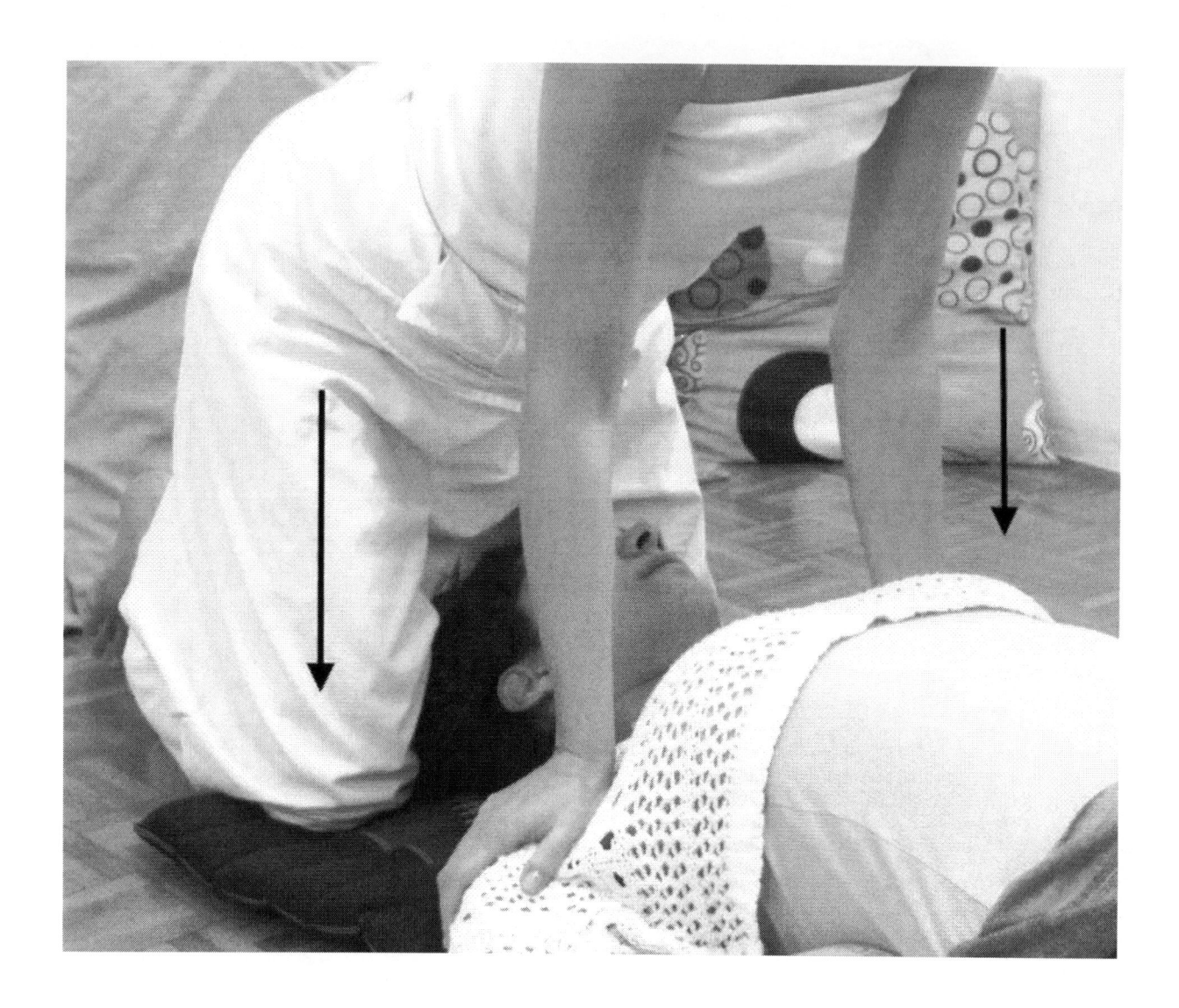

1. Kneel behind the receiver's head, and press down gently her shoulders, as she exhales. This technique promotes the proper alignment of the ribs.

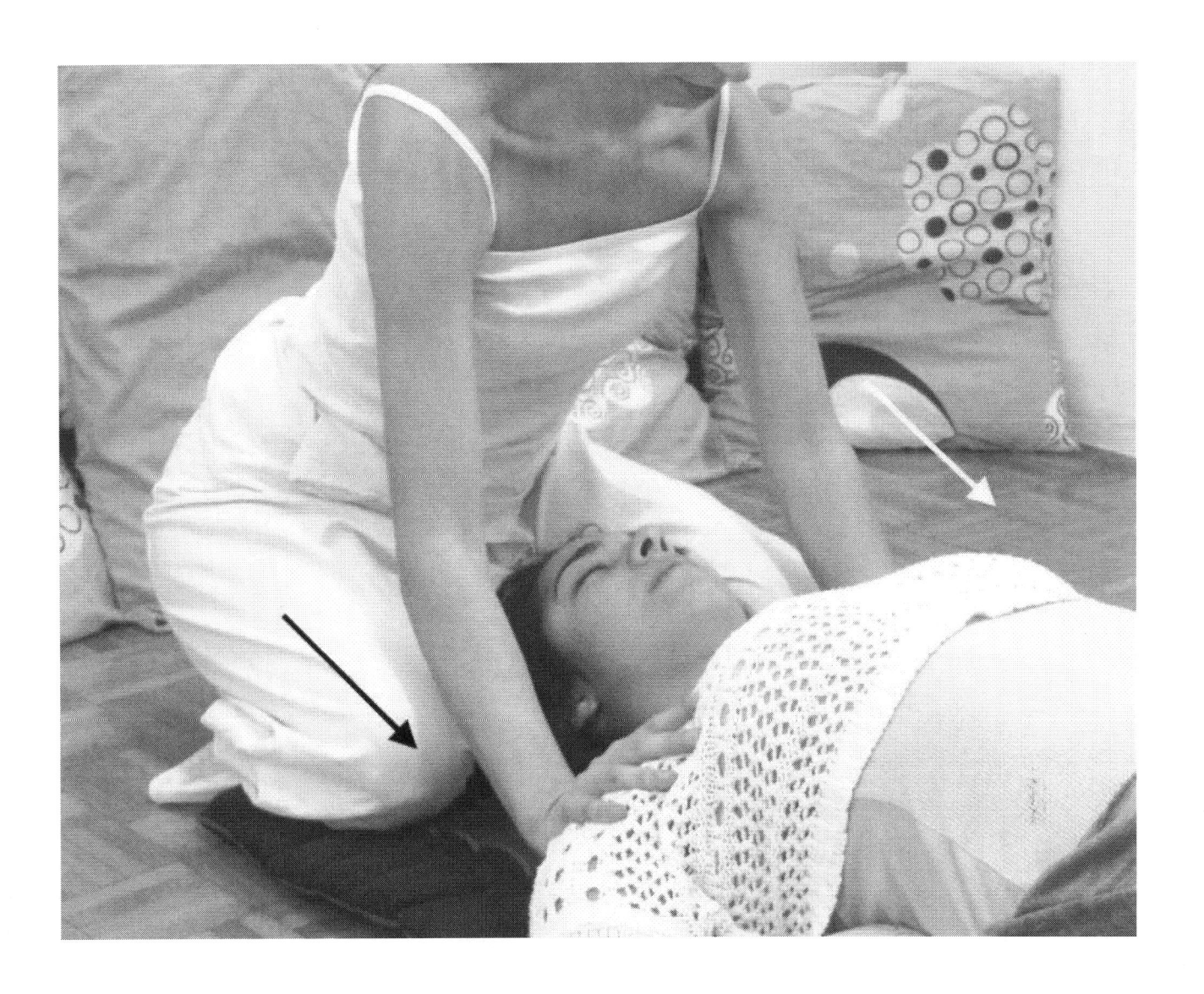

2. Then, press the receiver's shoulders alternatively, towards her feet.

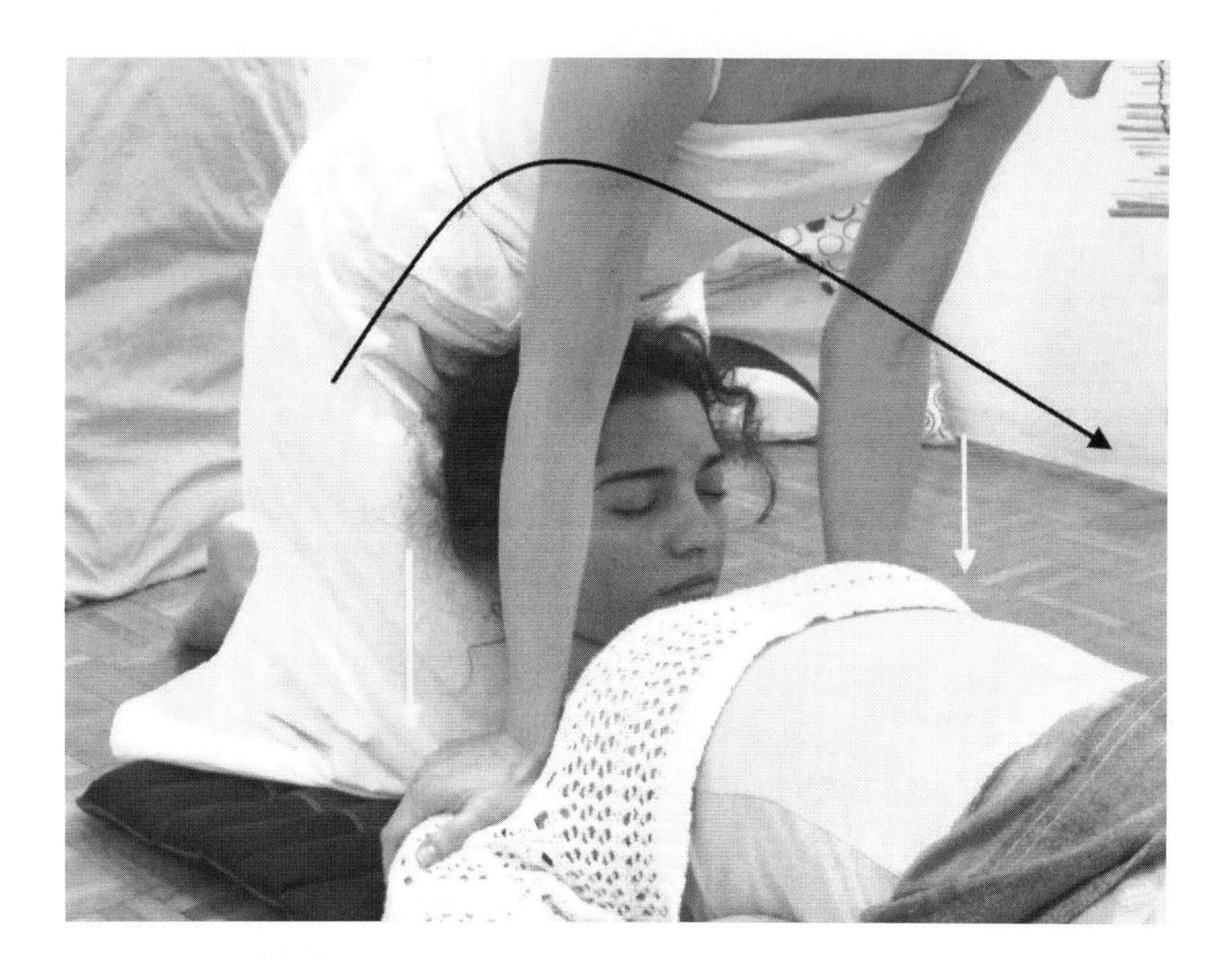

3. Now lift your thighs and place the receiver's head on them. Place your palms on her shoulders, and as she exhales, bring your pelvis forward, simultaneously pressing down her shoulder joint.

Never perform this technique on people with cervical degenerative disc disease.

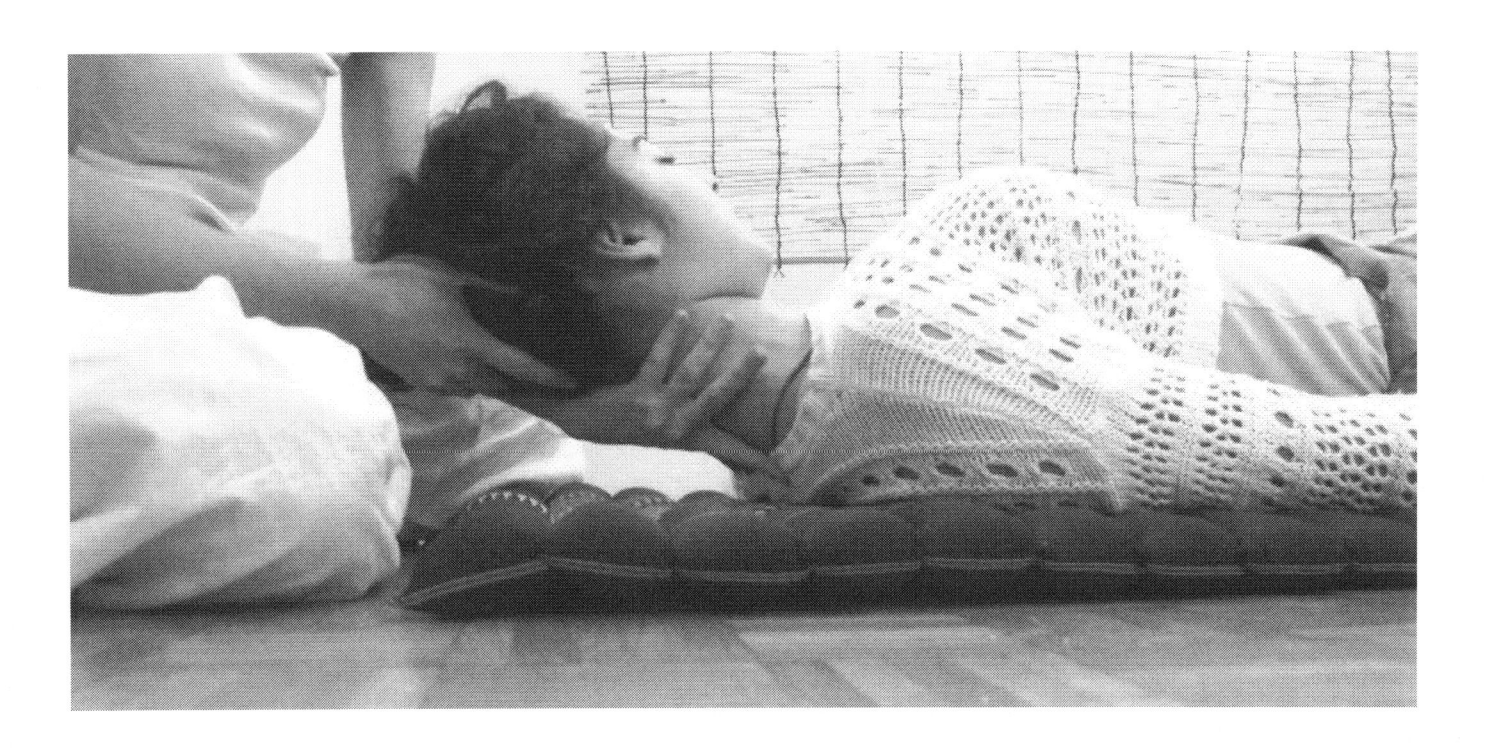

4. Then slide your palms gently on the receiver's neck.

Always keep one palm on the occipital bone, in order to stabilize the skull.

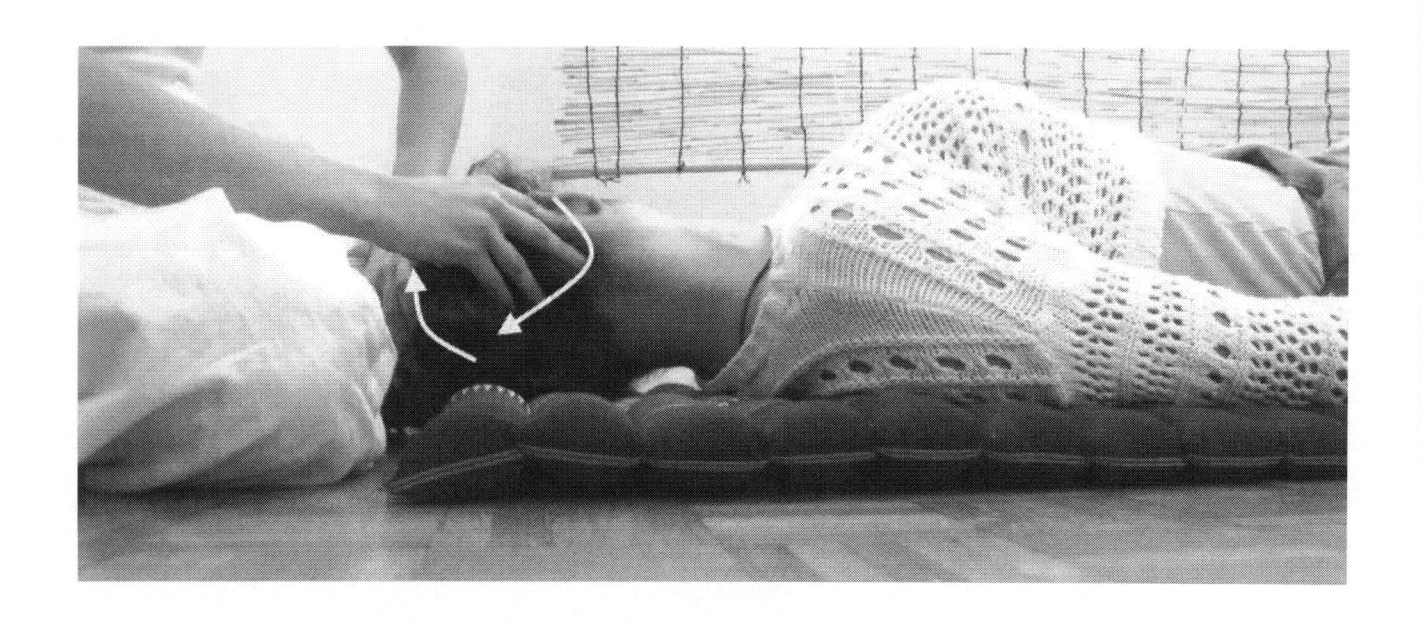

5. After that, massage the scalp thoroughly, performing deep tissue work on the epicranial aponeurosis.

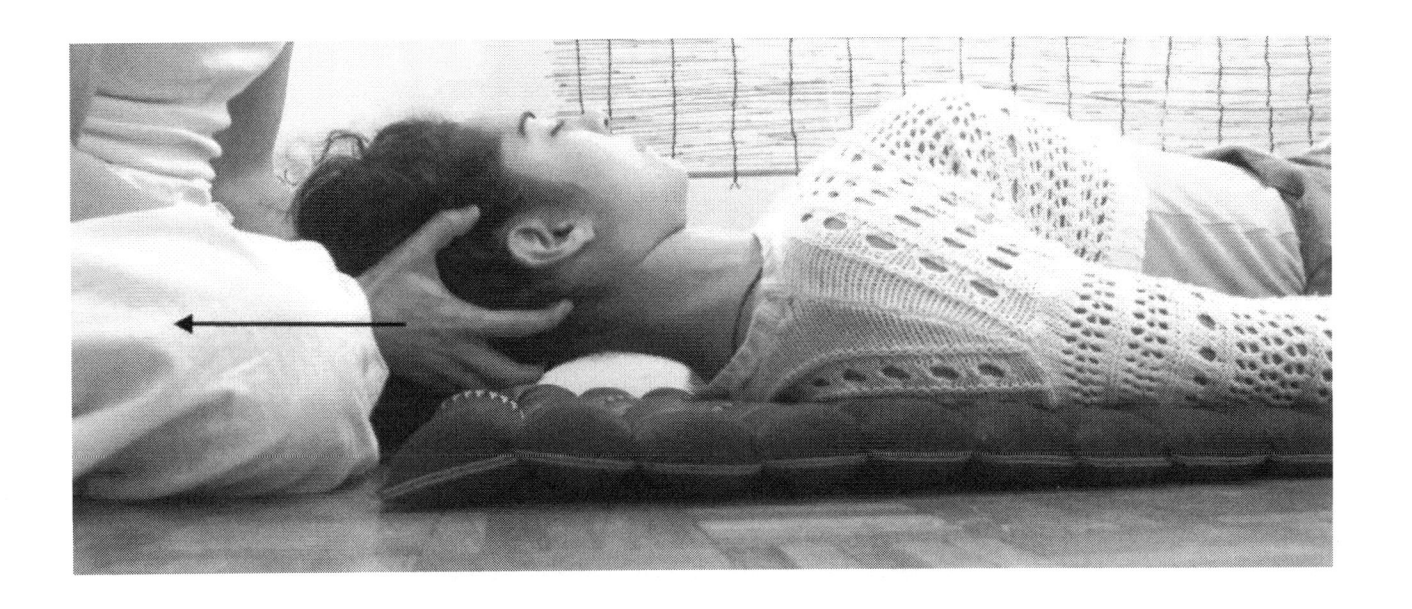

6. Then grasp firmly the atlanto-occipital joint, and pull it towards you. The head should be aligned with the spine.

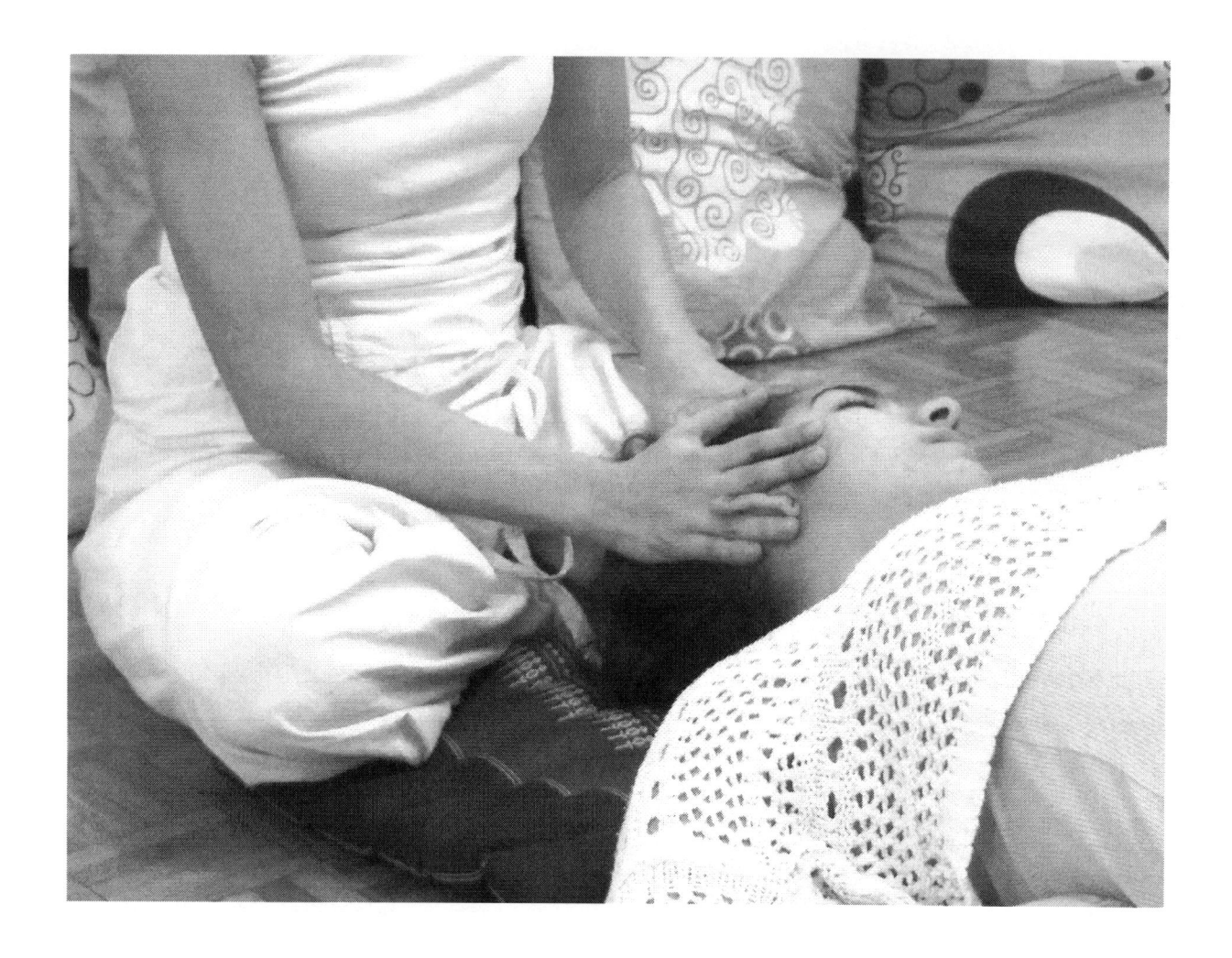

7. Place two fingers in front of the receiver's ear, and two fingers behind her ear. With your palm resting on her scalp, perform slow stationary circles.

Repeat on the other ear as well.

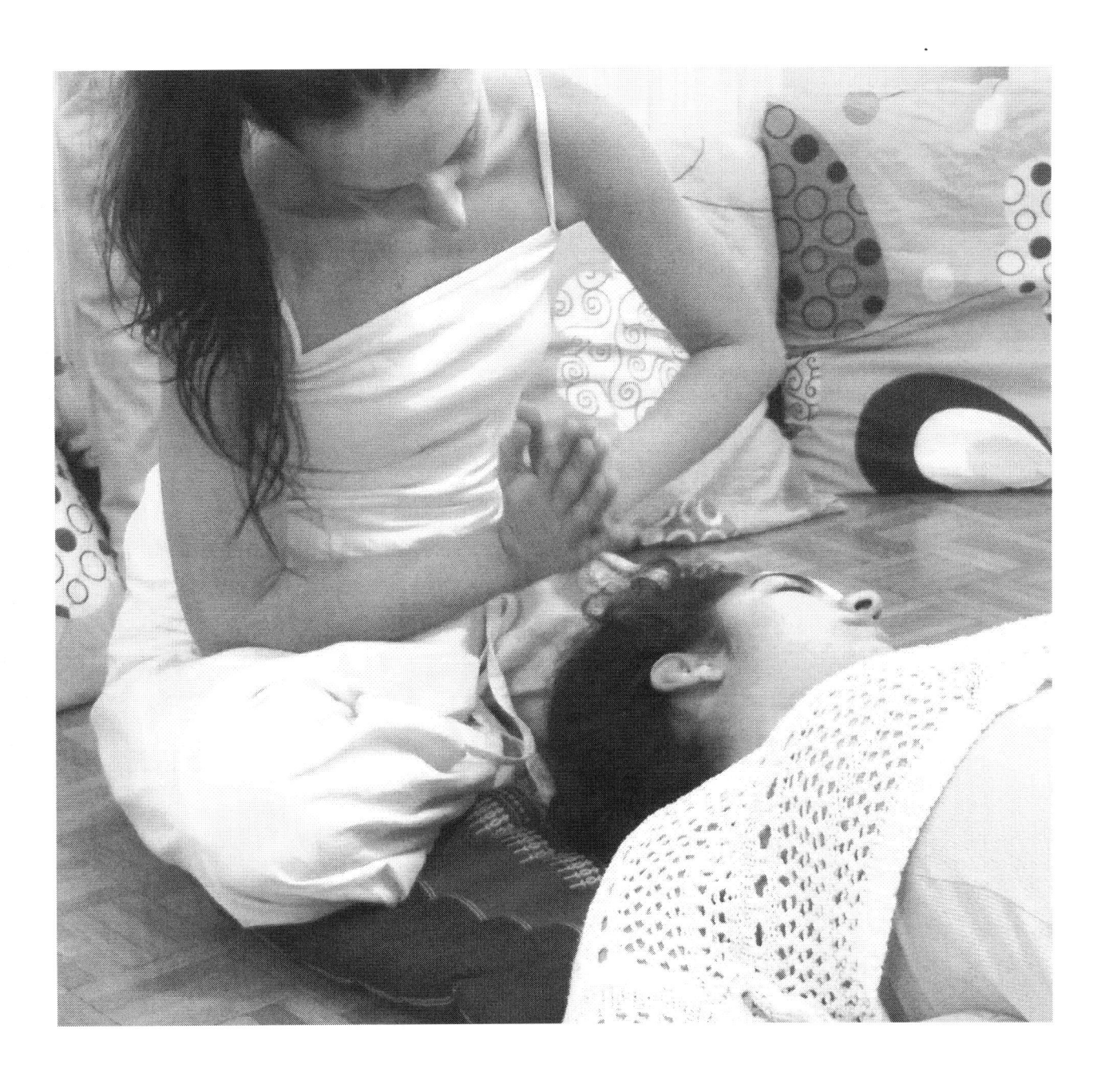

8. Do gentle tapotement techniques on the scalp.

face massage

Conclude the session with light facial massage. It is hard to take photos of these techniques, so I present a few diagrams.

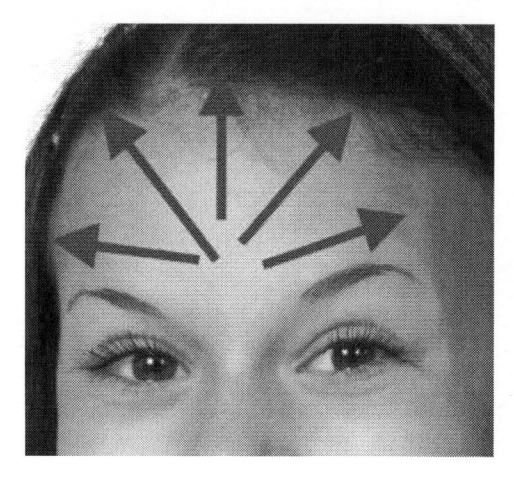

9. Slide your thumbs above the eyebrows, and then draw an "∧" shape – something like the peace sign.

When you slide your thumbs upwards on the central line of the forehead, go slowly and apply a bit of pressure.

This technique could be beneficial for sinusitis.

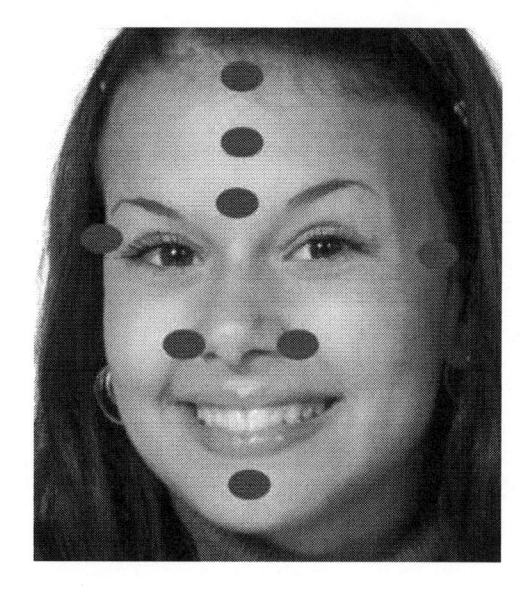

10. Using your thumbs, press the points shown at the photo.

Be more gentle below the forehead, and apply more pressure on the forehead.

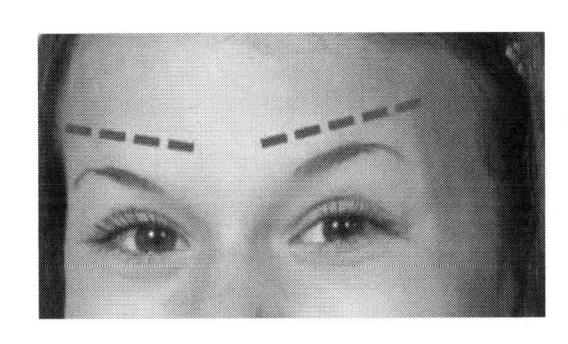

11. Make small circular movements with your thumbs, in opposite directions. Start above the nose and work your way towards the temples, on the *Itha & Pingkala Sen* lines above the eyebrows.

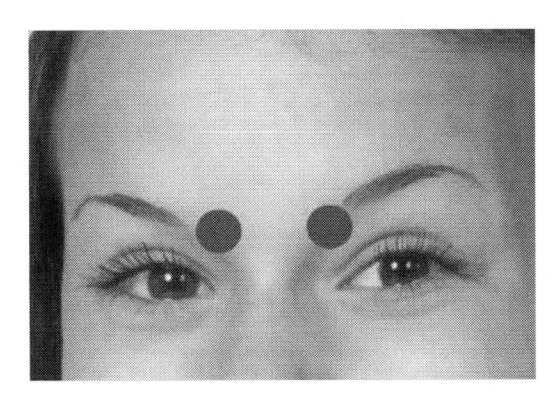

12. Press upwards the inner corner of the eye with the index finger. Do not apply too much pressure.

This is good acupressure point for headaches.

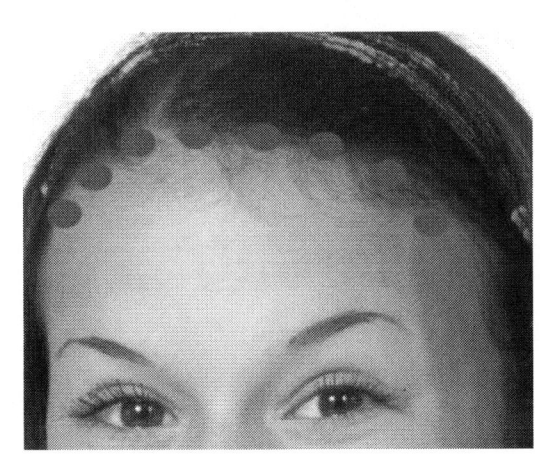

13. Using your thumbs, press these points below the hair line.

This is really relaxing…

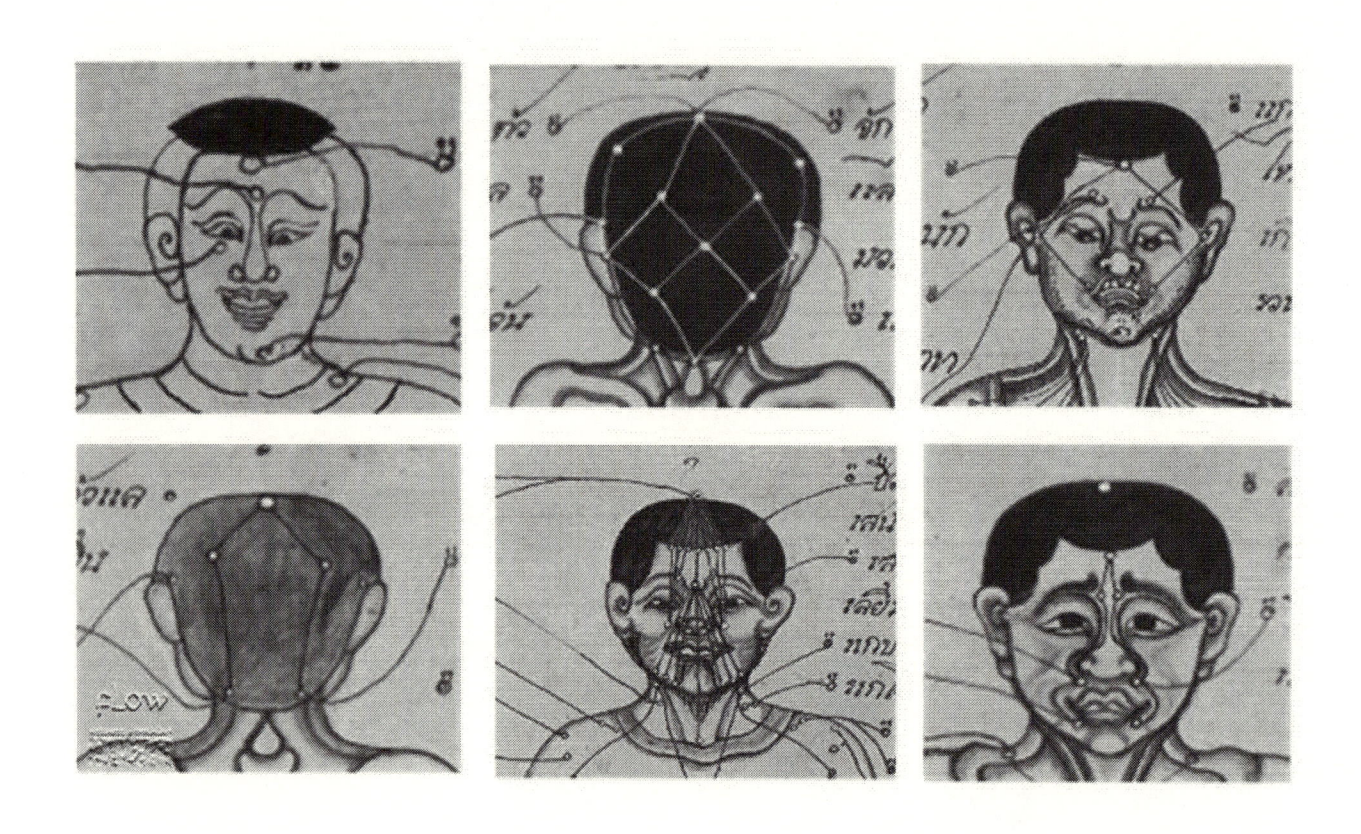

These are some traditional Thai acupressure points on the face and the scalp.

Source: British Library.

what lies underneath

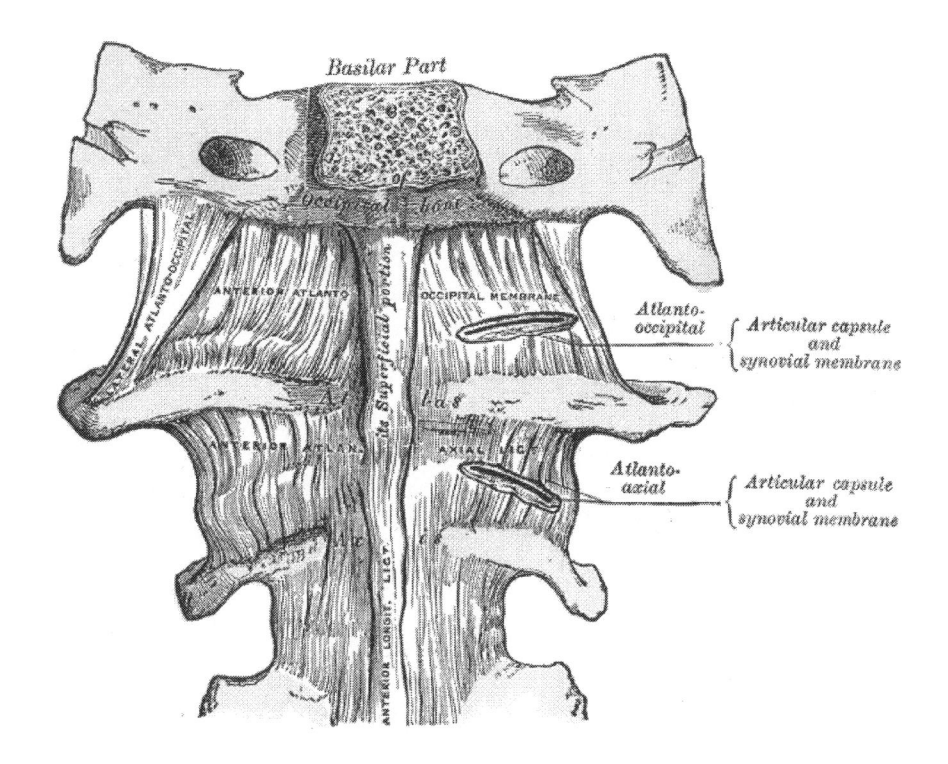

Anterior atlantoöccipital membrane and atlantoaxial ligament.

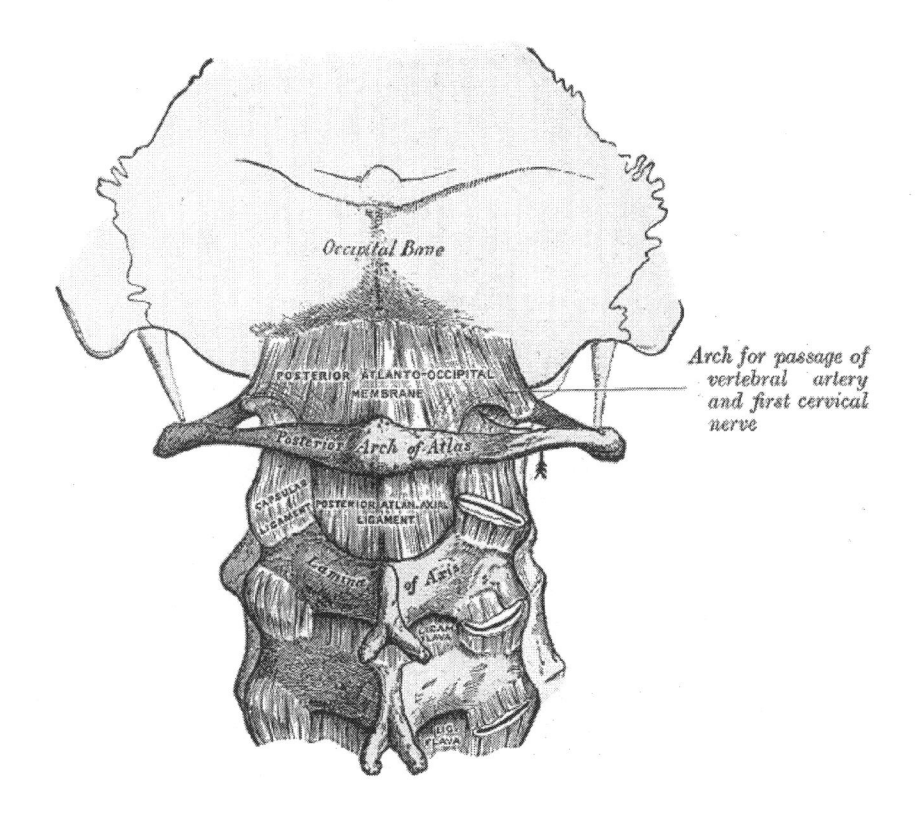

Posterior atlantoöccipital membrane and atlantoaxial ligament.

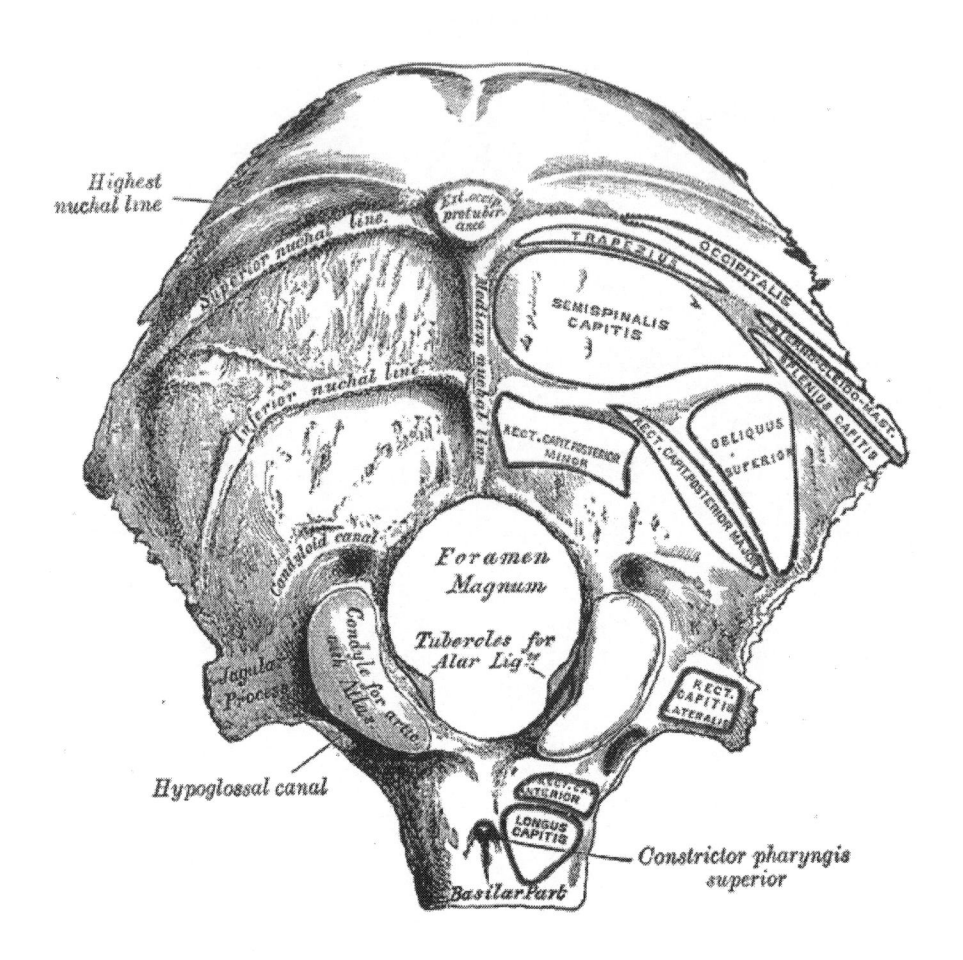

Outer surface of the occipital bone

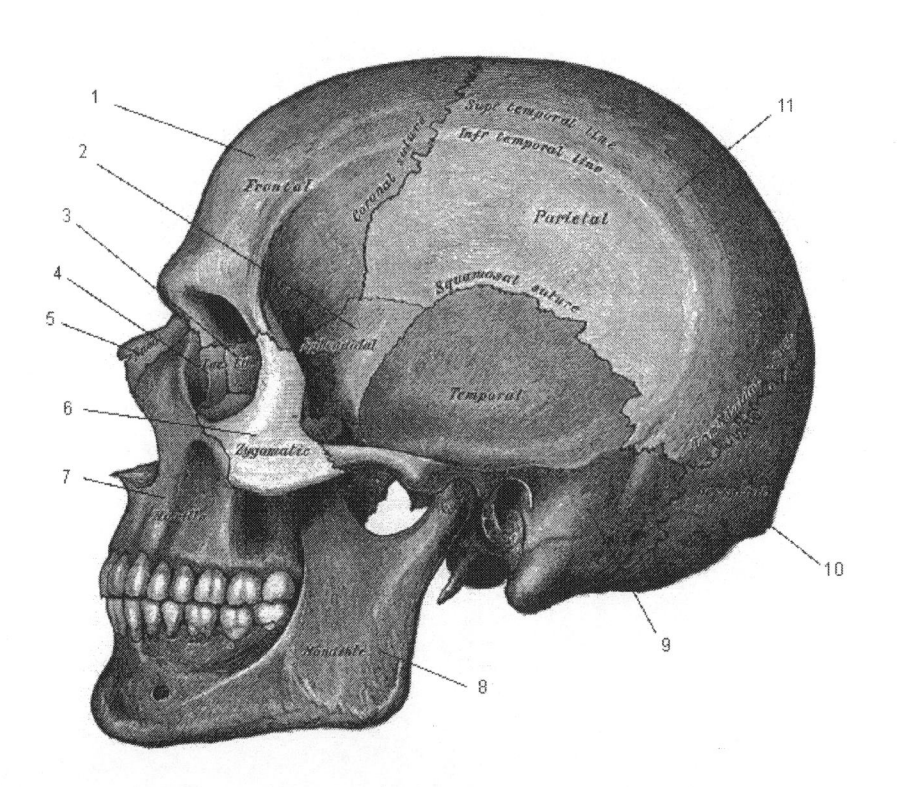

The skull

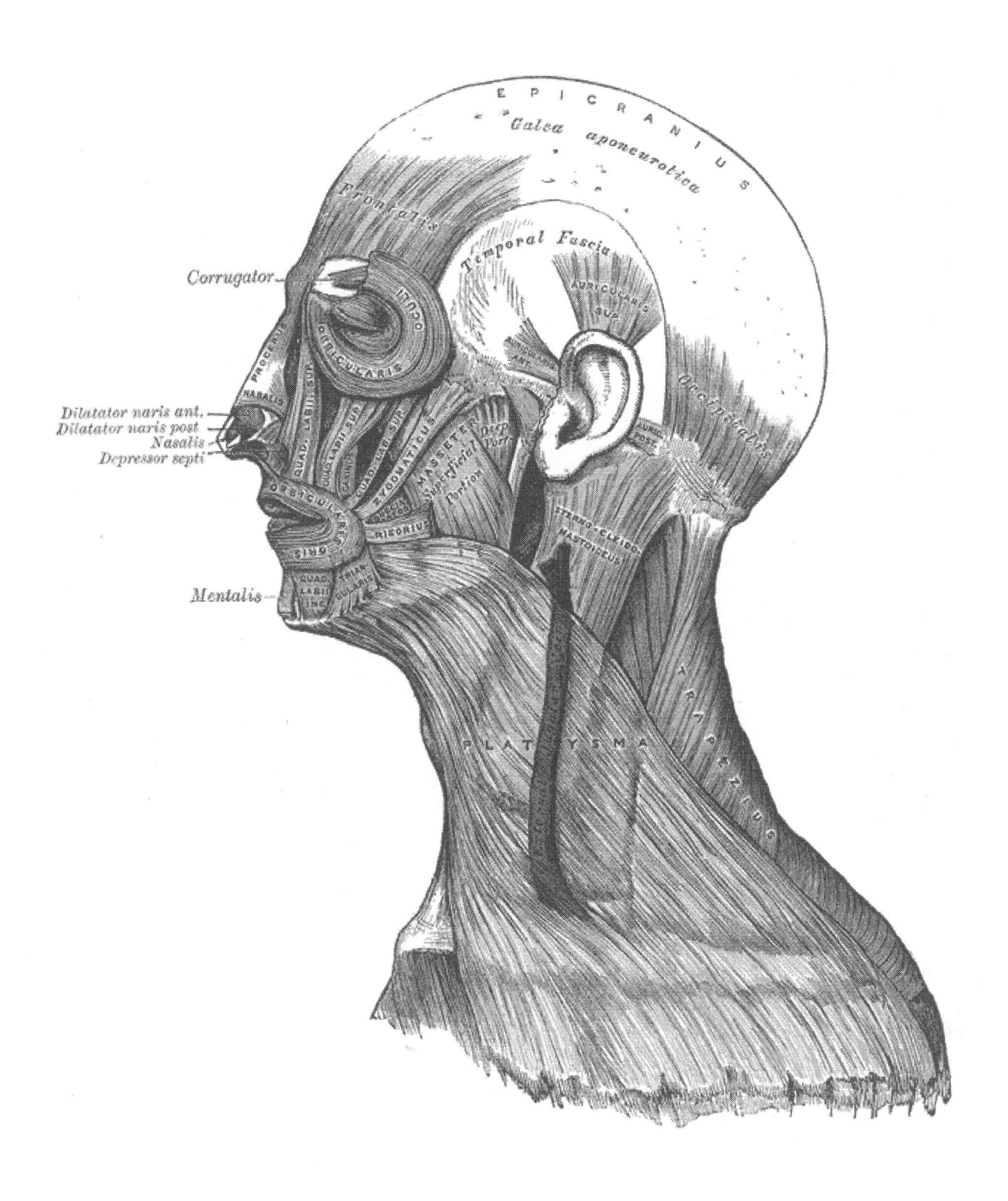

Face muscles and epicranial aponeurosis

tok sen

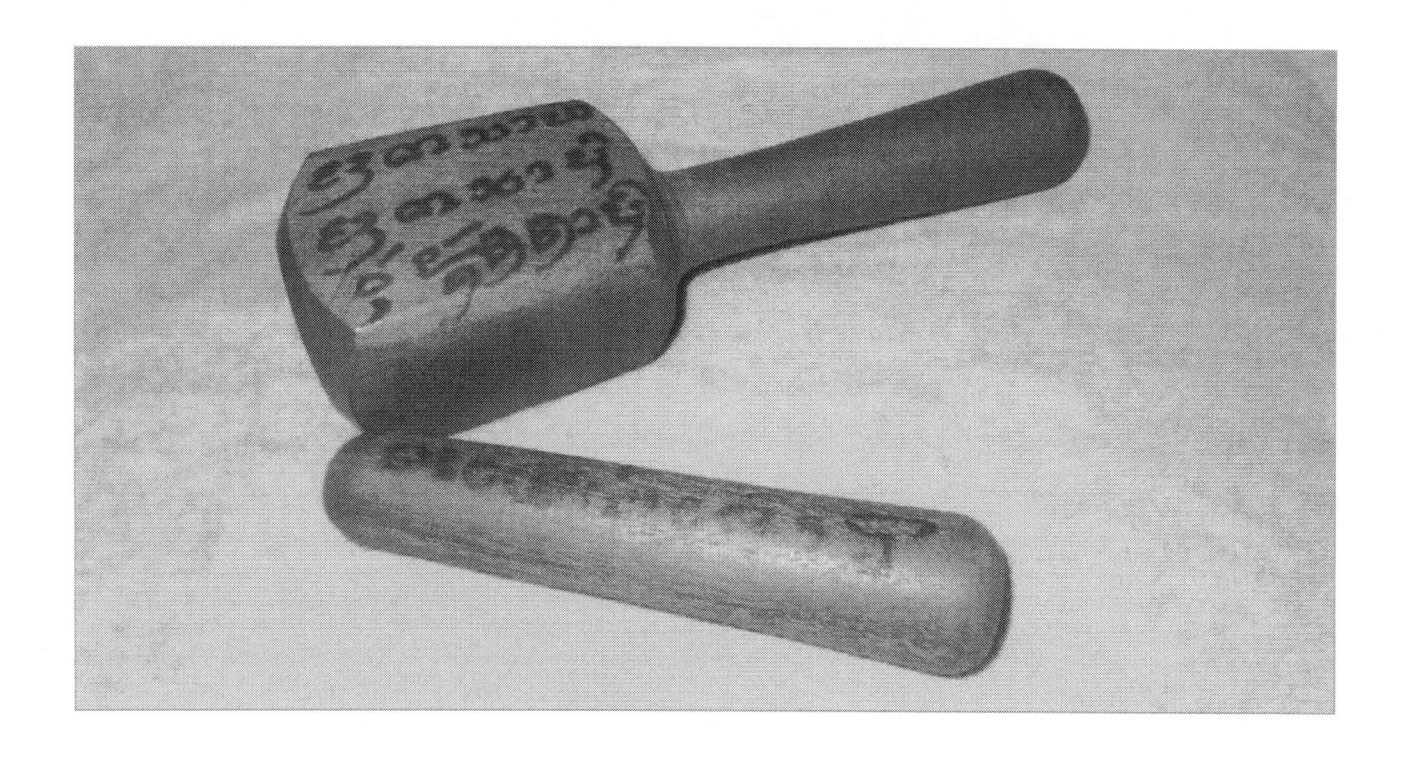

Tok Sen is an ancient, traditional technique, and it is unique to Northern Thailand . Essentially, it originates from the medicine that was applied in Lanna Kingdom (1292-1775 AD) and has its roots in ancient, shamanic traditions.

The therapist taps the receiver's body with the special wooden *Tok Sen* tools ("hammer" and "chisel") shown in the photo of the previous page. Traditionally, the tools were made from tamarind wood. According to some sources, the tamarind tree should have been struck by lightning.

The tools carry *mantra* - inscriptions written by a Buddhist monk, who has blessed them. As the therapist taps the body of the receiver with the tools (generally in sets of 3 gentle strikes), the blessing of the monk and the mantra vibration are transferred to the receiver.

Strike in sets of three rhythmical taps, in the course of the meridians. *Tok Sen* work should be applied at a specific rhythm and intensity; otherwise it may be annoying or even dangerous. Work mainly on the body of the muscle, avoiding the origin and insertion spots, and of course any tendons.

The following photos are just a short demonstration of the technique.

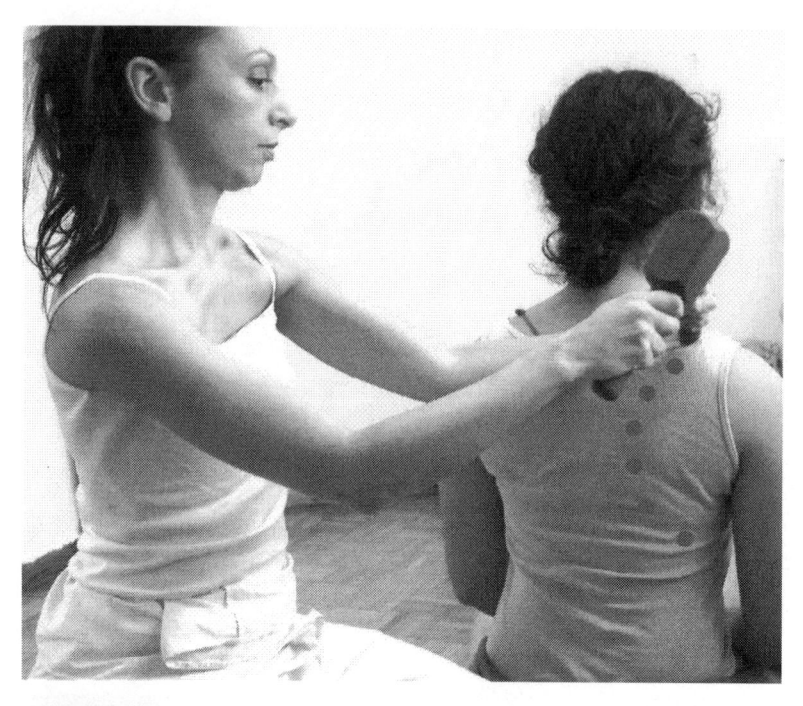

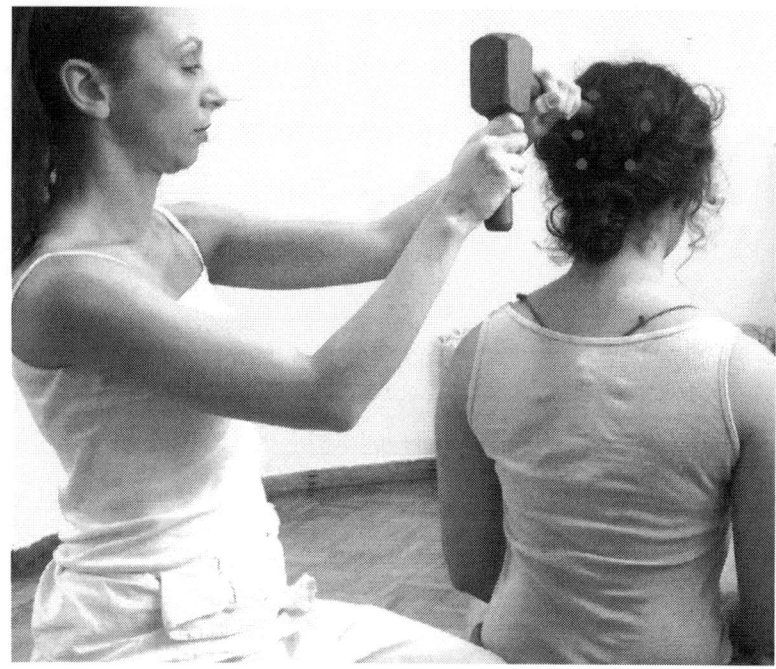

The technique can be applied in the seated position. Tap beside the scapula, and on the supraspinatus muscle.

You can also work on the scalp. Tap carefully and mildly.

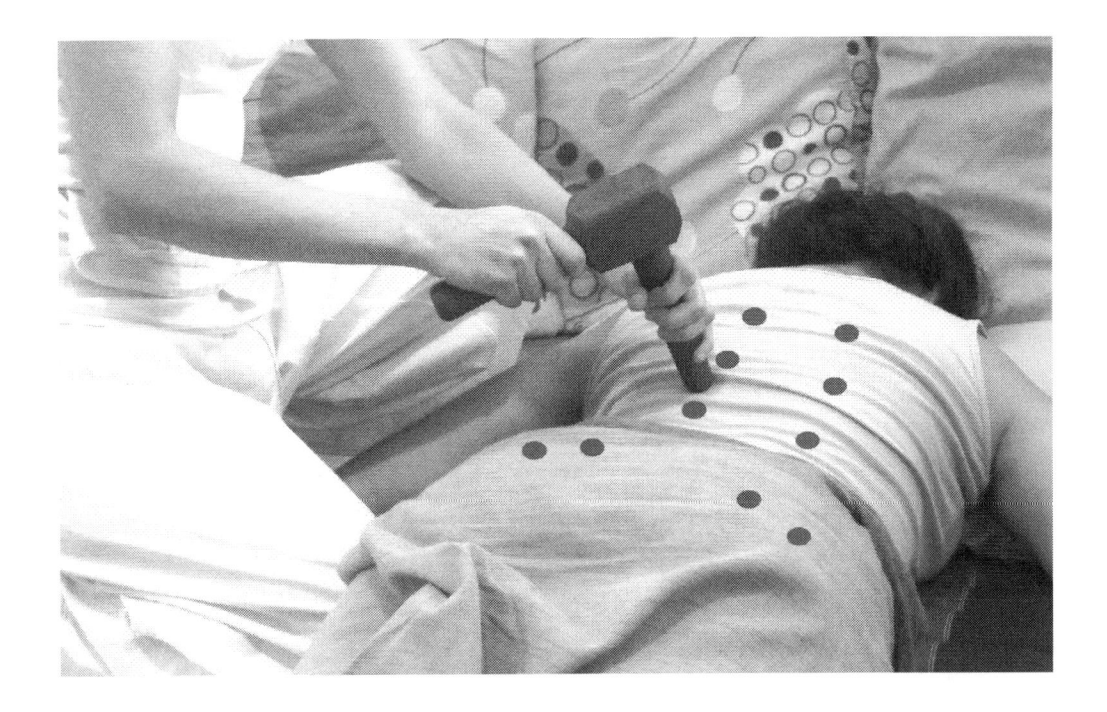

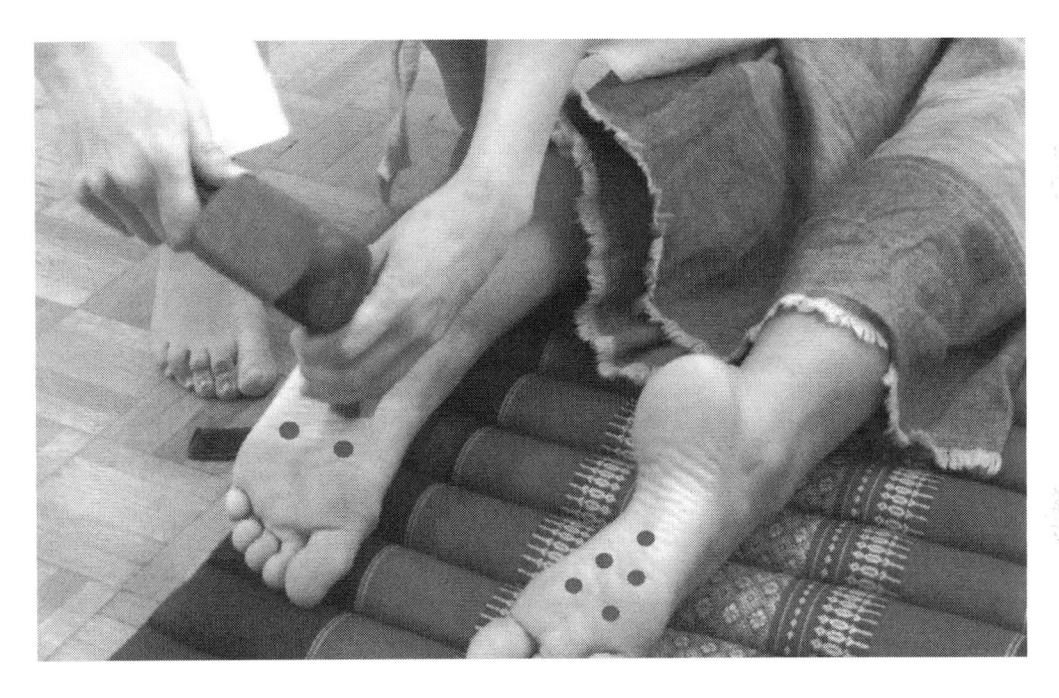

Apply Tok Sen on the supine position, in the course of *Itha & Pingkala Sen*.

Also, apply Tok Sen on the soles of the feet, by tapping the *Kalatharee Sen* lines. Do not tap on the dorsal surface of the feet.

Tok Sen can also be used on the side position, and it is especially pleasant on the iliotibial band.

luk pra kob

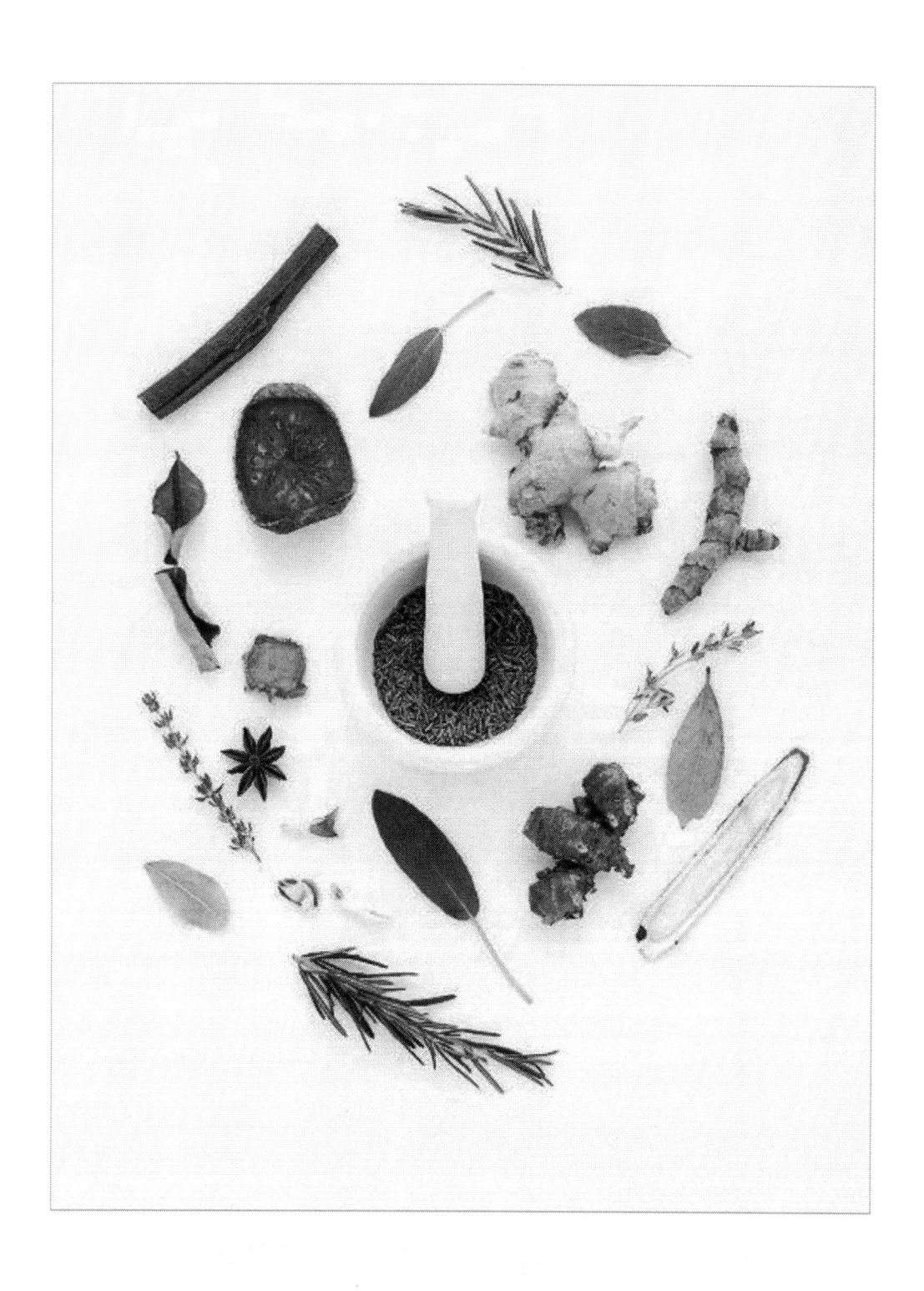

In Thailand, the herbal compresses (also known as "balls" or "packs") are called *Luk Pra Kob* – i.e. "pressure with a ball containing plants."

The compresses consist of a combination of medicinal herbs, which are placed in a piece of cloth. These compresses are steam-heated and placed directly on the skin. *Luk Pra Kob* is particularly beneficial for muscular pain and relief from stress. Depending on the combination of herbs, and suitable for the common cold.

In Thailand several traditional herbs are used, but some of them are difficult to obtain in Europe and USA.

The main herbs are as follows:

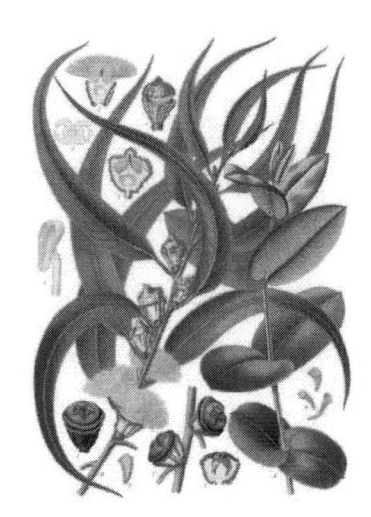

Eucalyptus (*Eucalyptus globulus*)

It is antipyretic and muscle relaxant. Excellent for treating sinusitis. Suitable for the common cold and cough (strong expectorant). In the compress, the leaves are cut into strips with scissors.

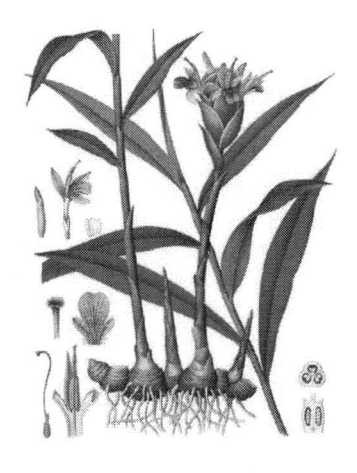

Ginger (*Zingiber officinale*)

In Thailand, therapists use a variety of yellow ginger called galangkal (*Alpinia galanga*). It is replaced satisfactorily by the common ginger. It is preferable to use fresh ginger, cut in small cubes or slices. Ginger, a wonderful anti-inflammatory herb, warms the body, is a cough suppressant and expectorant, and a muscle relaxant.

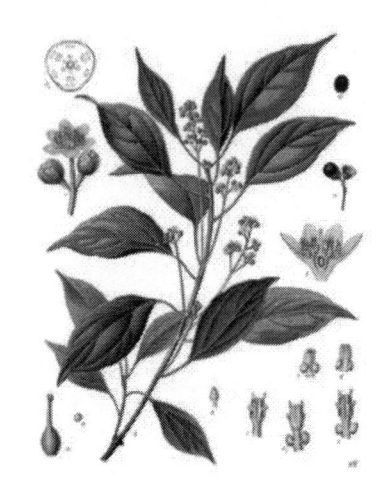

Camphor (Cinnamomum camphora)

Camphor is a very strong herb. It purifies the meridians, and has a definite effect on the energy body. The aroma is very pleasant. It is a basic herb for chronic pain (back pain, neck pain, etc.) and a muscle relaxant. It should not be used in epileptic patients or during pregnancy and breastfeeding (because of the ketones it contains). In compresses it is pulverized in a mortar. Use up to 1 tablet of camphor per session.

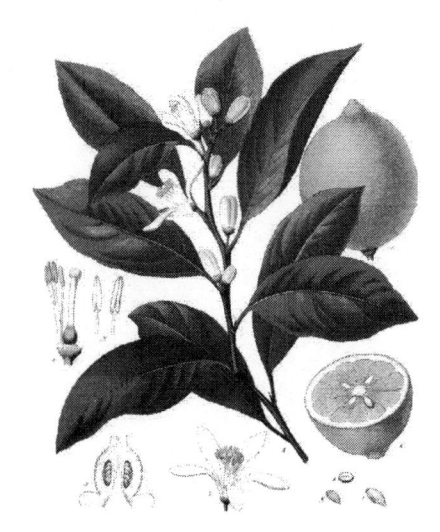

Lemon rind and leaves (Citrus limon)

Mainly used for its relaxing aroma. It is also beneficial for colds and coughs. It also promotes detoxification of the meridians and the physical body.

These four basic herbs suffice for Luk Pra Kob. Sometimes, it is even OK to use only eucalyptus and ginger.

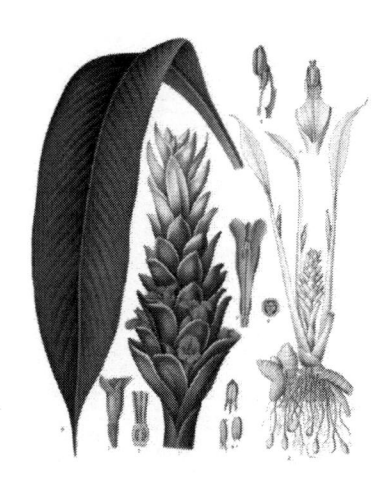

Additional herbs that can be used:

Turmeric (Curcuma longa)

In Thailand therapists use the fresh root, which is cut into thin slices. Turmeric powder (comes from the dried root) is also acceptable. This is an excellent anti-inflammatory herb. Use up to 1 teaspoonful for one treatment (otherwise the client's skin will turn yellow for a few days...)!

Lemongrass (Cymbopogon flexuosus)

The dried easily found in herbal medicine, rarely fresh. It looks like a leek in appearance and has a very sweet smell. In patches cut into slices. The lemongrass refreshes the body and promote detoxification. The pleasant smell is relaxing. The Thai name of the herb is *Ta khrai*.

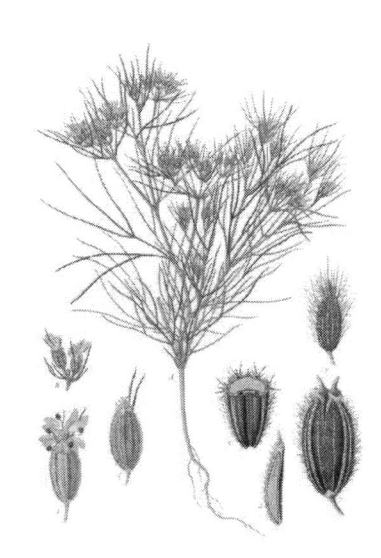

Cumin (*Cuminum cyminum*)

Use the seeds (pulverized or whole). It is beneficial for tight muscles. Use up to 1 teaspoonful for one treatment.

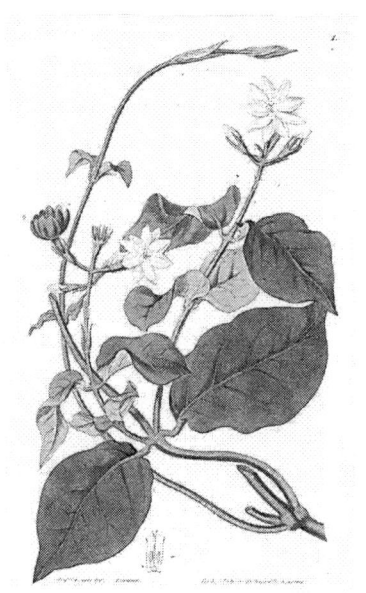

Jasmine flowers (*Jasmin arabicum*)

It is best to use flowers – however, the dried ones are also acceptable. Used primarily for bronchospasm (it can soothe chronic coughs, especially dry cough) and its deeply relaxing fragrance.

Thai herbs generally hard to find in Europe:

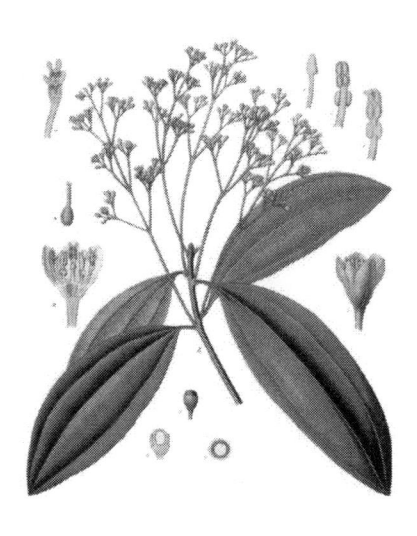

Cinnamon leaves (*Cinnamomum verum*)

Although cinnamon bark can be purchased anywhere, this is not the case with the leaves. They give a wonderful aroma to the compress, and have a deep warming effect on the muscles.

Never use cinnamon bark – the phenols it contains are highly irritating for the skin.

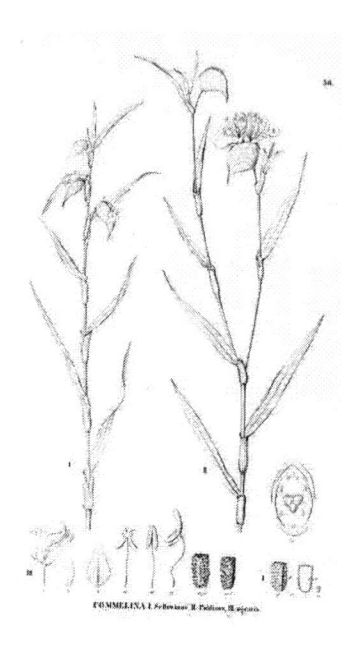

Watergrass (*Commelina diffusa*)

The Thai name of the plant is *Phak Plab*. It is an antipyretic, and a diuretic. It is added in the compress in case of fever.

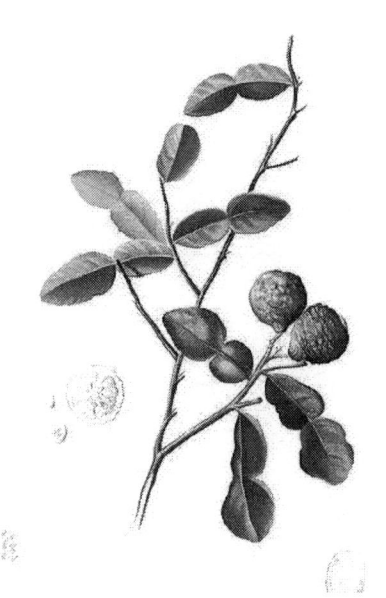

Kaffir lime (*Citrus hystix*)

The Thai name of the plant is *Ma krut*. In Thailand, its rind is frequently added in the compresses. The most distinctive feature of this citrus is its bumpy exterior.

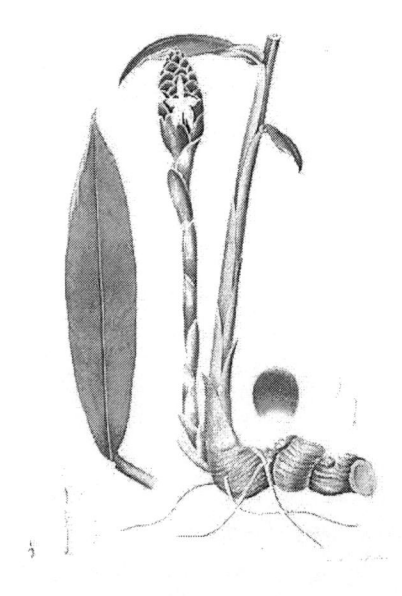

Cassumunar ginger (*Zingiber cassumunar*)

Its Thai name is *Phrai*. It is a potent bronchodilator, anti-inflammatory and antitussive herb. The root is frequently added in the compresses.

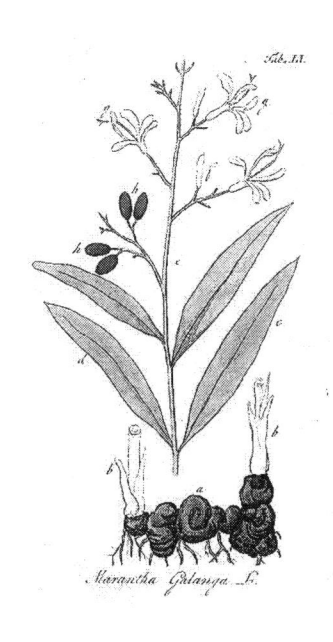

Alpinia galanga (*and / or the species A. Officinarum, A.nigra*)

This is a yellow, very hot herb and spice, widely used sin cooking. The Thai name is *Khaa* (internationally known as Siamese ginger, or Ginza). The root is frequently added in the compresses.

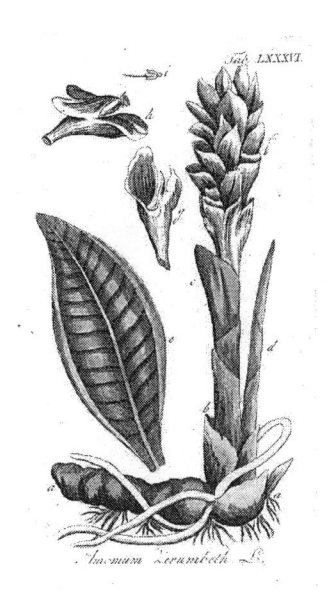

Zerumbet ginger (*Zingiber zerumbet*)

The Thai name of the herb is *Ka Thue*, and internationall it is known as Pinecone ginger. This is a potent herb. Very effective for tense muscles and injuries. The root is frequently added in the compresses.

This herb is also used in the indigenous medicine of Hawaii, for similar purposes.

A Thai compress may also contain Cardamom leaves. These are the species used (Thai names): Krawaan (*Amomum krervanh*), Wan Sao Lowng (*Amomum xanthioides*) & Reo krawaan (*Amomum uliginosum*).

preparation and use

First, prepare the mixture by mixing the herbs in a bowl. Then, place an amount roughly equal to a fist, on a square white cotton fabric, size 50 x 50 cm. Form a "ball" with the fabric and herbs, and then twist the remaining fabric. Tie it with a cotton string.

Then place the compresses m in a steamer to heat up. Once their aroma emerges (generally after 10 to 15 minutes), they are ready.

Before doing dynamic techniques in a region, heat it with the a compress. After kneading and stretching, apply the compress again.

At the end of the session, place them on the temples, forehead, chest, and below the shoulders.

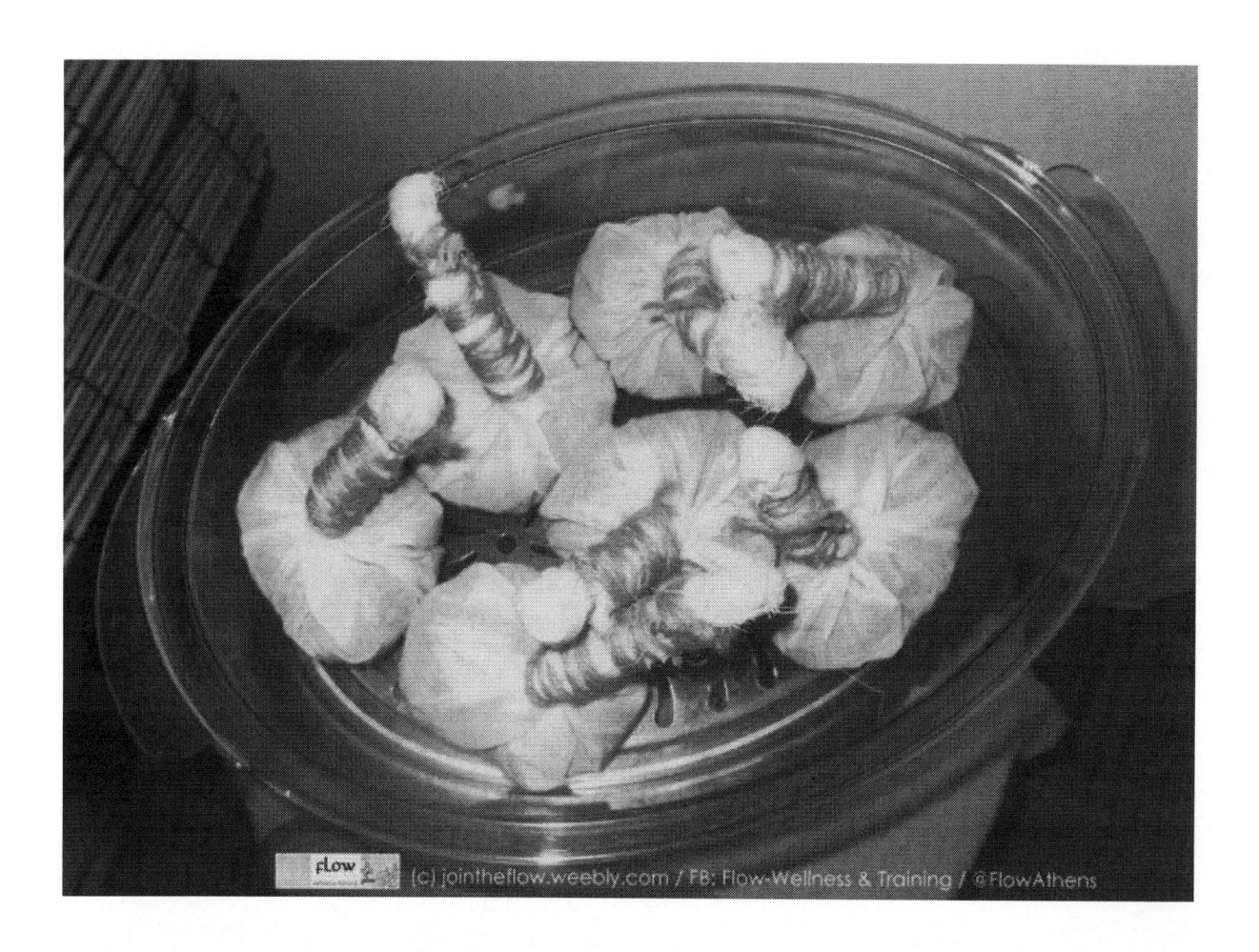

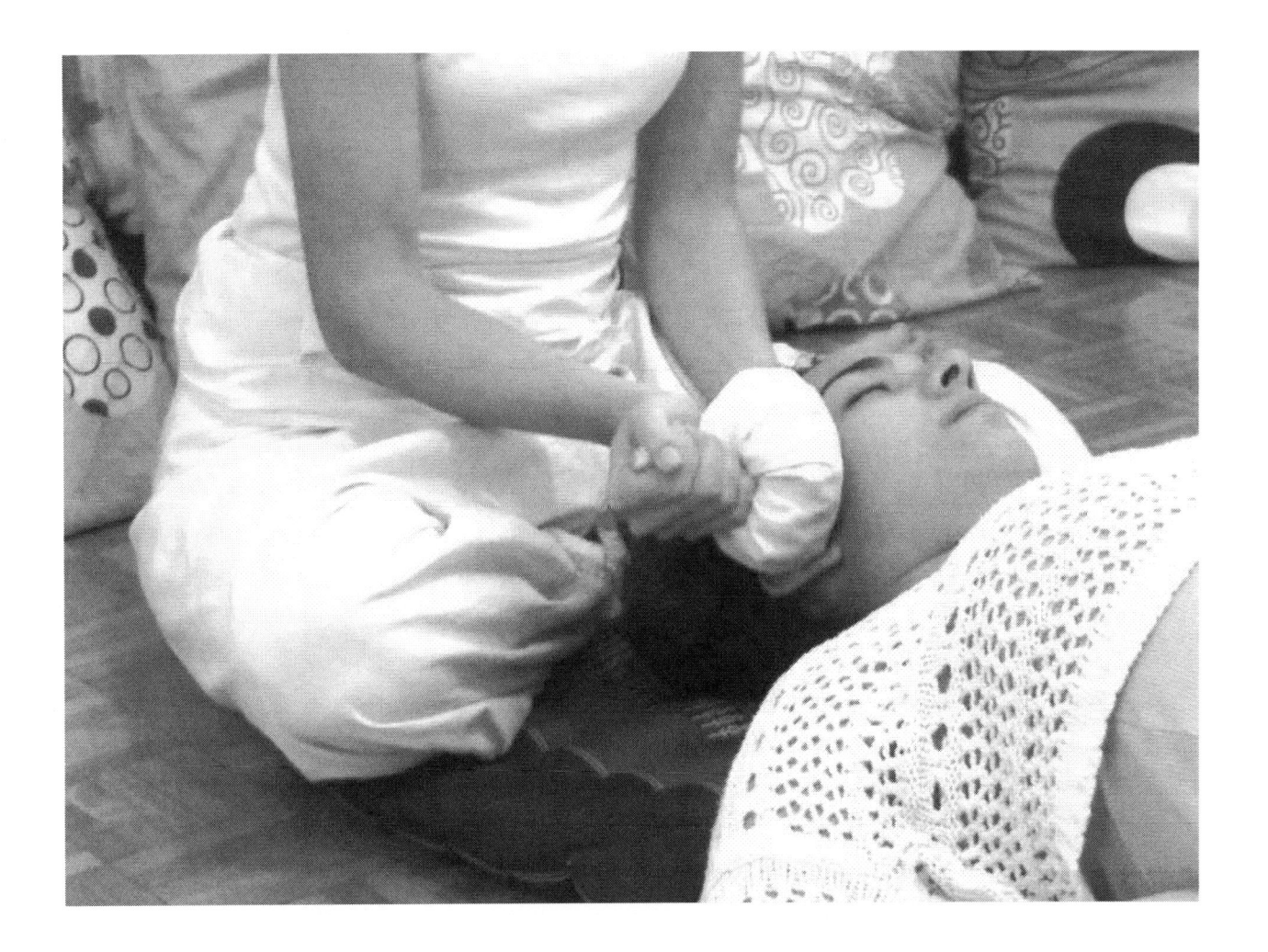

Points to remember

- You need at least two packs for each treatment, but you can use more if you so wish.
- Never apply heat on spider veins and acute injuries.
- The lower back area is very sensitive to heat – be very careful when applying *Luk Pra Kob* there.
- Work quickly when the packs are hot, and stay longer on a spot when they cool down a bit.
- Herbal packs leave stains on clothes. You may want to provide your clients with loose clothes, in order to protect their clothing.
- Discard the herbs after each treatment. The cloth used for them can be washed are reused (it will be stained however).
- It is best to receive training before applying herbal packs.

blending it all together

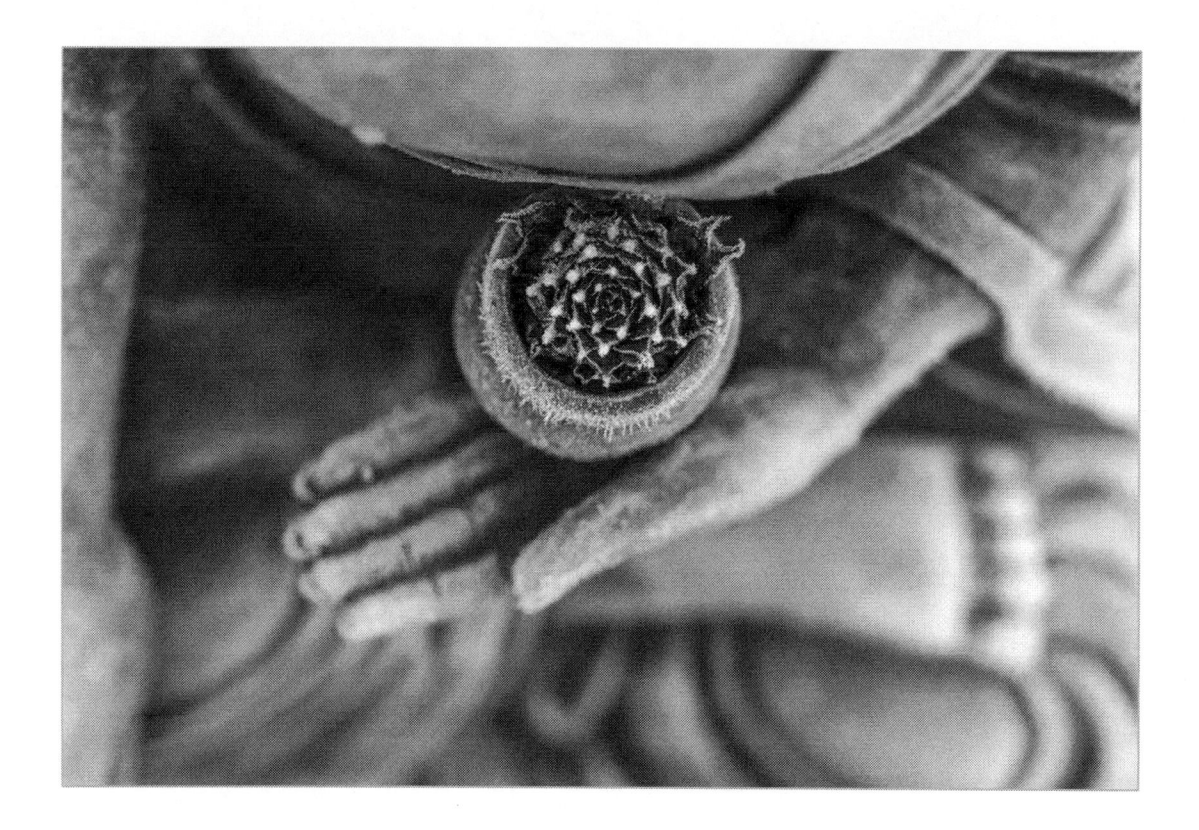

Traditionally, a Thai Massage session starts in the supine position, and then the therapist proceeds with the side position, the prone position, the sitting position, and concludes with the face techniques.

It takes a lot of time to apply all the techniques demonstrated in this book – about 6-7 hours! A skilled therapist is adept in all the techniques, and is able to pick immediately the appropriate ones for each case.

The key is to do some balancing techniques for the whole body, and then focus on the problematic area. I do not recommend protocols – I insist on creativity. However, this also needs training in a class, and a lot of practice!

I hope you enjoyed reading my book. Happy massaging!

Namaste,
Elefteria

Other books by Elefteria Mantzorou on Amazon

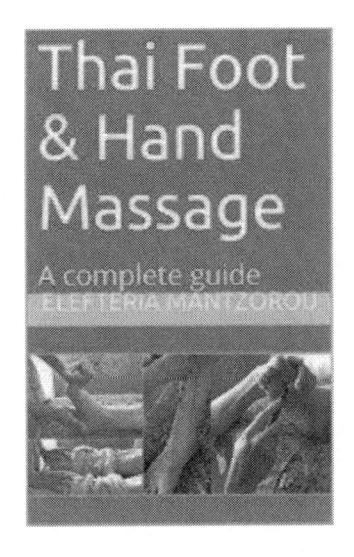

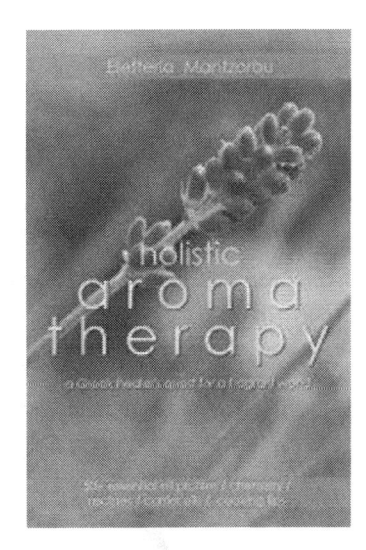

Follow Elefteria on social media:

Twitter: @FlowAthens
Facebook: Flow – Wellness and Training (mostly in greek).
YouTube: Flow – Wellness and Training (subscribe for lots of free massage videos)!

Credits
All photos that demonstrate Thai Massage techniques, as well as the 10 meridian plates, constitute copyrighted property of Elefteria Mantzorou. Their non-authorized use will be persecuted.
The photos at the beginning of each chapter are in the public domain, except the one at the beginning of the Tok Sen section, which is shot by Elefteria Mantzorou, and is copyrighted.
The anatomy plates are from Gray's Anatomy (taken from Bartleby.com) and are in the public domain.
The herb images are in the public domain.
The traditional Thai meridian illustrations are reproduced with the kind permission of the British Library.
Design, text and artwork by Elefteria Mantzorou.

Thai Massage is an ancient form of bodywork. It is considered sacred in Thailand, and it is practiced virtually everywhere - in temples, in luxurious spas, in crowded, noisy vegetable markets, and even in resorts in the jungle!

This book contains valuable information about the historical background of Thai Massage, and instructions for many techniques of the four positions (supine, side, prone and seated).

It is indispensable for the serious massage therapist, as well as anyone who studies any form of bodywork. Also, those who wish to learn massage, will find many useful techniques.

- 100 + photos with instructions
- Thai meridians illustrations
- Instructions for the preparation and application of the Thai herbal packs
- Indications and contraindications for for musculoskeletal disorders
- ... and much more!

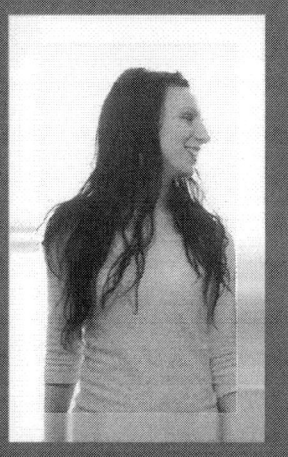

Elefteria Mantzorou was born in Greece, and was trained in traditional Thai Massage in Chiang Mai, Thailand.

Since 2004, she has taught Thai Massage, Thai Foot Massage and Thai Herbal Compresses to hundreds of students.

She is the director of FLOW - Wellness & Training, a massage therapy school located in Athens, Greece.

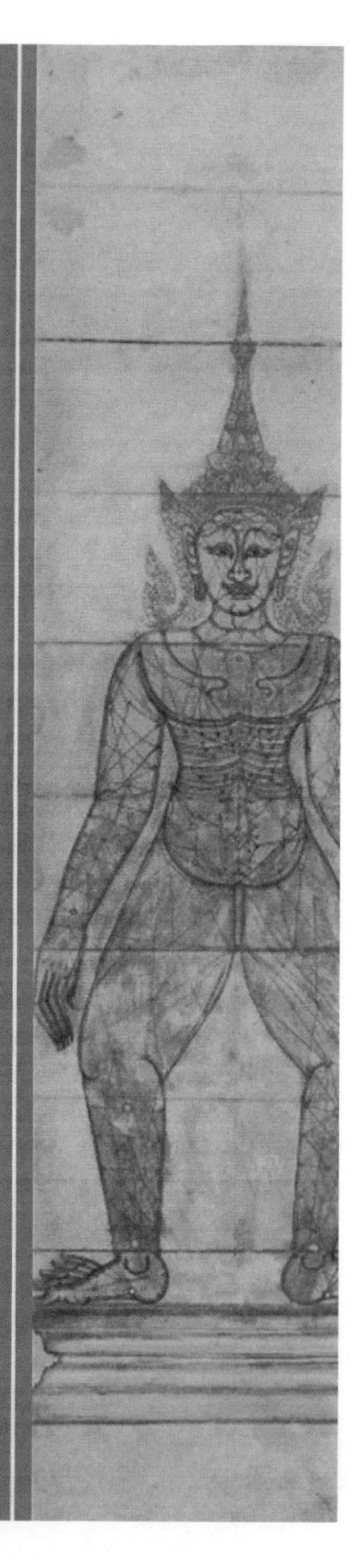

Made in the USA
Middletown, DE
06 April 2019